# SLEEP MEDICINE IN CLINICAL PRACTICE

# Dedication

Dr Silber dedicates this book to his wife Sandy
and his children, Bradley, Taryn and Ryan.


Dr Krahn dedicates this book to her husband Dr Eric Gordon
and her children Christina and Ian.


Dr Morgenthaler dedicates this book to his wife Robin
and his children Sarah, Kelsey, Zachary, Samuel and Olivia.

# SLEEP MEDICINE IN CLINICAL PRACTICE

## Michael H. Silber MBChB, FCP(SA)

Mayo Clinic College of Medicine
Rochester, MN, USA

## Lois E. Krahn MD

Mayo Clinic College of Medicine
Scottsdale, AZ, USA

## Timothy I. Morgenthaler MD

Mayo Clinic College of Medicine
Rochester, MN, USA

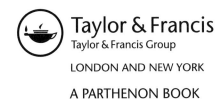

Taylor & Francis
Taylor & Francis Group

LONDON AND NEW YORK

A PARTHENON BOOK

First published in the United Kingdom in 2004
by Taylor & Francis,
an imprint of the Taylor & Francis Group,
11 New Fetter Lane,
London EC4P 4EE

Tel.:  +44 (0) 20 7583 9855
Fax.:  +44 (0) 20 7842 2298
Website:  www.tandf.co.uk

British Library Cataloguing in Publication Data

Data available on application

Library of Congress Cataloging-in-Publication Data

Data available on application

ISBN 1-84214-190-2

Distributed in North and South America by

Taylor & Francis
2000 NW Corporate Blvd
Boca Raton, FL 33431, USA

*Within Continental USA*
Tel.: 800 272 7737; Fax.: 800 374 3401
*Outside Continental USA*
Tel.: 561 994 0555; Fax.: 561 361 6018
E-mail: orders@crcpress.com

Distributed in the rest of the world by
Thomson Publishing Services
Cheriton House
North Way
Andover, Hampshire SP10 5BE, UK
Tel.: +44 (0) 1264 332424
E-mail: salesorder.tandf@thomsonpublishingservices.co.uk

Composition by Parthenon Publishing
Printed and bound by Antony Rowe Ltd., Chippenham, Wiltshire, UK

# Contents

# Disclaimer

Nothing in this publication implies that Mayo Foundation endorses any of the products mentioned in this book. Care has been taken to confirm the accuracy of the information presented and to describe generally accepted practices. However, the authors, editors and publisher are not responsible for errors or omissions or for any consequences from application of the information in this book and make no warranty, express or implied, with respect to the contents of the publication.

The authors, editors and publisher have exerted every effort to ensure that drug selection and dosage set forth in this text are in accordance with current recommendations and practice at the time of publication. However, in view of ongoing research, changes in government regulations and the constant flow of information relating to drug therapy and drug reactions, the reader is urged to check the package insert for each drug for any change in indications and dosage and for added warnings and precautions. This is particularly important when the recommended agent is a new or infrequently employed drug.

Some of the indications suggested for drugs described in this book may not have been approved by the US Food and Drug Administration (FDA). It is the responsibility of readers to ascertain which indications are 'off label' and to decide whether the medications should be prescribed for these purposes. Some drugs and medical devices presented in this publication may have FDA clearance for limited use in restricted research settings. It is the responsibility of health-care providers to ascertain the FDA status of each drug or device planned for use in their clinical practice.

# Preface

*Come, Sleep: O Sleep! the certain knot of peace,*
*The baiting place of wit, the balm of woe,*
*The poor man's wealth, the prisoner's release,*
*The indifferent judge between the high and low.*

**Philip Sidney,** *Astrophel and Stella*

In late June of 1995, the 9th annual meeting of the Associated Professional Sleep Societies was held in Nashville. To the amazement of the attending physicians and scientists, a special appearance by Dr Nathaniel Kleitman, then in his 100th year of life, had been arranged. Forty-two years had passed since the discovery of rapid eye movement (REM) sleep at the University of Chicago by Kleitman and his graduate student, Eugene Aserinsky. Many of us present were not even aware that the father of sleep medicine was still alive, and to see and hear him was a spine-chilling experience. Kleitman was the pioneer of sleep researchers in more ways than by discovering REM sleep. In 1938 he spent more than a month in Mammoth Cave, Kentucky, to study biological rhythms, and in 1939 he published the first modern book on sleep research, the classic *Sleep and Wakefulness*. However, the discovery of REM sleep was the seminal event in the investigation of sleep, and proved to be the beginning of an exponential explosion of knowledge that still continues. In a young field like this, the current generation of sleep physicians can still feel a direct link to the origins of our discipline.

Sleep medicine also has a long history at Mayo Clinic. As early as 1934, Lumen Daniels published a comprehensive review of the Mayo experience with narcolepsy[1]. In this lengthy article, he not only delineated all the clinical features of the disorder, but also described patients with what would later be called obstructive sleep apnea syndrome, although not recognizing its pathophysiology. In the 1950s, Dr Robert Yoss became one of the first specialists in narcolepsy, describing the tetrad of symptoms still recognized today, introducing pupillometry as the first test for the disorder and introducing methylphenidate as a treatment. Daytime sleep studies were performed in the 1970s, and in 1983 the Mayo Sleep Disorder Center was formally founded under the leadership of Dr Philip Westbrook. This center has remained a multidisciplinary clinic and laboratory, with currently 16 laboratory beds and a consultant staff of 13. A 1-year sleep medicine fellowship for physicians has been in place since 1990, as well as training programs for technologists. Active research continues in such fields as narcolepsy, the treatment of sleep apnea and parasomnias in neurodegenerative disorders.

Why have we chosen to write this book? There are already a number of large multiauthored textbooks of sleep medicine as well as smaller single-authored monographs.

However, we felt we could add a new perspective by writing a book coauthored by three colleagues working closely together in a large academic sleep center and representing the different perspectives of neurology, psychiatry and pulmonology. We have arranged the book around a clinical approach to the patient with a sleep disorder. We have included sufficient basic science to allow an understanding of the pathogenesis, diagnostic tools and treatments of sleep disorders, but predominantly emphasize the role of the clinician in diagnosing and managing disease. We have used tables, algorithms and figures to emphasize the approaches we advocate and have based these on what we hope has been a scholarly review of the literature as well as our own experience in a busy academic practise. We have used extensive case histories to personalize the text, describing both common and unusual clinical problems.

We have designed this book for a number of audiences. First, we hope it will be helpful to trainees studying sleep medicine as well as those in neurology, pulmonology, psychiatry and other residencies who would like to explore the world of sleep in more depth than is covered in general textbooks. We have also considered the needs of practising sleep physicians who might appreciate reading about the approaches of a different sleep center, especially in areas aligned to a primary specialty different from their own. We also hope the book may be beneficial to the faculty of sleep medicine training programs as a basis for an organized curriculum. Finally, we would be delighted if the book were to spur the interest of medical students and physicians not working in sleep medicine, and stimulate them to make this enticing field a part of their professional lives.

We would like to thank the many people who have directly or indirectly made this book possible. We work in the most collegial of sleep centers, and all of our colleagues have contributed to our thinking about sleep. We have also learned from our nurses, technologists and trainees. In particular we must thank Drs Peter Hauri and John Shepard, past directors of our center, for imparting their knowledge and wisdom. Cameron Harris, co-ordinator of the Mayo Sleep Disorders Center, and Dan Herold, supervisor of our sleep laboratory, shared their extensive technical expertise and helped in the production of many of the illustrations. Bryce Bergene of the Mayo Division of Media Support Services was responsible for the artwork. Les Ottjes, Annette Schmidt and Julie Stamschror provided secretarial support. Dr Leila Arens read much of the manuscript and provided valuable advice. Roberta Schwartz of the Mayo Department of Publications guided us through the intricacies of producing a book. Finally, we must thank Jonathan Gregory of Parthenon Publishing Group who first suggested that we write this book, overcame our objections and supported us through many months of hard but enjoyable work.

## REFERENCE

1.  Daniels LE. Narcolepsy. *Medicine* 1934;13: 1–21

# Section I
# Basics of sleep medicine

# Chapter 1

# Physiological basis of sleep

*I met at eve the Prince of Sleep,*
*His was a still and lovely face,*
*He wandered through a valley steep,*
*Lovely in a lonely place.*

*Dark in his pools clear visions lurk,*
*And rosy, as with morning buds,*
*Along his dales of broom and birk*
*Dreams haunt his solitary woods.*

*INTERNATIONAL*
*10–20 SYSTEM*

*SINGLE TRACING = DERIVATION*
*BIPOLAR*
*REFERENTIAL*

*ARRANGEMENT OF*
*DERIVATION = MONTAGE*

**Walter de la Mare, *I Met at Eve***

Sleep can be defined in behavioral terms as a normal, recurring, reversible state of loss of the ability to perceive and respond to the external environment. Voluntary motor activity largely ceases, and a quiescent posture, specific to each species, is adopted. Sleep is present in mammals and birds, probably in reptiles, amphibians and fish, and possibly in some invertebrate species. It may be present in only one cerebral hemisphere at a time in dolphins, porpoises, whales and some species of birds, presumably as a defense against predators. Sleep is generated by the brain, but is associated with profound changes in physiology elsewhere in the body. Contrary to early belief, the neurophysiology of sleep involves active and dynamic changes in neural functioning and is far from a passive state characterized by absence of wakefulness.

## ELECTROENCEPHALOGRAPHY

The human scalp electroencephalogram (EEG) was first recorded by Hans Berger of Germany in 1929. Understanding sleep physiology requires some knowledge of the basis of the EEG and the manner in which it is recorded. The EEG is recorded by electrodes that are attached to multiple areas of the scalp. These record summated electrical activity from synapses in the uppermost levels of the cerebral cortex. Electrodes are applied according to the international 10–20 system, a method for finding the correct electrode sites by attention to certain anatomical landmarks. The electrodes used most often in monitoring sleep are discussed in Chapter 4.

A single tracing of EEG is known as a derivation; in a full EEG 16 or more derivations are recorded simultaneously from multiple areas of the scalp. Two forms of recording are used, bipolar and referential. In a bipolar derivation, the difference in electric potentials recorded by two adjacent electrodes is displayed, while in a referential derivation, the electric potential recorded from a single scalp electrode compared with that recorded from a relatively inactive electrode at a distance from the scalp, such as over the ear (Figure 1.1). An arrangement of derivations in a specified order is known as a montage.

The various frequency ranges of electrical activity recorded on an EEG are arbitrarily divided into four categories (Table 1.1). Alpha rhythm consists of alpha frequency activity in sinusoidal trains recorded over the occipital head region during wakefulness when a subject's eyes are shut (Figure 1.2).

**Table 1.1** Electroencephalogram (EEG) wave frequencies

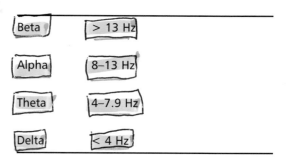

| | |
|---|---|
| Beta | > 13 Hz |
| Alpha | 8–13 Hz |
| Theta | 4–7.9 Hz |
| Delta | < 4 Hz |

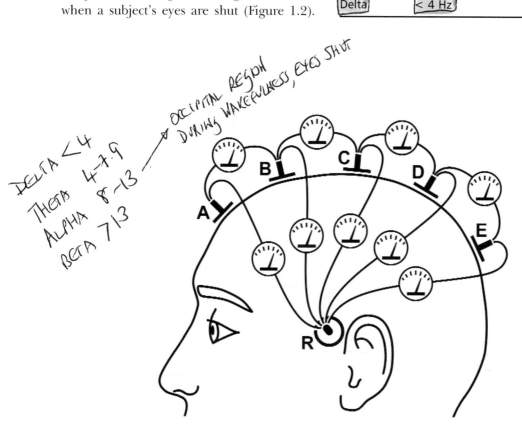

**Figure 1.1** Bipolar and referential electroencephalogram (EEG) derivations. The difference between the scalp potentials underlying electrodes A and B is compared in a bipolar derivation, A–B. The chain of derivations A–B, B–C, C–D and D–E constitute a bipolar montage. In contrast, the potential underlying electrode A is compared with the potential (assumed to be close to zero) recorded from the distant electrode R attached to the ear. This derivation (A–R) is known as a referential derivation and the chain of derivations A–R, B–R, C–R, D–R and E–R constitute a referential montage

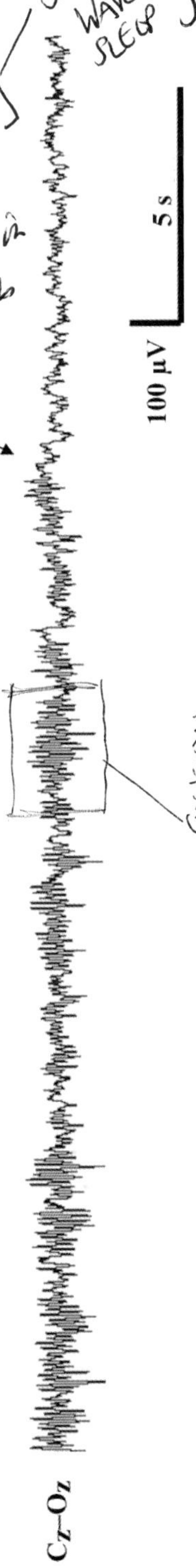

*[Handwritten margin notes around figure: "Most slow wave occurs in the earlier sleep cycles"; "NREM 1 2 3 4 — SLOW WAVE SLEEP"; "REM — Most REM occurs in late cycles"; "B A T D >13 8-13 4-7.9 <4"; "BETA >13, ALPHA 8-13, THETA 4-7.9, DELTA <4"; "REM 25%, STAGE1 5%, 2 50%, 3&4 20%"; "SINUSOIDAL"; "5 s"; "100 µV"; "Cz–Oz"]*

**Figure 1.2** Alpha rhythm. This tracing shows occipital alpha rhythm, attenuating with eye opening (arrow). $C_z$–$O_z$ derivation is explained in more detail in Chapter 4

Opening the eyes attenuates alpha rhythm, as does the development of drowsiness.

## SLEEP STATES AND CYCLES

Human sleep is not a uniform process but comprises two states, non-rapid eye movement sleep (NREM sleep) and rapid eye movement sleep (REM sleep). A night's sleep in an adult consists of between four and six sequential cycles, each lasting approximately 90 min, during which a longer period of NREM sleep is followed by a generally shorter period of REM sleep. NREM sleep is divided into four stages of increasing depth of unresponsiveness, known as stages 1–4 NREM sleep. Stages 3 and 4 are often combined, and referred to as slow wave or delta sleep. Figure 1.3 illustrates schematically the progression of sleep through the different states. It can be seen that most slow-wave sleep occurs during earlier sleep cycles, whereas most REM sleep occurs during later cycles. Transitions from NREM to REM sleep usually occur via stage 2 NREM sleep. It is normal for sleep cycles to be interrupted by occasional brief arousals, often associated with position changes and usually without full return to consciousness. Approximately three-quarters of a night's sleep in a young adult comprises NREM sleep (5% stage 1, 50% stage 2 and 20% stages 3 and 4), while REM sleep comprises one-quarter (Figure 1.4).

## NREM sleep

NREM sleep is characterized by synchronized, rhythmic EEG activity, partial relaxation of voluntary muscles and reduced cerebral blood flow. Heart rate, blood pressure

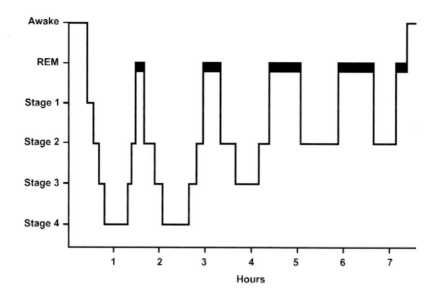

**Figure 1.3** Schematic representation of the cycles of a night's sleep. This figure is a representation of a typical night's sleep in a young adult, demonstrating five sleep cycles with most slow-wave sleep in earlier cycles and most rapid eye movement (REM) sleep in later cycles. Brief periods of wakefulness, which are normally present during the night, have been omitted

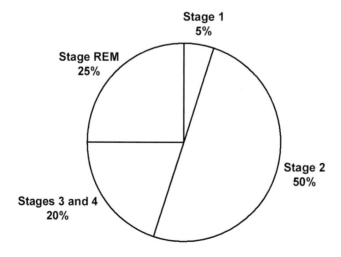

**Figure 1.4** Percentage of sleep stages in a young adult. REM, rapid eye movement

and respiratory tidal volume fall. Some mental imagery persists during NREM sleep, but on waking this is more often described as fragmentary thoughts or simple images than as vivid dreams.

Stage 1 NREM sleep is characterized by the disappearance of occipital alpha rhythm and its replacement by low-amplitude theta activity. Sharply contoured vertex waves (V-waves) may appear over the frontocentral head regions, and positive occipital sharp transients of sleep (POSTS) may be seen posteriorly (Figure 1.5). Slow, horizontal, rolling eye movements develop, voluntary muscles relax and response to environmental sensory stimuli lessens or ceases. The onset of sleep is usually preceded by a poorly defined period of drowsiness (see Chapter 5). The onset of behavioral sleep differs from the arbitrarily defined onset of

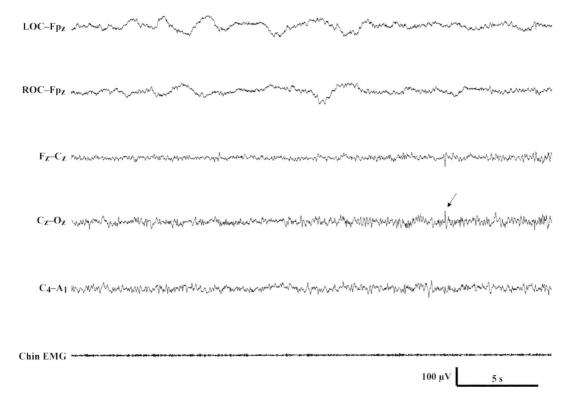

LOC–Fp$_z$

ROC–Fp$_z$

F$_z$–C$_z$

C$_z$–O$_z$

C$_4$–A$_1$

Chin EMG

100 µV         5 s

**Figure 1.5** Stage 1 non-rapid eye movement (NREM) sleep. This 30-s epoch shows the characteristics of stage 1 NREM sleep. The LOC–Fp$_z$ and ROC–Fp$_z$ derivations record eye movements. The Fp$_z$–C$_z$, C$_z$–O$_z$ and C$_4$–A$_1$ derivations record electroencephalogram (EEG) activity. All these derivations are explained in more detail in Chapter 4. The EEG is low-amplitude, mixed-frequency. A single rudimentary vertex wave is present (see arrow). Slow, rolling horizontal eye movements of drowsiness are present on the eye movement channels. Electromyogram (EMG) amplitude is low

*[handwritten: K-COMPLEXES ARE ASSOCIATED WITH ↑ SYMP. ACTIVITY]*

electrophysiological sleep, with responsiveness to the environment progressively declining from drowsiness preceding stage 1 sleep to early stage 2 sleep.

Two EEG phenomena, K-complexes and sleep spindles, characterize stage 2 NREM sleep (Figure 1.6). K-complexes are high-amplitude, diphasic waves, and sleep spindles are chains of rhythmic 12–14-Hz activity. Both are recorded over the vertex and last at least 0.5 s. Although they may occur

independently, often a spindle follows a K-complex. K-complexes occur both spontaneously with a periodicity of about 30 s, and in response to external auditory stimuli. They are associated with transient increases in sympathetic activity, and may have evolved as a mechanism for inducing protective partial arousals during sleep in hazardous environments. Slow eye movements and POSTS may sometimes persist into stage 2 sleep. Slow-wave sleep (stages 3

*[handwritten: A SPINDLE OFTEN FOLLOWS A K COMPLEX]*

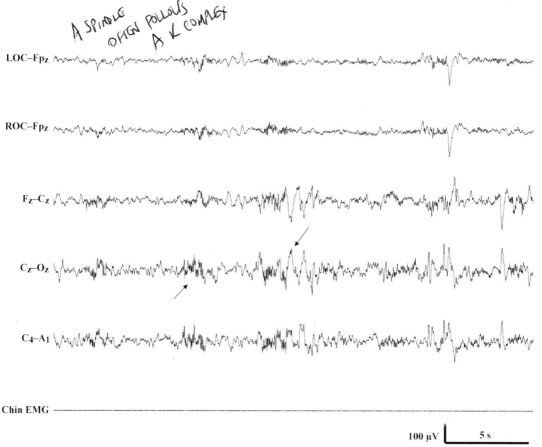

**Figure 1.6** Stage 2 non-rapid eye movement (NREM) sleep. This 30-s epoch shows the characteristics of stage 2 NREM sleep. Derivations are described in Figure 1.5 and in Chapter 4. Eye movements have ceased. K-complexes (high-amplitude diphasic waves maximal over the vertex) and sleep spindles (12–14-Hz activity) are indicated by arrows. EMG, electromyogram

and 4 NREM sleep) is characterized by increasing quantities of synchronized, high-amplitude delta activity with frequency of 2 Hz or less, occurring over wide areas of the cortex (Figure 1.7). This is the deepest stage of sleep, requiring the greatest sensory stimuli to induce an arousal.

## REM sleep

REM sleep (Figure 1.8), also known as paradoxical sleep, can be conceptualized as a state of internal arousal, sharing some features of NREM sleep and some of wakefulness. REM sleep phenomena can be classified as tonic and phasic, tonic persisting throughout a REM sleep period, and phasic occurring intermittently (Table 1.2). The tonic phenomena include a desynchronized, low-amplitude, mixed-frequency cortical EEG, resembling the EEG of wakefulness with the eyes open, and rhythmic hippocampal theta activity. Voluntary muscles become

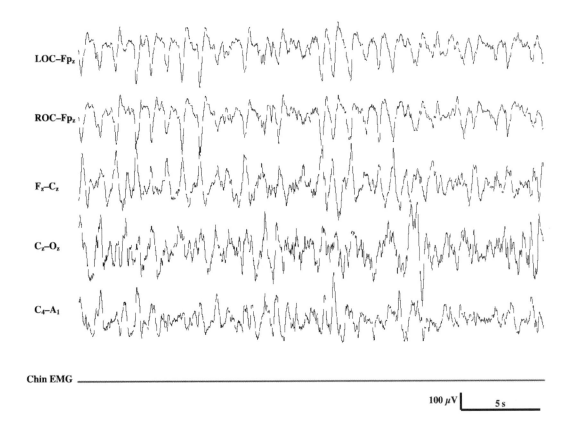

**Figure 1.7** Stage 4 non-rapid eye movement (NREM) sleep. This 30-s epoch shows the characteristics of stage 4 NREM sleep. Derivations are described in Figure 1.5 and in Chapter 4. High-amplitude slow delta waves are the predominant finding. EMG, electromyogram

largely atonic with only the extraocular muscles and diaphragm retaining activity. Cerebral blood flow increases relative to NREM sleep. Thermal regulation is impaired, resulting in near poikilothermia. Penile erections occur in men and clitoral engorgement in women. The most characteristic REM sleep phenomenon is that of dreaming. Subjects woken during REM sleep will report dreaming in about 85% of awak-

enings, but dreams are rarely recalled after a period of REM sleep has ended. REM dreams are vivid, surrealistic, emotionally charged, multicolor experiences with frequent auditory accompaniments and perceptions of movement.

Superimposed phasic events include rapid eye movements. These are conjugate, irregular, predominantly horizontal or oblique eye movements that occur in clusters

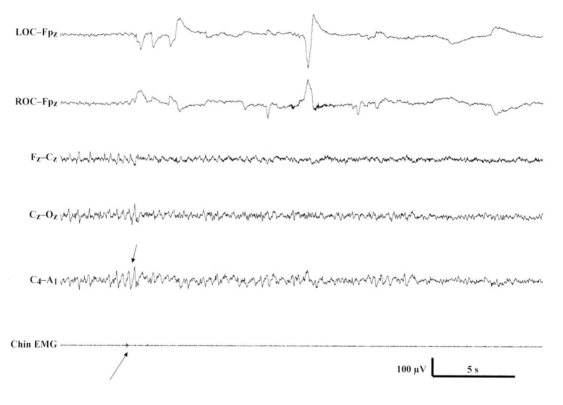

**Figure 1.8** Rapid eye movement (REM) sleep. This 30-s epoch shows the characteristics of REM stage sleep. Derivations are described in Figure 1.5 and in Chapter 4. Irregular, conjugate, horizontal rapid eye movements are present in the eye movement channels. Sawtooth waves (arrow) precede rapid eye movements, but the remainder of the electroencephalogram (EEG) consists of low-amplitude mixed-frequency rhythms. Electromyogram (EMG) tone is absent apart from a single short phasic twitch (arrow)

**Table 1.2** Phenomena of rapid eye movement (REM) sleep

---

*Tonic phenomena*
Desynchronized, mixed-frequency electroencephalogram (EEG)
Hippocampal theta activity
Atonic voluntary muscles
Increased cerebral blood flow
Impaired thermal regulation
Penile erections and clitoral engorgement
Dreams

*Phasic phenomena*
Rapid eye movements
Phasic muscle twitches
Irregular accelerations of heart and respiratory rate
Ponto-geniculo-occipital waves
Sawtooth waves

---

during a period of REM sleep. Superimposed on the skeletal muscle atonia are irregular short bursts of muscle activity, known as phasic muscle twitches. Irregular accelerations of heart rate and respiration occur. In animals, intermittent ponto-geniculo-occipital (PGO) waves can be recorded from the pontine tegmentum, the lateral geniculate body of the thalamus, and the cerebral cortex, especially the occipital lobe. The human scalp EEG may show sawtooth waves, trains of triangular 2–4-Hz waves recorded over the vertex, often preceding bursts of rapid eye movements.

The transition between NREM and REM sleep is not an abrupt process. Experimental studies with intracellular electrodes in pontine reticular formation neurons show that there is a gradual membrane depolarization of these cells prior to the onset of REM sleep. This is mirrored in the human polysomnogram by such phenomena as K-complexes or spindles intruding into early REM sleep, or muscle atonia developing several seconds before any other REM sleep phenomena. In obstructive sleep apnea syndrome (see Chapter 8), it is common to see a distinct worsening of apneas as the first sign that REM sleep is approaching. In patients with neurodegenerative disorders, periods of sleep can be recorded with an intermixture of NREM and REM phenomena, often referred to as ambiguous sleep. The most extreme form of this (status dissociatus) occurs when it is impossible to distinguish wakefulness, NREM and REM sleep on a polysomnogram.

## Case 1.1

A 68-year-old man presented with a 4-year history of nocturnal hallucinations. He would wake from sleep seeing vivid images of snakes, spiders or Arabian palaces in his bedroom. On one occasion he was convinced he saw the dead body of his wife next to him, and was actually phoning for help when his wife walked into the bedroom. The images lasted several minutes, and at times he would jump out of bed to avoid them. The patient was aware of mild, short-term memory problems. Neurological examination confirmed difficulties with learning and recall, but was otherwise normal. A polysomnogram showed markedly abnormal sleep architecture. During most of the night, alpha rhythm with variable amounts of theta and delta activity was seen. Occasional sleep spindles were present. No REM sleep was recorded, but at one time rapid eye movements were seen coincident with sleep spindles and not associated with muscle atonia. The patient aroused from sleep once and reported seeing a bear. Initially a definitive diagnosis was not possible, but with the passage of time moderate cognitive impairment developed, and a diagnosis of dementia with Lewy bodies was made.

This case illustrates dissociation of the phenomena of wakefulness, NREM and REM sleep resulting in ambiguous sleep states and manifesting clinically by vivid nocturnal hallucinations. Severe sleep abnormalities preceded other manifestations of a neurodegenerative illness. These issues are discussed at greater length in Chapters 16 and 17.

## CHANGES IN SLEEP PHYSIOLOGY WITH AGE

The two states of sleep are present in neonates, but are known as quiet (NREM) and active (REM) sleep. Active sleep may constitute 50% of total sleep time, with a shorter cyclical periodicity of 50–60 min and frequent transitions from wakefulness directly into active sleep. Daily total sleep time in a neonate is at least 16 h (Figure 1.9). Sleep spindles develop by 3 months of age, and K-complexes by 5 months. Sleep spindles in the first year of life may be asynchronous, occurring alternately over each hemisphere. During the first decade, the percentage of REM sleep falls, and the time

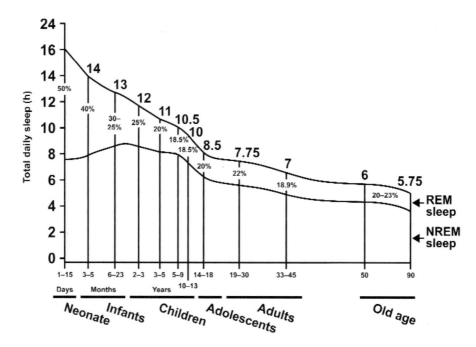

**Figure 1.9** Schematic representation of changes in sleep with age. This graph shows schematically the changes in sleep time and sleep stages from birth to old age. REM, rapid eye movement; NREM, non-rapid eye movement. Modified with permission from reference 1

of the first REM sleep period from sleep onset (REM latency) increases.

REM sleep latency again shortens in the elderly. The percentage of slow-wave sleep begins to fall in adolescence, and continues to decline with advancing age. Sleep in the elderly is also characterized by increased awakenings during sleep, reduced total sleep time and daytime napping. Periodic limb movements of sleep (see Chapter 15) become commoner, and an increased tendency to sleep-disordered breathing is noted.

The timing of sleep also varies with age. First-decade children tend to go to sleep earlier than adults, and often wake earlier as well. During adolescence, sleep onset becomes delayed, with 15–25-year-olds preferring to sleep from after midnight to late in the morning. This delayed sleep phase pattern is a physiological change, and is not simply due to social factors[2]. Some older persons develop an advanced sleep pattern, with sleep onset at 7–8 p.m. and waking in the early hours of the morning (Figure 1.10).

**FUNCTIONS OF SLEEP**

We sleep for almost one-third of our lives, and yet the functions of sleep remain enigmatic. Many functions have been proposed (Table 1.3), and all may be

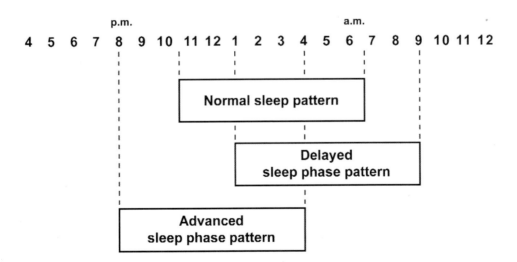

**Figure 1.10** Different sleep phase patterns. This diagram illustrates different sleep phase patterns with alterations in the timing of sleep in the 24-h cycle

partially correct. It has been proposed that sleep, especially NREM sleep, is necessary for protein synthesis, cell division and growth, thus allowing for repair of the body or brain. REM sleep appears to consolidate memory, and may serve a role in deleting unnecessary memory files[3]. Sleep may be necessary to maintain immunocompetence[4]. Species with a high metabolic rate have longer sleep times, suggesting that sleep may be required to conserve energy[5]. However, there is no accepted model linking these varied effects, and the fundamental role of sleep at cellular and molecular levels has yet to be elucidated.

## NEUROANATOMICAL LOCALIZATION OF SLEEP AND WAKEFULNESS

### REM sleep

#### The REM sleep generator

The search for the generator of REM sleep has involved many different mammalian experimental models, including transection, tissue ablation and unit recording studies[6]. After transection of the midbrain, electro-physiological features of REM sleep can be recorded caudal, but not rostral, to the transection. In contrast, after transection at the junction between the medulla and the pons, REM phenomena can be recorded rostral, but not caudal, to the transection. Following transections both above and below the pons, REM sleep can be recorded from the isolated pons, but not from structures rostral or caudal to it. Thus, transection experiments demonstrate that the principal REM sleep

**Table 1.3** Proposed functions of sleep

| |
|---|
| Body repair theory |
| Brain restoration theory |
| Memory and learning theory |
| Unlearning theory |
| Immunocompetence theory |
| Thermoregulation and energy conservation theory |

generator is localized in the pons (Figure 1.11).

The dorsal portion of the pons (pontine tegmentum) contains a network of neurons and ascending fiber tracts known as the ascending reticular formation. Ablation of the more rostral portion of the pontine tegmentum, known as the nucleus reticularis pontis oralis (NRPO), eliminates REM sleep. More precise experiments have shown that the critical area for REM sleep generation consists of a small area in the lateral portions of the NRPO ventral to the locus ceruleus (Figure 1.12). Application of kainic acid, a cytotoxin, to this area has demonstrated that cell loss rather than nerve fiber damage is responsible for the disruption of REM sleep.

Unit recording studies with microelectrodes have detected a population of neurons in the lateral NRPO that have a high rate of discharge only during REM sleep (REM sleep-on cells). At least some of these cells produce acetylcholine. REM sleep-off cells have been found in the noradrenergic locus ceruleus and in the serotonergic raphe system. These cells

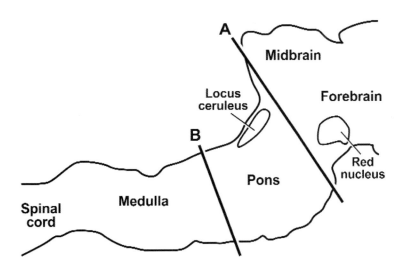

**Figure 1.11** Brainstem transection experiments to determine the generator of rapid eye movement (REM) sleep. Transections at point B result in REM phenomena being recorded only rostral to the cut. Transections at point A result in REM phenomena only caudal to the cut, while transections at both points A and B result in REM phenomena recordable only from the pons. Modified with permission from reference 6

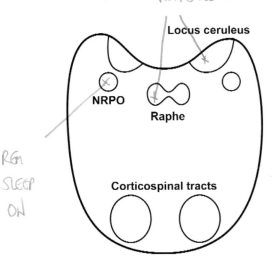

**Figure 1.12** Schematic transverse section through the pons. Dorsal is at the top of the figure, ventral at the bottom. NRPO, nucleus reticularis pontis oralis

discharge regularly during wakefulness and slowly during non-REM sleep, and are silent during REM sleep.

*Effector pathways in REM sleep*

With the principal REM sleep generator being localized to a small number of cells in the rostral pontine tegmentum, extensive axonal pathways are required to produce the range of REM sleep phenomena, such as skeletal muscle atonia, rapid eye movements and dreams. Muscle atonia can be produced by electrical stimulation of a number of areas in the brainstem, including the pedunculo-pontine nucleus of the pons, the retrorubral nucleus of the lower midbrain and the nucleus magnocellularis of the medial medulla. The pathway involves axons probably arising from the dorsolateral pedunculo-pontine nucleus, which travel in the tegmen-toreticular tract to synapse on cell bodies in the nucleus magnocellularis and nucleus paramedianus in the ventromedial medulla (Figure 1.13). Neurochemical studies have shown that the neurotransmitter of the axons of the tegmentoreticular tract ending on cells in the nucleus magnocellularis is glutamate, while that of axons ending on the

nucleus paramedianus is acetylcholine. Axons from these nuclei run in the ventro-lateral reticulospinal tract, terminating on spinal-cord anterior horn cells. Release of glycine produces hyperpolarization and thus postsynaptic inhibition, resulting in muscle atonia. The glutamate receptors in the nucleus magnocellularis involved in the muscle atonia pathway are of the non-NMDA (*N*-methyl-D-aspartate) type, but stimulation

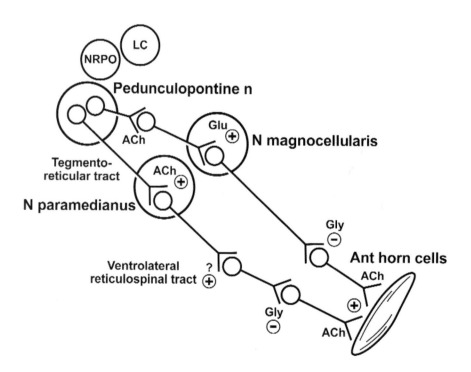

**Figure 1.13** Schematic diagram of the neural pathways mediating rapid eye movement (REM) sleep atonia. The pedunculopontine nucleus (n) is in the pons, nucleus (N) magnocellularis and paramedi-anus in the medulla, and anterior (Ant) horn cells in the ventral horn of the spinal cord. NRPO, nucleus reticularis pontis oralis; LC, locus ceruleus; ACh, acetylcholine; Glu, glutamate; +, excitatory neuro-transmitter; –, inhibitory neurotransmitter; ?, unknown neurotransmitter

of glutamate NMDA receptors in the same region produces muscle twitching. This phenomenon may explain the paradoxical association of muscle atonia and phasic muscle twitching observed during REM sleep.

This physiology helps to explain the pathogenesis of some of the pathological phenomena associated with REM sleep (Figure 1.14). Atonia without other phenomena of REM sleep can be produced experi-

mentally by the injection of cholinergic agonists into the dorsal pons, or by electrical stimulation or injection of glutamate into the medial medulla. This is a model of cataplexy, the sudden loss of muscle tone with emotion occurring in patients with narcolepsy (see Chapter 7). A population of medullary cells has been detected in narcoleptic dogs that fire only during REM sleep and cataplectic attacks. In contrast, REM sleep without atonia can be produced

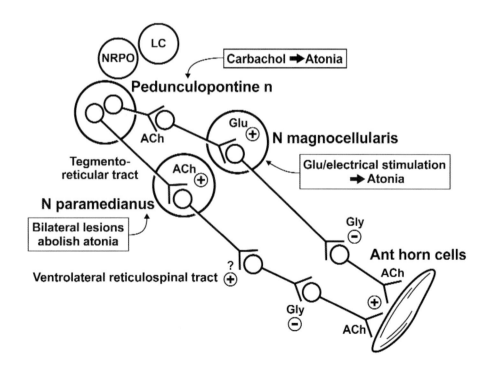

**Figure 1.14** Experimental intervention in the neural pathway mediating rapid eye movement (REM) sleep atonia. These experimental interventions produce experimental models for the human conditions of cataplexy and REM sleep behavior disorder (see text). Abbreviations as in Figure 1.13

by lesions of the dorsal pons in cats, which presumably interrupt the tegmentoreticular tract. Depending on the exact site of the lesion, the animal's behavior ranges from slight raising of the head to elaborate aggressive motor activity[7]. This experimental preparation is a model for the condition of REM sleep behavior disorder, in which patients lose the muscle atonia of REM sleep and act out their dreams, often in a violent manner (see Chapter 16).

PGO waves, generated in the cholinergic peribrachial area of the pontine tegmentum, project to the lateral geniculate body and other thalamic nuclei as well as the occipital cortex. They serve as the physiological correlate of the neural pathways mediating REM phenomena rostral to the pons. PGO waves precede rapid eye movements, and may play a role in the generation of dream imagery in the occipital cortex.

## NREM sleep

### NREM sleep networks

In contrast to REM sleep, animals with brainstem transections demonstrate NREM type neuronal activity both rostrally and caudally. There is no single generator of

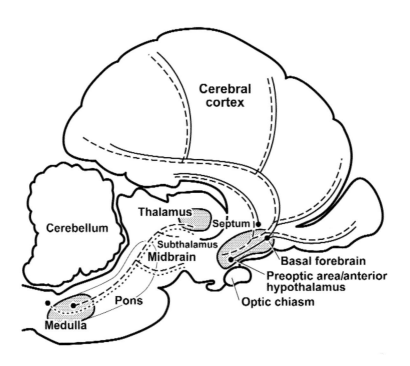

**Figure 1.15** Midline sagittal section through the brain demonstrating the networks involved in NREM sleep generation. Shaded areas indicate major nuclei involved in NREM sleep generation (nucleus of the solitary tract in the medulla, nucleus reticularis in the thalamus, anterior hypothalamus, preoptic area and basal forebrain). Modified with permission from reference 8

NREM sleep, but rather a widespread inter-connecting network of cell groups in the brain stem, diencephalon and forebrain that control this state[8] (Figure 1.15). In the medulla, the nucleus of the solitary tract includes a population of neurons that discharge more actively during NREM sleep than during wakefulness, while electrical stimulation of the region produces sleep. Fibers from this nucleus project to the pons, midbrain, thalamus, hypothalamus and the frontal cortex. The thalamic reticular nucleus is responsible for the generation of spindle activity and for deafferentation of the cortex during sleep by inhibition of ascending sensory pathways.

Electrical stimulation of the anterior hypothalamic and preoptic areas results in sleep. In the encephalitis lethargica outbreak associated with the influenza pandemic following World War I, patients with severe insomnia were found to have lesions in these areas. Anterior to the preoptic nuclei lies the basal forebrain area, including the nucleus of the diagonal band and the substantia innom-inata (Figure 1.16). Electrical stimulation here also produces sleep, and single unit recordings demonstrate a population of cells that fire more rapidly during NREM sleep than during wakefulness. Basal forebrain neurons project to wake centers in the posterior hypothalamus, and may induce sleep by inhibiting these cells.

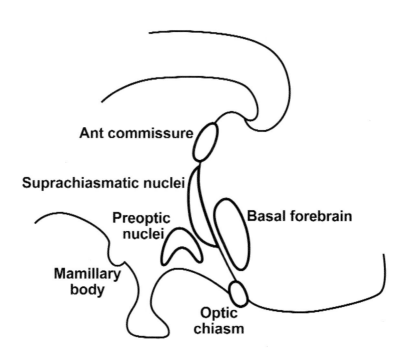

**Figure 1.16** Midline sagittal section through the hypothalamus and basal forebrain. This figure illustrates the anatomy of the preoptic nuclei and basal forebrain nuclei involved in the generation of non-rapid eye movement (NREM) sleep. Ant, anterior

### Spindle generation and cortical synchronization

One of the electrophysiological characteristics of NREM sleep is the presence of highly synchronized cortical activity in the form of sleep spindles and high-amplitude delta waves. Spindle activity depends on some unusual properties of thalamic neurons. During waking and REM sleep, thalamic reticular neurons show tonic activity, but during NREM sleep they alter their electrical activity to produce a burst-firing pattern. The mechanism involves initial hyperpolarization with superimposed depolarization, resulting in bursts of rhythmic action potentials at the frequency of sleep spindles. Reticular neurons project to other thalamic nuclei, and by releasing γ-hydroxybutyrate (GABA), an inhibitory neurotransmitter, induce widespread hyperpolarization and subsequent rhythmic burst firing. These thalamic nuclei in turn project to the cortex and initiate cortical spindle activity. Similar mechanisms are thought to underlie delta wave generation in slow-wave sleep. The important role of the thalamus in the initiation of sleep is illustrated by the rare prion disorder, fatal familial insomnia, in which degeneration of the anteroventral and dorsomedial thalamic nuclei results in profound insomnia (see Chapter 10).

### Wakefulness

Similar to NREM sleep, the state of wakefulness is controlled by a network of neuronal systems. These are concentrated in the central brainstem reticular formation and its projections to diencephalic and frontal regions. The major areas involved are the ascending reticular formation of the midbrain and pons, the non-specific thalamic nuclei, the posterior hypothalamus and the basal forebrain area. In addition to neurons firing preferentially during sleep, the latter region also includes a population of cells firing during wakefulness. Histamine-releasing neurons in the tuberomamillary hypothalamic nuclei are especially important in the generation of alertness. In contrast to patients with the form of encephalitis lethargica characterized by insomnia, those with profound hypersomnia were often found to have lesions in the posterior hypothalamus.

## BIOCHEMISTRY OF SLEEP

### Acetylcholine

There are two major cholinergic neural systems, one originating in the pontine tegmental reticular formation and the other in the basal forebrain. Acetylcholine appears to be responsible for intrinsic activation processes in wakefulness and in REM sleep. Cholinergic cells of the reticular formation are active during wakefulness and REM sleep but silent during NREM sleep (Table 1.4). The inhibition of these neurons at the onset of sleep is believed to be the trigger for the change in firing pattern of thalamic nuclei responsible for spindle generation. Basal forebrain cholinergic cells discharge during wakefulness and not during NREM sleep. Acetylcholine is involved in the executive pathways controlling REM phenomena such as REM atonia and PGO spikes.

### Catecholamines

Catecholamines are involved in maintenance of the wake state. Noradrenergic neurons of

**Table 1.4** Neurotransmitter systems in sleep and wakefulness. Modified with permission from reference 9

|  | Wake | NREM sleep | REM sleep |
| --- | --- | --- | --- |
| Cholinergic neurons | active | silent | active |
| Noradrenergic neurons | active | partially active | silent |
| Serotoninergic neurons | active | partially active | silent |

the locus ceruleus project widely to the cerebral cortex, and fire actively during wakefulness. They continue to discharge during NREM sleep but at a slower frequency, and are silent during REM sleep. Dopaminergic neurons arising in the ventral tegmentum of the brainstem innervate the septal nuclei and the frontal cortex, resulting in arousal. Drugs increasing catecholamines at the synaptic cleft, including amphetamines and cocaine, cause cortical activation.

**Serotonin**

The serotoninergic midline raphe nuclei in the brainstem tegmentum fire rapidly in wakefulness and less rapidly in NREM sleep, while they are silent in REM sleep. This pattern is very similar to that of the locus ceruleus discussed above. The exact role of serotonin in sleep generation has not been fully elucidated.

**Histamine**

Histaminergic neurons in the tuberomamillary nucleus in the posterior hypothalamus promote cortical arousal. Sedation is a major side-effect of the histamine-1 antagonists.

**Hypocretins (orexins)**

Hypocretins (also known as orexins) are recently identified peptide neurotransmitters secreted by a small group of cells in the posterolateral hypothalamus[10]. Hypocretin-releasing axons project widely to the limbic system, thalamus, brainstem reticular core and neocortex (Figure 1.17). A precursor molecule, preprohypocretin, is converted into hypocretin-1 (hcrt-1) (orexin A) and hypocretin-2 (hcrt-2) (orexin B). There are two hypocretin receptors, hypocretin receptor 1 with a high affinity for hcrt-1, and hypocretin receptor 2 with a high affinity for both hcrt-1 and hcrt-2. The first indication of a relationship of the hypocretin system to sleep and alertness was the discovery that narcolepsy in dogs, an autosomal recessive disorder, was due to a deletion in the hypocretin 2 receptor gene[12]. At about the same time, researchers studying hypocretin knock-out mice noted that they developed sleep attacks and falls very reminiscent of cataplexy[13]. Most human narcoleptics tested have shown undetectable levels of hypocretin-1 in the cerebrospinal fluid (see Chapter 7). Intraventricular infusion of hypocretins

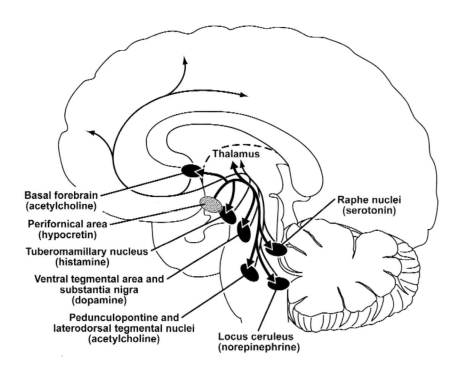

**Figure 1.17** Widespread projections of hypocretin (orexin)-synthesizing neurons. The figure demonstrates how hypocretin (orexin)-synthesizing neurons from the perifornical area of the hypothalamus project to many other neurons involved in a wide range of neurotransmitter systems. Modified with permission from reference 11

in rats causes increased alertness. The hypocretin system appears to act primarily to promote wakefulness by facilitating the release of wake-producing monoamines.

## Other sleep factors

Many other humoral substances found within the brain or cerebrospinal fluid appear to modulate sleep. Adenosine concentration in the brain increases during prolonged wakefulness and decreases with subsequent recovery sleep[14]. This suggests that it may play a role as a sleep-inducing chemical. Caffeine produces alertness by blocking adenosine receptors. Prostaglandin $D_2$ promotes sleep while prostaglandin $E_2$ inhibits sleep. A number of substances enhance slow-wave sleep, including the cytokines interleukin-1 and tumor necrosis factor; a nonapeptide, delta sleep-inducing peptide; and growth hormone-releasing hormone.

## Melatonin

Melatonin, a peptide hormone secreted by the pineal gland, plays a role in control of the circadian system. Its synthesis and actions are discussed in Chapter 13.

## REFERENCES

1. Roffwarg HP, Muzio JN, Dement WC. Ontogenic development of the human sleep–dream cycle. *Science* 1966;152:604–19

2. Carskadon MA, Vieira C, Acebo C. Association between puberty and delayed sleep preference. *Sleep* 1993;16:258–62

3. Crick F, Mitchison G. The function of dream sleep. *Nature (London)* 1983;304: 111–14

4. Toth LA, Opp MR. Sleep and infection. In Lee-Chiong TL, Sateia MJ, Carskadon MA, eds. *Sleep Medicine*. Philadelphia: Hanley & Belfus, 2002:77–84

5. Zepelin H, Rechtschaffen A. Mammalian sleep, longevity, and energy metabolism. *Brain Behav Evol* 1974;10:425–470

6. Siegel JM. Brainstem mechanisms generating REM sleep. In Kryger MH, Roth T, Dement WC, eds. *Principles and Practice of Sleep Medicine*. Philadelphia: WB Saunders, 2000:112–33

7. Hendricks JC, Morrison AR, Mann GL. Different behaviors during paradoxical sleep without atonia depend on pontine lesion site. *Brain Res* 1982;239:81–105

8. Jones BE. Basic mechanisms of sleep–wake states. In Kryger MH, Roth T, Dement WC, eds. *Principles and Practice of Sleep Medicine*. Philadelphia: WB Saunders, 2000:134–54

9. Garcia-Rill E. Mechanisms of sleep and wakefulness. In Lee-Chiong TL, Sateia MJ, Carskadon MA, eds. *Sleep Medicine*. Philadelphia: Hanley & Belfus, 2002:31–9

10. Mignot E, Taheri S, Nishino S. Sleeping with the hypothalamus: emerging targets for sleep disorders. *Nature Neurosci* 2002;5:S1071–5

11. Silber MH, Rye DB. Solving the mysteries of narcolepsy: the hypocretin story. *Neurology* 2001;56:1616–17

12. Lin L, Faraco J, Li R, *et al*. The sleep disorder canine narcolepsy is caused by a mutation in the hypocretin (orexin) receptor 2 gene. *Cell* 1999;98:365–76

13. Chemelli RM, Willie JT, Sinton CM, *et al*. Narcolepsy in orexin knockout mice: molecular genetics of sleep regulation. *Cell* 1999; 98:437–51

14. Porkka-Heiskanen T, Strecker RE, Thakkar M, Bjorkum AA, Greene RW, McCarley RW. Adenosine: a mediator of the sleep-inducing effects of prolonged wakefulness. *Science* 1997;276:1265–8

# Chapter 2

# Classification of sleep disorders

*"The time has come," the Walrus said,*
*"To talk of many things;*
*Of shoes–and ships–and sealing wax–*
*Of cabbages–and kings–"*

**Lewis Carroll, *Through the Looking-Glass***

Sleep medicine is a young field and its nosology is far from fixed. The idea that the study of sleep physiology might evolve into a branch of medicine devoted to disorders of sleep arose during the 1960s. The first attempt to classify sleep disorders had its origin in a workshop at the 1972 annual meeting of the Association for the Psychophysiological Study of Sleep (APSS), resulting in the establishment of a Nosology Committee in 1976. Since then, two major classifications of sleep disorders have been published and a third is currently in preparation. This ongoing process results from a need to find a common terminology and diagnostic system that are widely accepted and reflect current practice and research.

and predicted that there would be considerable changes as the field evolved. Like subsequent nosologies, the division of the subject was based on a combination of the best available scientific data and the shared judgment of experienced clinicians. Sleep and arousal disorders were divided into four categories (Table 2.1), the first two based on patient complaints, and the third and fourth on presumed pathophysiology. The authors recognized that the harmoniously named DIMS (disorders of initiating and maintaining sleep) and DOES (disorders of excessive somnolence) were not clearly separable, with some conditions presenting at times with insomnia and at other times with excessive sleepiness.

## THE DIAGNOSTIC CLASSIFICATION OF SLEEP AND AROUSAL DISORDERS: 1979

In 1979, a 137-page classification of sleep disorders sponsored by the Association of Professional Sleep Disorders Centers and the APSS was published in the newly formed journal *Sleep*[1]. This remarkable document remained the framework for the study of sleep disorders for more than a decade. The authors, led by Dr Howard Roffwarg, readily admitted that this was a work in progress,

**Table 2.1** Classification of Sleep and Arousal Disorders: 1979

| | |
|---|---|
| A | DIMS: Disorders of initiating and maintaining sleep (insomnias) |
| B | DOES: Disorders of excessive somnolence |
| C | Disorders of the sleep–wake schedule |
| D | Dysfunctions associated with sleep, sleep stages or partial arousals (parasomnias) |

## THE INTERNATIONAL CLASSIFICATION OF SLEEP DISORDERS (ICSD)

By 1985 it had become apparent that knowledge had progressed to the point that a new classification was needed. The American Sleep Disorders Association (ASDA), in collaboration with the European Sleep Research Society, the Japanese Society of Sleep Research and the Latin American Sleep Society, commissioned a new nosology that was published in 1990, under the leadership of Dr Michael Thorpy[2]. The classification comprised 84 disorders and utilized a somewhat different grouping of topics based on pathophysiological concepts (Table 2.2). The term 'dyssomnia' was introduced to define disorders producing a complaint of either insomnia or sleepiness. The dyssomnias were subdivided into intrinsic sleep disorders (arising from dysfunction of the body or mind), extrinsic sleep disorders (arising from the external environment) and circadian rhythm disorders. Parasomnias were split into four categories, reflecting the states of sleep from which they arose. Two new categories were introduced: sleep disorders associated with other medical or psychiatric disorders, and proposed sleep disorders. Formal diagnostic, severity and duration criteria were devised. The nosology was revised in minor details in 1997, but remained essentially unchanged.

In 2002 the American Academy of Sleep Medicine, the successor to the ASDA, set up a committee to revise once again the classification of sleep disorders. More than 10 years had passed since the last major revision, and advances in the field had again dictated the need for a new approach. Under the direction of Dr Peter Hauri, the committee has proposed a more pragmatic classification, based on current clinical concepts of the grouping of sleep disorders. Table 2.3 is a preliminary version of the proposed classification. The full nosology is expected to be published in 2004.

**Table 2.2** The International Classification of Sleep Disorders: 1990

*Dyssomnias*
Intrinsic sleep disorders
Extrinsic sleep disorders
Circadian rhythm sleep disorders

*Parasomnias*
Arousal disorders
Sleep–wake transition disorders
Parasomnias usually associated with REM sleep
Other parasomnias

*Sleep disorders associated with other medical or psychiatric disorders*
Associated with mental disorders
Associated with neurological disorders
Associated with other medical disorders

*Proposed sleep disorders*

REM, rapid eye movement

## OVERVIEW OF SLEEP DISORDERS

This book discusses sleep disorders using a clinical approach to symptoms, rather than following a catalog of disorders. However, an overview of some of the disease categories is now presented to provide a broad framework for the chapters that follow. Although the International Classification of Sleep Disorders-2 (ICSD-2) nosology is still in preparation, this description follows the proposed outline as summarized in Table 2.3.

**Table 2.3** Proposed International Classification of Sleep Disorders-2 (ICSD-2): 2004*

*Insomnias*
Psychophysiological insomnia
Idiopathic insomnia
Paradoxical insomnia
Inadequate sleep hygiene
Behavioral insomnia of childhood
Insomnia related to a mental condition or
substance abuse
Insomnia related to a medical condition or
medication

*Sleep-related breathing disorders*
Obstructive sleep apnea syndrome and variants
Central sleep apnea syndrome
Sleep-related central alveolar hypoventilation
syndrome
Sleep-related breathing disorders related to
medical conditions

*Hypersomnias not related to respiratory issues*
Narcolepsy
Idiopathic hypersomnia
Recurrent hypersomnia
Insufficient sleep syndrome
Hypersomnia related to a mental disorder or
substance abuse
Hypersomnia related to a medical condition or
medication

*Circadian rhythm disorders*
Delayed sleep phase syndrome
Advanced sleep phase syndrome
Non-24-h sleep–wake syndrome
Jet lag syndrome
Shift work sleep disorder

*Parasomnias*
Disorders of arousal
Parasomnias associated with REM sleep
Other parasomnias
Parasomnias related to a mental disorder or
substance abuse
Parasomnias related to a medical condition or
medication

*Sleep-related movement disorders*
Restless legs syndrome
Periodic limb movement disorder
Sleep-related bruxism
Sleep-related rhythmic movement disorder

*Other sleep disorders*

*Isolated symptoms, apparently normal variants
and unresolved issues*

* These categories should be regarded as preliminary. Only some of the common disorders in each
category have been included in this table; REM, rapid eye movement

## Insomnias

Insomnia is a symptom of perceived reduction in the quantity or quality of sleep and is not a single clinical entity. However, certain causes of chronic insomnia are believed to be due to intrinsic disturbances of brain function (Chapter 10). The commonest is psychophysiological insomnia, also known as learned or conditioned insomnia. This disorder originates following a period of stress associated with sleep difficulties. Despite resolution of the stress, the insomnia persists as an abnormal conditioned response to going to bed. Idiopathic insomnia, sometimes termed primary insomnia, is a form of insomnia that starts in early childhood and persists through life. Its pathogenesis is unknown. Paradoxical insomnia (previously known as sleep state misperception) exists when a patient complains of difficulty initiating or maintaining sleep, but a polysomnogram shows normal sleep architecture and efficiency.

Inadequate sleep hygiene is a cause of insomnia related to poor sleep habits, such as drinking caffeinated beverages close to bedtime, sleeping with the TV on or exercising just prior to going to bed (Chapter 10). Insomnia is very common in a range of psychiatric disorders, including mood disorders, anxiety disorders and psychoses (Chapter 14). Medical conditions causing insomnia include chronic pain of any kind (Chapter 10). Environmental sleep disorder refers to insomnia or resultant daytime sleepiness induced by external noise, such as a bed partner's snoring (Chapter 5). Medications, alcohol and illicit drugs can affect sleep both during use and after withdrawal (Chapter 14). Two causes of insomnia seen in first-decade children are sleep-onset association disorder in which children are only able to initiate sleep in the presence of a specific object or person, and limit-setting sleep disorder in which inadequate enforcement of bedtimes leads to children refusing to go to bed at appropriate times (Chapter 10).

## Sleep-related breathing disorders

This category includes disorders of sleepiness caused by dysfunction of the upper airway or respiratory control mechanisms. Obstructive sleep apnea, obstructive sleep hypopnea and upper airway resistance syndromes are a spectrum of disorders characterized by hypotonia of upper airway muscles during sleep, resulting in varying degrees of reduced airflow with resultant hypoxemia and recurrent arousals. These disorders are highly prevalent, increasing in incidence with age and body mass index (Chapter 8). Central sleep apnea syndrome is a rarer form of sleep-disordered breathing in which dysfunction of respiratory control results in recurrent apneas with open airway. Causes include left ventricular failure (in which central apneas are a poor prognostic sign) and sleeping at high altitudes (Chapter 8). Central alveolar hypoventilation syndrome includes conditions of reduced respiratory drive during sleep related to neuromuscular diseases or brainstem dysfunction, and results in nocturnal hypoxemia and hypercapnia (Chapter 9). Other respiratory disorders with sleep-related symptoms include asthma, in which attacks of bronchospasm may occur in the early hours of the morning, and chronic obstructive pulmonary disease with nocturnal hypoxemia (Chapter 9).

## Hypersomnias not related to respiratory issues

Certain disorders of excessive daytime somnolence are believed to be caused by intrinsic brain dysfunction. Narcolepsy, recognized for over a century, consists of excessive daytime sleepiness usually associated with weakness of muscles with emotion (known as cataplexy) and the premature occurrence of rapid eye movement (REM) sleep. In most instances, this appears to be due to dysfunction of the hypocretin (orexin) neurotransmitter system (Chapter 7).

Idiopathic hypersomnia is a similar, but less well-defined disorder, with hypersomnolence but no cataplexy and no disturbance in the timing of REM sleep (Chapter 7). Recurrent hypersomnia is a very rare disorder with periods of sleep lasting days to weeks, often associated with behavioral disturbances (Chapter 7). Insufficient sleep syndrome is a major societal problem in which voluntary sleep deprivation can result in impairment of alertness and cognitive abilities. Medications and illicit drug use can cause excessive daytime sleepiness. Hypersomnia may also be due to medical conditions, such as Parkinson's disease and dementias (Chapter 17).

## Circadian rhythm sleep disorders

This group of conditions includes both intrinsic and environmental disorders in which the timing of sleep within the 24-h circadian cycle becomes disturbed (Chapter 13). Delayed-sleep phase syndrome is a pathological exaggeration of the normal tendency of teenagers to go to bed later and wake later than first-decade children or adults. This may result in school or college failure or inability to succeed in the workplace. Advanced sleep phase syndrome is a rarer condition with initiation of sleep early in the evening and thus waking earlier than desired. It is usually seen sporadically in the elderly, but a familial form of the disorder has been described. Non-24-h sleep–wake disorder occurs when the biological clock fails to entrain to the 24-h geosynchronous cycle, resulting in the sleep period slowly rotating around the clock. This may be seen in blind patients with inadequate light stimulation of the hypothalamic suprachiasmatic nuclei.

Shift work sleep disorder occurs especially in shift workers who rotate shifts, with frequent changes in work times between day, evening and night. Insomnia and other physical and psychological disturbances are common. Jet lag syndrome occurs with air travel across time zones from east to west or the reverse. Several days are needed for the biological clock to adapt to such alterations and travellers develop insomnia, excessive sleepiness and mood and somatic symptoms.

## Parasomnias

Parasomnias are undesirable physical phenomena that occur predominantly during sleep (Chapter 16). Arousal disorders, comprising sleepwalking, sleep terrors and confusional arousals, are a spectrum of conditions in which a sudden arousal from slow-wave sleep is associated with abnormal behavior due to the patient's inability to make a rapid transition to complete wakefulness. They are common in childhood but can persist or even develop in adulthood, and may be associated with potentially injurious behavior.

Parasomnias usually associated with REM sleep include nightmares, which are frightening dreams during REM sleep resulting in awakening. Sleep paralysis, occurring at sleep onset or on wakening, is an inability to move for seconds to minutes. It is believed to be due to the muscle atonia of REM sleep developing inappropriately, and may occur both as a normal phenomenon and in patients with narcolepsy. REM sleep behavior disorder occurs when the normal muscle atonia of REM sleep is lost, allowing the enactment of dreams. Patients flail their arms, kick and vocalize, frequently resulting in injuries to themselves or their bed partners. The condition occurs predominantly in older men, and is often associated with neurodegenerative diseases, especially Parkinsonian syndromes. Other parasomnias (not state-related) include sleep enuresis, the continued occurrence of bedwetting in children beyond the age when it normally ceases. Parasomnias related to a known psychiatric disorder include nocturnal panic attacks and nightmares in post-traumatic stress disorder. Parasomnias related to medical conditions include confusional behavior at night in patients with dementia.

### Sleep-related movement disorders

Restless legs syndrome, a very common cause of insomnia, is characterized by an overwhelming urge to move the legs while sitting or lying and relief by movement. It is often familial and appears to be due to central dopaminergic dysfunction. It is usually associated with rhythmic kicking of the legs during sleep, but periodic limb movements of sleep may also accompany other sleep disorders and may occasionally alone be a cause of insomnia or hypersomnia (Chapter 15). Rhythmic movement disorder can occur during any stage of sleep, but is commonest during drowsiness. It consists of large rhythmic movements, usually of the axial musculature, and includes the conditions previously known as body rocking and head banging. Bruxism (tooth grinding)

may occur during any stage of sleep and can result in jaw pain and damage to teeth (Chapter 16).

### Other sleep disorders

This category includes sleep-related epilepsy (Chapter 18), headaches (Chapter 18), gastroesophageal reflux disease (Chapter 10) and laryngospasm (Chapter 17). These conditions can occur predominantly or exclusively during sleep.

### Isolated symptoms, apparently normal variants and unresolved issues

This category includes a number of miscellaneous entities whose clinical significance is uncertain. Sleep starts, also known as hypnic jerks, are sudden muscle contractions at sleep onset that are noted at times by most people, but can occasionally cause initial insomnia (Chapter 16). Primary snoring is also included in this section (Chapter 8).

### REFERENCES

1.  Association of Professional Sleep Disorders Centers. Diagnostic classification of sleep and arousal disorders. *Sleep* 1979;2:1–137

2.  American Sleep Disorders Association. *The International Classification of Sleep Disorders.* Rochester, MN: Davies Printing Co., 1990

# Chapter 3

# Assessing the patient with a sleep disorder

*Sleep is that golden chain that ties
health and our bodies together*

**Thomas Dekker, *The Gull's Handbook***

## THE SLEEP HISTORY

Sleep medicine is primarily a clinical discipline. The most important diagnostic methodology used is not polysomnography, but rather the sleep history. All physicians are trained in the skills of eliciting a history, but the technique and emphasis vary from specialty to specialty. A sleep history involves more than a description of a patient's sleep. It is actually a sleep–wake history, the drawing of a picture of a 24-h day from the viewpoints of alertness and tiredness, occupation and leisure hours, rest and sleep. Both the patient's external activities and internal moods are equally important in understanding how the quality of sleep and waking can be compromised. Environmental, social and medical influences all need to be understood.

In addition, the elicitation of a collateral history is crucial in reaching an accurate formulation of the problem. The patient's bed partner can provide vital information regarding sleep behavior of which the patient is unaware, such as snoring, acting out of dreams and sleep position. An observer can also provide valuable independent input regarding perceptions of the patient's daytime sleepiness and confirmation of the patient's description of bed-and wake-times. In the case of children, a collateral history from parents and sometimes teachers is essential, and care-givers play a similar role in patients with dementia. For patients who live alone, companions on overnight excursions may provide valuable information.

While there are many components of the sleep history that are common to all sleep complaints, some disorders require special questions. The physician should be constantly formulating and testing hypotheses of diagnosis as the history evolves, and should tailor questions to the picture that emerges. It should be borne in mind that there are often multiple causes of a sleep-related symptom, and a model that is based on a formulation of the patient's problem may be more appropriate than one based on identifying a single diagnosis.

A characteristic aspect of the sleep history has been completion by the patient of a usually lengthy questionnaire before interview with the clinician. This appears to have developed because of the cross-disciplinary nature of sleep medicine, resulting in symptoms crossing a number of traditional specialty boundaries. The questionnaire ensures that all areas are covered, and serves

**Table 3.1** Epworth sleepiness scale. Reproduced with permission from reference 1

How likely are you to doze off or fall asleep in the following situations, in contrast to feeling just tired? This refers to your usual way of life in recent times. Even if you have not done some of these things recently, try to work out how they would have affected you. Use the following scale to choose the most appropriate number for each situation:

0 = no chance of dozing
1 = slight chance of dozing
2 = moderate chance of dozing
3 = high chance of dozing

| Situation | Chance of dozing |
| --- | --- |
| Sitting and reading | . . . . . . . . . . . . . |
| Watching TV | . . . . . . . . . . . . . |
| Sitting inactive in a public place (e.g. a theater or a meeting) | . . . . . . . . . . . . . |
| As a passenger in a car for an hour without a break | . . . . . . . . . . . . . |
| Lying down to rest in the afternoon when circumstances permit | . . . . . . . . . . . . . |
| Sitting and talking to someone | . . . . . . . . . . . . . |
| Sitting quietly after a lunch without alcohol | . . . . . . . . . . . . . |
| In a car, while stopped for a few minutes in traffic | . . . . . . . . . . . . . |

as a possible road-map for planning the direction of the encounter. It often includes a scale of alertness, such as the Epworth sleepiness scale[1], which can also be useful in monitoring the response to therapeutic interventions (Table 3.1). Especially in the assessment of insomnia, patients may be asked to complete a sleep log for 1–2 weeks before the interview (see Figure 11.2). This includes indicating bedtime, rising time, time asleep, daytime naps, degree of alertness on waking and consumption of substances that may affect alertness.

### Case 3.1

A 38-year-old woman presented with a 2-year history of difficulty in sleeping at night and daytime fatigue. She would go to bed at 11 p.m. but be unable to fall asleep until after midnight. She would then wake at least three times during the night, taking 30–60 min to fall asleep on each occasion. Her night sleep terminated at 6 a.m. with a bedside alarm. She was unrefreshed on wakening and remained tired all day, but did not nap. On weekends she would go to bed an hour later, still have difficulty initiating and maintaining sleep, and would wake spontaneously at 9 a.m., feeling slightly more refreshed. She described a number of factors disturbing her sleep. First, 3–4 times a week on lying down to sleep she would experience a crawling-type discomfort in her calves with a strong desire to move them, but not troubling her later during the night. Second, she would frequently watch the clock while lying awake, worrying about her inability to sleep and her husband's difficulty finding work. Finally, she described pain over the left hip whenever she rolled on that side. She did not snore.

This case indicates how multiple organic and psychosocial factors can interact in the causation of a sleep problem. The problem was formulated as insomnia and daytime tiredness due to a combination of restless legs syndrome, poor sleep hygiene, situational stress, trochanteric bursitis and insufficient sleep. Medication for restless legs syndrome was prescribed and a steroid injection into the left trochanteric bursa organized. Counseling on sleep hygiene was provided, including recommendations to move the clock away from the bedside and to read rather than lie awake in the bedroom worrying. The patient realized she could wake 30 min later in the morning and still be in time for work. With these multiple interventions, the patient's symptoms improved markedly.

## Case 3.2

A 48-year-old man presented with daytime sleepiness. He did not snore and had no other features to suggest an intrinsic disorder of sleepiness. When asked his occupation, he described his work as an automobile mechanic, working from 7:30 a.m. to 5:00 p.m. He described his weekday sleep pattern as going to bed at 11 p.m. and waking at 5:45 a.m. with no problem initiating or maintaining sleep. Towards the end of the interview, his wife

arrived. As part of a general discussion of the problem, she revealed that her husband had a second job, running a mail-order business, which he did from 6 p.m. to at least 11 p.m. every night. She was asked to confirm her husband's bedtime and expressed amazement that he had stated it as 11 p.m. 'You are never in bed until at least midnight and usually later!', which her husband sheepishly agreed was nearer the truth than his initial assertion. Further discussion revealed that, in addition, he was a part-time firefighter and emergency medical technician, and was called out at night about twice a week. It was clear that the correct diagnosis was insufficient sleep syndrome and life-style changes were advised.

This case illustrates the importance of obtaining a collateral history. The patient did not intentionally deceive the physician but either was embarrassed by the need to have several jobs or failed to appreciate their relevance.

The following outline provides a framework for the sleep history.

### Overview of a typical night's sleep

The physician should ascertain whether the patient's sleep–wake cycle is regular. If it differs at weekends or with varying work shifts, then each condition should be described separately. If it has changed recently, then the premorbid sleep pattern should also be ascertained. The patient should be asked for a preferred time of going to bed and rising if a schedule could be set without societal restraints.

*Sleep initiation*

Activities before bed should be described, as these can affect sleep onset. Bedtime, any behaviors while awake in bed, such as reading or watching television, the time the light is switched off and the estimated time to fall asleep should be ascertained. If sleep latency is prolonged, the patient should be asked the reasons and their relative importance. Any noise or light in the bedroom should be described. For young children with insomnia, a detailed description of how the child is put to bed should be obtained, as well as any requirements the child has for initiation of sleep, such as a bottle, a stuffed toy or the presence of a parent.

*Sleep maintenance*

The number of awakenings that the patient perceives each night should be ascertained. An attempt should be made to determine the causes of these arousals, including external factors, such as a restless or snoring bed partner, pets sleeping on the bed or noise outside the bedroom. Possible medical causes include nightmares, jerks of the legs, snort arousals, dyspnea, gastroesophageal reflux, diaphoresis and urge to urinate. Waking from the need to urinate should be differentiated from urination after waking from another cause. Multiple causes of pain or discomfort can arouse patients from sleep, including muscle cramps, headaches, arthritis, fibromyalgia, angina, restless legs, peripheral neuropathy and carpal tunnel syndrome. The length of time before returning to sleep, and activities while awake, such as worrying or clock-watching in bed, read-ing, watching TV, eating or surfing the Internet should be described. The patient should be asked to estimate the total time spent asleep.

*Sleep termination*

The time of waking in the morning should be determined, as well as whether the patient awakes spontaneously or with the help of a bed partner, parent or alarm clock. How tired or refreshed the patient feels on waking should be assessed, as well as early morning symptoms such as dry mouth, sore throat, headache or confusion. Early-morning headaches associated with obstructive sleep apnea syndrome are generally short-lasting and do not fulfil criteria for any specific headache type such as migraine or tension headache[2].

## Specific nocturnal symptoms

*Respiration*

The duration and frequency of snoring should be ascertained from an observer, as well as any changes with time. Its intensity should be gauged by whether it is audible outside the bedroom with the door open or closed, and whether it can be heard in another room or on another floor of the house. The sleeping positions associated with snoring should be determined, as well as approximately what percentage of the night the patient spends in each position. The occurrence of episodes of waking with a choking sensation in the throat should be noted. An attempt should be made to deter-mine the frequency and duration of apneas

**Table 3.2** Causes of nocturnal dyspnea

| Cause | Clinical features |
| --- | --- |
| Asthma | noise is an expiratory wheeze |
| Laryngospasm | noise is described as a harsh strangulated inspiratory sound; sometimes associated with symptoms of gastroesophageal reflux |
| Obstructive sleep apnea syndrome | snoring, snort arousal or observed apnea |
| Central sleep apnea syndrome | periodic respiratory pattern observed |
| Paroxysmal nocturnal dyspnea | dyspnea sleeping flat with relief by sitting up; sometimes associated chest pain |
| Alveolar hypoventilation syndrome due to diaphragmatic weakness | dyspnea lying flat even when awake; observed paradoxical movement of the diaphragm |
| Nocturnal panic attacks | dyspnea associated with severe anxiety, palpitations, diaphoresis, paresthesias; usually associated daytime panic attacks |

and in what sleep position they occur. To assess whether they are central or obstructive, the physician sometimes needs to imitate types of apnea for the bed partner. The patient's own awareness of snoring or snort-related arousals should be noted. The presence of stridor, wheeze or perception of dyspnea should be ascertained as well as the number of pillows used under the head. Nocturnal dyspnea can have many causes (Table 3.2) and details on historical inquiry can narrow the differential diagnosis.

*Movements*

Any history of restless legs syndrome should be elucidated. The bed partner or parent, in the case of children, should be asked whether the patient is a restful or restless sleeper, and whether periodic limb movements of sleep, bruxism, sleepwalking, sleep terrors or seizure-like activity occur. Does the patient eat at night with or without recollection? Any dream enactment behavior, such as shouting, flailing the arms or kicking the legs, should be described. Sleep-talking alone is common and not particularly helpful diagnostically. If abnormal motor behavior is present, the time of night the events occur and whether the patient relates them to periods of dreaming should be noted, as well as the occurrence of any injuries to the patient or others. Although the best possible description of motor activity at night should be obtained, it should be recognized that this is often vague or inaccurate when the observer is half asleep or suddenly woken.

## Daytime symptoms

### General

The occupational and leisure activities of typical week and weekend days should be described. Details of present or past shift work are important. Knowing any particular time of maximal alertness – late at night ('owl') or early in the morning ('lark') – may be helpful in assessing whether circadian factors might contribute to insomnia or sleepiness.

### Excessive daily sleepiness

An attempt should be made to distinguish sleepiness from mental or physical fatigue (Chapter 6). If the predominant symptom is sleepiness, situations resulting in inappropriate sleep should be identified. The patient should be asked about sleepiness while working at a desk, reading, watching television, sitting in an audience such as in a theater or during a conference, or while talking to friends or relatives. Sleepiness while driving should be delineated in terms of the time or distance before lapses of alertness occur. Any drifting of the car onto the rumble strips, off the road or across the median should be noted, as well as any motor vehicle accidents from falling asleep. Patients should be asked about planned naps, their frequency, duration and restorative value.

### Cataplexy, sleep paralysis and hypnagogic hallucinations

Cataplexy is the sudden, bilateral loss of muscle strength due to emotion, especially laughter, and less frequently anger, excitement, sadness or fear. Occasional episodes of an internal sense of body weakness from profound laughter, or a subjective feeling of weakness with sudden terror or hearing disastrous news, should be differentiated as far as possible from true loss of muscle tone. Cataplexy can be generalized, affecting most voluntary muscles with the patient falling to the ground, unable to talk or move but with full consciousness. More often it is partial, but bilateral, with buckling of the knees, sagging of the face or drooping of the jaw. Superimposed twitching of facial muscles may occur. Any history of transient paralysis or hallucinations, most often visual, occurring before sleep or on awakening should be obtained. Hallucinations at sleep onset are described as hypnagogic, while those on awakening as hypnopompic, but often the term hypnagogic is used loosely to describe both phenomena.

## Background history

### Psychosocial

A history of psychiatric disease should be documented. Questions should be directed to symptoms of depression, such as anhedonia, feelings of hopelessness, loss of appetite and thoughts of death or suicide. The patient's present and past marital status and relationships should be probed, as social circumstances and the stresses arising from them can have profound effects on sleep. Other stressors should be identified and any history of past abuse delineated. Details of tobacco, alcohol, caffeine or illicit drug use should be obtained. Knowing the frequency of physical exercise and degree of exposure to sunlight can be relevant in understanding mechanisms of insomnia.

### Medical

A past or current history of hypertension, cardiorespiratory or neurological disorders, or upper airway disease or surgery may be relevant. A history of changes in weight over time should be obtained. Any sexual dysfunction should be noted. All medications should be reviewed. Obstructive sleep apnea syndrome (OSAS) is a risk factor for hypertension, ischemic heart disease and stroke, and can result in impotence. Enlarged tonsils (especially in children), nasal obstruction and obesity can predispose to OSAS. Various lung diseases, especially chronic obstructive pulmonary disease, may cause nocturnal hypoventilation. Many sleep disorders accompany Parkinson's disease and dementia, while peripheral neuropathy may cause nocturnal foot pain and predispose to restless legs syndrome. A history of epilepsy may increase the probability that nocturnal spells are seizures.

### Family history

Any family history of snoring, OSAS, insomnia, excessive daytime sleepiness, narcolepsy, restless legs syndrome, sleep walking or sleep terrors, circadian rhythm disorder, vascular disease, epilepsy, dementia, Parkinson's disease, psychiatric disease or substance abuse should be obtained.

## PHYSICAL EXAMINATION OF THE PATIENT WITH A SLEEP DISORDER

There is no uniform physical examination for patients with sleep disorders, and clinicians need to be familiar with examinations spanning a range of specialties, depending on the specific clinical problem. For suspected sleep apnea, general, upper airway, pulmonary and cardiac examinations are important. For problems of insomnia, a psychiatric mental state examination is required, while for restless legs syndrome, a neurological examination for peripheral neuropathy is needed. An examination for Parkinsonism or dementia may be needed in older patients with nocturnal movement disorders.

### Examination for suspected sleep-disordered breathing

The patient's height and weight should be measured and the body mass index calculated. Attention should be paid to any features suggesting endocrinopathies that predispose to OSAS, such as hypothyroidism, acromegaly or Cushing's syndrome. The neck should be examined and its circumference measured. Any abnormalities of the facial or jaw structure resulting in dental malocclusion, overbite or overjet should be noted (Figure 3.1). The oropharynx should be examined for tonsillar tissue, size and appearance of the uvula and soft palate, and adequacy of the anteroposterior and lateral diameters of the oropharynx. A swollen, red uvula or erythematous soft palate may indicate repetitive trauma from heavy snoring. A large base of the tongue may contribute to upper airway obstruction. The nose should be examined for degree of patency of the

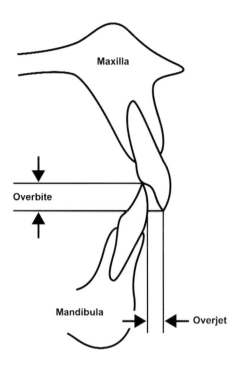

**Figure 3.1** Overbite and overjet. This figure illustrates the differences on physical examination of the jaw between overbite and overjet. Modified with permission from reference 3

anterior nasal passages and any septal deviation. If the question of possible nasopharyngeal obstruction arises (such as might be caused by adenoidal hypertrophy in a child), then a nasal endoscopic examination may be necessary.

A pulmonary examination is especially necessary if sleep-related hypoventilation is suspected. Abnormalities of respiratory rate or rhythm should be noted, and the chest examined for degree of inspiratory movement, and abnormalities of percussion and auscultation. Any chest deformities and kyphoscoliosis should be noted. A low-volume cough, inability to lie flat without dyspnea and paradoxical inward movement

of the abdomen with inspiration may indicate diaphragmatic weakness. Causes of diaphragmatic weakness include idiopathic phrenic neuropathies, myopathies, myasthenia gravis and amyotrophic lateral sclerosis. A cardiovascular examination should be performed to assess for systemic hypertension and signs of left ventricular failure or cor pulmonale.

## Case 3.3

A 6-year-old boy was referred for heavy snoring, observed apneic pauses during sleep and daytime hyperactivity. He was known to have multiple congenital malformations, characteristic of

Hajdu–Cheney syndrome[4]. These included cleft lip and palate, which had been repaired with the creation of a pharyngeal flap to ensure velopharyngeal competence. He also had mid-face anomalies, platybasia (congenital flattening of the skull base), syringobulbomyelia and hydrocephalus, for which a ventriculoperitoneal shunt had been placed. Physical examination revealed macrocephaly, a short, kyphotic neck typical of craniocervical junction anomalies, mid-face retrusion with maxillary hypoplasia and an open bite malocclusion. The palate was high-arched, with scars from previous cleft palate repair. The pharyngeal flap was visible. Polysomnography revealed 45 apneas and hypopneas per hour, the majority obstructive, but some mixed with both central and obstructive components. Oxyhemoglobin saturation fell to a minimum of 72%. A number of anatomical factors were considered to be responsible for the patient's sleep-disordered breathing, including the mid-face anomalies, the short, kyphotic neck and the surgically constructed pharyngeal flap. Syringobulbia may have contributed to the central component of the apneas. The surgeon was reluctant to remove the pharyngeal flap, so a second sleep study with nasal continuous positive airway pressure (nCPAP) was performed. An air pressure of 6 cmH$_2$O eliminated all disordered breathing events. After some difficulty with nasal interfaces, the patient tolerated a full-face mask very well, and was compliant with treatment. Snoring and apneas ceased and daytime behavior improved. He was still wearing nCPAP and doing well 7 years after the initial presentation.

This case illustrates the importance of the physical examination in determining the anatomical factors that can predispose to sleep-disordered breathing. These can sometimes be corrected surgically, but often nCPAP remains the treatment of choice.

## Examination for suspected restless legs syndrome

In cases of suspected restless legs syndrome, the lower extremities should be examined for evidence of peripheral neuropathy, local causes which might trigger the symptoms or any other cause of leg discomfort. Foot deformities, varicose veins, arthritis, absent peripheral pulses and limitation of straight leg raising should be noted. Perception of light touch, pinprick, temperature and vibration should be tested over the feet. Strength of the leg muscles should be determined and quadriceps and gastrocnemius deep-tendon reflexes assessed. Gait should be examined.

## Examination for parkinsonism and dementia

Sleep disorders are common in neurodegenerative diseases, and parkinsonism and dementia may occasionally present with

**Table 3.3** Four basic signs of parkinsonism

| Positive signs | Negative signs |
| --- | --- |
| Rest tremor | Bradykinesia |
| Cogwheel rigidity | Loss of postural reflexes |

**Table 3.4**  The short test of mental status.  Modified with permission from reference 5

| Questions | Points |
|---|---|
| *Orientation* Give name, address, location (building), city, state day or date, month, year | 8 (1 for each name) |
| *Attention* Repeat lists of digits, maximum seven | 7 (maximum number of digits correctly repeated) |
| *Learning* Learn 4 words (apple, Mr Johnson, charity, tunnel) Offer up to 4 trials to learn all 4 words | 4 (1 for each word learned, subtract 1 for each trial needed after the first) |
| *Arithmetic calculation* Multiply 5 by 13, subtract 7 from 65, divide 58 by 2, add 11 and 29 | 4 (1 for each correct calculation) |
| *Abstraction* How are the following similar? orange/banana, horse/dog, table/bookcase | 3 (1 for each abstract similarity: fruit, animal, furniture) |
| *Information* Name current US president, name first US president, state number of weeks in a year, define an island | 4 (1 for each correct answer) |
| *Construction* Draw the face of a clock showing 11:15, copy a picture of a cube | 4 (2 per picture) |
| *Recall* Recall the 4 words from the learning subtest | 4 (1 per word) |
| Total | 38 |

disturbances of sleep and wakefulness. Nocturnal confusion and symptoms suggestive of rapid eye movement (REM) sleep behavior disorder should in particular raise suspicion of these disorders. A brief, targeted neurological examination can easily detect parkinsonism (Table 3.3). The coarse, pill-rolling, rest tremor is typical of the diseases. Cogwheel rigidity should be tested by passive flexion–extension or supination–pronation movements of the wrists. Asking the patient to shake the head slowly or wave the other arm in a circle in the air while tone is being assessed can result in accentuation of rigidity. Reductions in the speed of rapid alternating movements of the tongue, hands, fingers and feet may indicate bradykinesia, which can also be assessed by inspecting facial movements, including the rate of spontaneous blinking, and by listening to the patient's speech. Postural reflexes are examined by the pull test, in which the patient is asked to maintain stance while being suddenly pulled backwards by an arm around the chest. Inspection of gait may reveal a forward-stooped, festinating gait, with reduced arm swing and accentuation of the rest tremor.

A number of brief office tests of global cognitive functioning have been developed. These include the mini-mental status examination[4] and the short test of mental status[5] (Table 3.4). For the latter test, a score of 29/38 or less predicts dementia with a sensitivity of 0.92 and a specificity of 0.91[5].

## Examination for psychiatric disease

A brief examination of the patient's mental state may be necessary to understand underlying psychiatric disorders that could cause or contribute to insomnia and other sleep problems (Table 3.5). Mood is the predominant emotion that underlies the patient's perception of the world, and includes depression, anxiety, euphoria and emptiness. Affect is the patient's external expression of mood. A patient's speech can be rapid or slow, pressured or hesitant. Disturbances of thought content include obsessions, compulsions, phobias, delusions and hallucinations. Hypnagogic and hypnopompic hallucinations, which are usually visual, should be differentiated from hallucinations more characteristic of psychosis, which are most often auditory and occur during full wakefulness. Table 3.4 illustrates the assessment of cognition, and includes tests of orientation, attention, learning, recall, language and construction. Judgment refers to the patient's ability to react appropriately in social circumstances, and insight includes the ability to understand the illness and its consequences. Motivation, closely related to judgment and insight, indicates the patient's effort to achieve a goal.

**Table 3.5** Psychiatric mental state examination

Appearance and behavior

Mood and affect

Speech

Thought

Cognition

Judgment, insight and motivation

## THE CLINICAL ASSSESSMENT

At the end of a history and appropriate physical examination, the physician should be able to formulate an explanation of the patient's sleep complaints in terms of probable mechanisms and diagnoses. A decision needs to be made whether further tests are needed and especially whether polysomnography should be performed. Sleep studies are expensive, and physicians should be clear how the results of laboratory testing will influence their therapeutic decision-making before studies are ordered. If no investigations are warranted, then the physician should be comfortable offering the patient an explanation of the symptoms and a plan of management.

## REFERENCES

1. Johns MW. A new method for measuring daytime sleepiness: the Epworth sleepiness scale. *Sleep* 1991;14:540–5

2. Loh NK, Dinner DS, Foldvary N, Skobieranda F, Yew WW. Do patients with obstructive sleep apnea wake up with headaches? *Arch Intern Med* 1999;159:1765–8

3. Fritsch KM, Iselo A, Rush EW, Bloch KE. Side effects of mandibular advancement devices for sleep apnea treatment. *Am J Respir Crit Care Med* 2001;164:813–18

4. Brennan AM, Pauli RM. Hajdu-Cheney syndrome: evolution of phenotype and clinical problems. *Am J Med Genet* 2001;100: 292–310

5. Kokmen E, Naessens MPH, Offord KP. A short test of mental status: description and preliminary results. *Mayo Clin Proc* 1987; 62:281–8

# Chapter 4

# Diagnostic testing for sleep disorders

*For some must watch, while some must sleep:*
*So runs the world away*

**William Shakespeare,** *Hamlet*

## POLYSOMNOGRAPHY

Polysomnography, the recording of multiple physiological parameters during sleep, is the fundamental tool of sleep physicians. The technique evolved from electroencephalography (EEG) recordings, and made possible the discovery of rapid eye movement (REM) sleep by Aserinsky and Kleitman in 1953. By the 1970s, the technique had been adapted to the diagnosis of disease, and when the first examinations in Sleep Medicine were offered in the USA in 1978, successful candidates were known as Accredited Clinical Polysomnographers. Today, polysomnography is the major activity of all clinical sleep laboratories.

Clinical sleep studies are performed in both EEG and sleep laboratories. The electroencephalographer is predominantly interested in abnormalities in cortical rhythms during sleep that may indicate the presence of a seizure disorder. The polysomnographer, on the other hand, uses the sleep EEG as a method to determine the duration, depth and continuity of nocturnal sleep and the relationship between arousals and sleep disorders. This requires the study of sleep over an entire night, with the monitoring of multiple neurological, respiratory

and cardiac parameters. Table 4.1 summarizes some of the differences between nocturnal polysomnography and a sleep EEG performed by an EEG laboratory.

### Indications for polysomnography

Not all patients assessed in a sleep disorders center require polysomnography[1] (Table 4.2). Probably the commonest indication is sleep-disordered breathing, including suspected obstructive sleep apnea or hypopnea syndrome and central sleep apnea syndrome. Polysomnography is also indicated for titration of nasal continuous positive airway pressure in patients with diagnosed sleep-disordered breathing. Nocturnal hypoxemia due to chronic lung disease can be assessed by oximetry alone, and is not an indication for full polysomnography unless sleep-related upper airway obstruction is also suspected. In the absence of other symptoms suggestive of sleep-disordered breathing such as observed apneas, snort arousals or excessive daytime sleepiness, the presence of snoring, obesity, systemic hypertension or suspected nocturnal cardiac arrhythmias do not warrant polysomnography.

**Table 4.1** Comparison of sleep electroencephalography (EEG) and polysomnography

|  | *Sleep EEG* | *Polysomnography* |
| --- | --- | --- |
| Study duration | 30 min | 6–8 h |
| Sleep states recorded | predominantly NREM | NREM and REM |
| EEG derivations | 16–20 | 1–3 |
| Other polygraphic derivations | usually none | multiple |
| EEG low-frequency filter | 1 Hz | 0.5 Hz |
| Usual display windows | 10 s | 30–120 s |
| Scoring of stages | not scored | rigorously scored |

NREM, non-rapid eye movement; REM, rapid eye movement

**Table 4.2** Indications for polysomnography

Evaluation of suspected sleep-disordered breathing

Evaluation of excessive daytime sleepiness of uncertain cause

Evaluation of suspected narcolepsy and idiopathic hypersomnia

Evaluation of suspected periodic limb movement disorder

Evaluation of some suspected parasomnias

Evaluation of selected cases of persistent insomnia

Polysomnography can confirm a suspicion that periodic limb movements of sleep are the cause of insomnia or excessive daytime sleepiness, especially if restless legs syndrome is not present. It is important to determine not only the frequency of periodic limb movements but also the percentage causing arousals, as the movements themselves are common findings, especially in the elderly, and are often of little clinical significance. Restless legs syndrome is usually diagnosed on clinical history, and polysomnography is generally not helpful (see Chapter 15). Parasomnias should be investigated by polysomnography if the associated behavior is violent, injurious or highly disturbing to the sleep of others. Another indication in suspected parasomnias is diagnostic uncertainty, especially if nocturnal seizures are a possibility and a routine EEG is unhelpful. A modified study is usually performed, with time-synchronized video and additional EEG and electromyographic monitoring (see Chapter 16).

In addition to polysomnography, the evaluation of excessive daytime sleepiness due to suspected narcolepsy or idiopathic hypersomnia requires a multiple sleep latency test (see Chapter 6). Polysomnography is not indicated for the routine evaluation of insomnia. However, indications for a sleep study include uncertainty whether the primary symptom is disturbed nocturnal sleep or daytime somnolence, suspicion that an organic cause for insomnia may be present, such as a movement or respiratory disorder, or if behavioral or pharmacological treatment has been unsuccessful[2].

## A night in the sleep laboratory

Patients scheduled to undergo polysomnography usually report at 7–8 p.m. They complete a questionnaire about their activities on the day preceding the study and their intake of alcohol, caffeinated beverages and medications. A technician applies electrodes and other sensors, and patients then read or watch television until they are sleepy. Rooms in a sleep laboratory are designed to look like bedrooms, and are furnished with comfortable beds different from those usually found in a hospital. A bell-pull is provided to summon the technician if needed.

After the patient is connected to the polysomnography acquisition unit, biocalibrations are performed. The patient is asked to look in all directions and blink the eyes, close the eyes for a time to record alpha rhythm, dorsiflex the ankles, breathe deeply and perform an isovolume maneuver to optimize the recording of chest and abdominal movements. Lights are switched off apart from an infrared lamp needed to provide illumination for video recording, and the patient is asked to try to sleep. A sleep study lasts for 6–8 h, depending on the indication and the time the patient went to bed.

A technician monitors the patient throughout the night, through video monitoring and observation of the recorded data. Notes are kept on significant events during the night, including changes in position, trips to the bathroom and unusual motor activity. During some studies, the patient may be asked to change position to assess the effect on sleep-disordered breathing. In some laboratories, nasal continuous positive airway pressure is applied during the night (a 'split-night' study). After the study is terminated, electrodes are removed unless a multiple sleep latency test is planned, and the patients are offered the opportunity to shower and wash their hair.

## Recording sleep data

Until the 1990s, polysomnographic instruments recorded data in analog form, displaying it on paper using galvanometers and ink recorders. The usual paper speed was 10 mm/s, one-third as slow as a conventional EEG. Even at this paper speed, large piles of paper were generated during a single night study, making review unwieldy and long-term storage impractical. It was also not possible to vary the time base, sensitivity, filter settings or montage during data review. Today, almost all sleep laboratories use digital systems, displaying data on a monitor and allowing for alteration in study parameters during review of the record. In particular, varying time bases can be used, ranging from a 10-s window to review EEG to a 180-s or slower window to display periodic respiratory events such as Cheyne–Stokes respiration. Thirty- and 60-s windows are most commonly used in routine studies. The number of available amplifiers determines the number of recording channels, while the number of display channels varies from system to system but is usually 16–32. Data are archived on electronic media, allowing a huge reduction in storage space.

Polysomnography involves the monitoring of neurological, respiratory and cardiac function during sleep (Table 4.3). To deter-

**Table 4.3** Variables monitored during routine polysomnography

---

*Neurological*
EEG
EOG
EMG
    submental
    anterior tibial

*Respiratory*
Airflow
Respiratory effort
Oxyhemoglobin saturation
Upper airway sound

*Cardiac*
ECG

---

EEG, electroencephalography; EOG, electro-oculography; EMG, electromyography; ECG, electrocardiography

mine sleep state, a minimum of a single derivation of EEG, one derivation recording submental electromyography (EMG) and two derivations to record eye movement potentials (electro-oculography, or EOG) are required. In practice, most polysomnograms will include 3–4 EEG derivations. One or two EMG derivations recorded from the anterior tibial muscles are needed to assess for periodic limb movements. Respiratory monitoring required includes a measure of airflow, channels recording respiratory effort, oxyhemoglobin saturation and a visual representation of snoring intensity. A single channel of electrocardiography (ECG) is also needed. Other physiological functions monitored on occasion include EMG from arm muscles in suspected parasomnias, additional EEG derivations for possible seizure disorders, esophageal pressure as a marker of transthoracic pressure and esophageal pH for nocturnal esophageal reflux. A typical standard polysomnogram montage is shown in Figure 4.1.

*EEG*

The most important EEG derivation for scoring sleep is $C_3$–$A_2$ or $C_4$–$A_1$, named according to the international 10–20 system (Figure 4.2). This referential derivation links the vertex area just lateral to the midline to the opposite ear, thus providing optimal monitoring of the cortical regions that maximally generate K-complexes, sleep spindles and sawtooth waves. The use of a reference electrode on the opposite ear provides a long interelectrode distance to increase waveform amplitude. Formal scoring of sleep is performed using this derivation. However, other derivations are commonly used, including $O_1$–$A_2$ or $O_2$–$A_1$, to provide

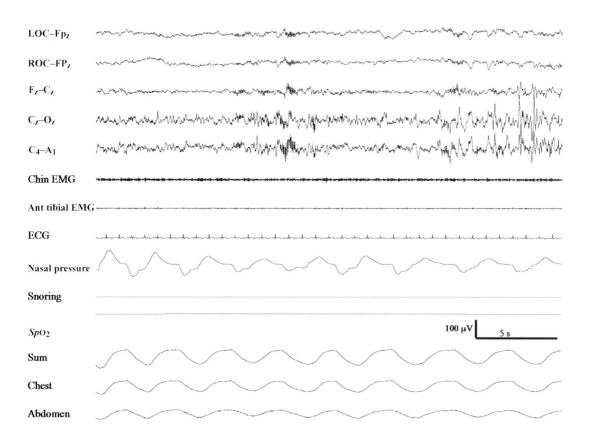

**Figure 4.1** Typical polysomnogram (PSG) montage. This 30-s fragment of a PSG shows stage 2 non-rapid eye movement (NREM) sleep. Typical derivations recording neurological, respiratory and cardiac function are illustrated. The first two channels display the electro-oculogram (EOG) (LOC, left outer canthus; ROC, right outer canthus). The third to fifth channels record the electroencephalogram (EEG) and the sixth and seventh the submental surface electromyogram (EMG) and the surface EMG recorded from both anterior tibial muscles. A nasal pressure monitor estimates nasal airflow. The sonogram is the integrated signal of upper airway noise. The $SpO_2$ channel records oxyhemoglobin saturation by pulse oximetry. The electrocardiogram (ECG) is recorded from lead I. Respiratory effort is estimated by chest and abdominal impedance plethysmography. The 'sum' channel is the arithmetic sum of the chest and abdominal changes. See text for further details

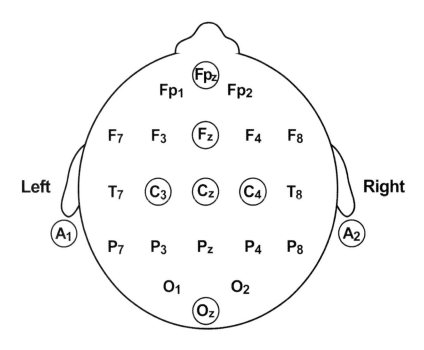

**Figure 4.2** International 10–20 system of electroencephalogram (EEG) electrode placement. This figure illustrates the approximate placement of EEG electrodes used in the international 10–20 system. Electrodes commonly used in routine polysomnograms (PSGs) are circled. See text for further details of derivations used

a record of alpha activity from occipital brain regions, as well as bipolar derivations also centered on the vertex. Our laboratory uses three EEG derivations, $C_3$–$A_2$, $F_z$-$C_z$ and $C_z$-$O_z$, allowing both referential and bipolar coverage of the vertex and monitoring of the frontal and occipital areas. When studying patients with suspected parasomnias or nocturnal seizures, extensive additional EEG derivations are used in association with time-synchronized video recording, a technique known as video-EEG polysomnography[3] (Chapter 16). A low-frequency filter setting of 0.5 Hz and a high-frequency filter setting of 70 Hz should be used in all EEG channels.

*EOG*

The eyeball is polarized with a negative retinal and a positive corneal potential. Therefore, eye movements can be visualized by monitoring changes in the electrical potentials recorded on the face and scalp. Horizontal, slow eye movements of drowsiness can easily be differentiated from rapid eye movements of REM sleep. During blinking, the eyeballs turn upwards (Bell's phenomenon), and this is a useful sign of alertness. Two systems of EOG derivations are in common use (Figure 4.3). The Rechtschaffen and Kales (R and K) derivations link

# EOG

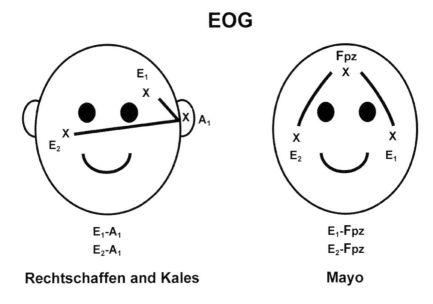

**Rechtschaffen and Kales**          **Mayo**

**Figure 4.3** Systems for recording the electro-oculogram (EOG). This figure demonstrates electrode placement for the two commonly used systems for recording the EOG. See text for details. Reproduced with permission of the American Academy of Neurology from reference 4

electrodes below and lateral to each eye to a single ear electrode, while the Mayo derivations reference similar electrodes below the eyes to the $Fp_z$ EEG electrode over the central forehead. The R and K derivations are designed so that all eye movements are represented by out-of-phase signals, while the Mayo derivations allow eye movement direction to be determined. Vertical eye movements (such as blinks) are displayed as in-phase deflections, whereas horizontal eye movements seen in drowsiness or REM sleep are out-of-phase (Figure 4.4). However, in the Mayo system, more skill is required to differentiate eye movements from cortical EEG activity and electrode artifacts.

*EMG*

The submental surface EMG is routinely recorded using two electrodes, one located beneath and the other above the chin. These record electromyographic activity from a number of muscles, including the mentalis, mylohyoid and digastric. At the onset of REM sleep, submental muscle tone is lost, and this provides an important marker of the change in state. Electrodes are placed over the center of the anterior tibial muscles and either referenced to each other or to further electrodes on the tendon of the muscles. In contrast to EEG recordings, a low-frequency filter of 10 Hz is used to eliminate

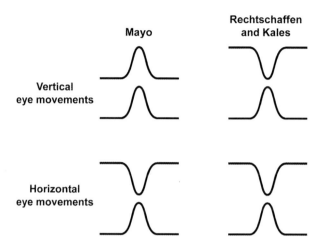

**Figure 4.4** Direction of eye movement deflections. This figure illustrates the direction of the deflections in the electro-oculogram (EOG) associated with eye movements in different directions using the Mayo and Rechtschaffen and Kales recording systems

gross movement artifact. Abnormally increased EMG activity can be seen during REM sleep in REM sleep behavior disorder, and rhythmic bursts of activity in the anterior tibial derivation(s) are characteristic of periodic limb movements of sleep.

*Airflow*

Airflow can be measured directly by using a pneumotachometer, but this requires a tight-fitting mask over the face of the patient and is not practical in clinical studies. Instead, one of two indirect techniques are generally used, namely thermal sensors or nasal pressure monitors. Thermocouples or thermistors placed in front of the mouth and each nostril record temperature changes between inspired and expired air. Airway pressure

variations can be measured with a cannula placed in the nostrils and connected to a pressure transducer. These techniques do not measure airflow quantitatively, but changes in the amplitude of the signals reflect relative alterations in flow.

*Respiratory effort*

The most direct measure of respiratory effort is to determine the changes in pressure that occur in the thoracic cavity, relative to the atmosphere, during inspiration and expiration. This can be achieved by measuring esophageal pressure, which is directly related to transpleural pressure. With quiet inspiration, esophageal pressure of a normal adult will decline by approximately $5 \, \mathrm{cmH_2O}$. A balloon-tipped, transducer-tipped or water-filled catheter can be placed via the nose into the esophagus, but patients often find the technique uncomfortable, and sleep continuity can be disrupted. A number of indirect measures are available and more often used, but esophageal pressure monitoring remains the gold standard for the diagnosis of upper airway resistance syndrome and the definitive differentiation of obstructive and central apneas or hypopneas (Chapter 8).

Inductive plethysmography is a technique for indirectly detecting respiratory effort by measuring changes in the dimensions of the thoracic cavity. Wires embedded in elastic bands placed around the chest and abdomen measure changes in the cross-sectional area of these cavities. Arithmetic summation of the signals from the rib cage and abdomen provides an estimate of respiratory tidal volume. Normally, the thoracic and abdominal cavities both expand during inspiration. In upper airway obstruction, diaphragm paralysis, mid- to low-cervical spinal cord transection and chronic obstructive pulmonary disease, the cavities may move in opposite directions, producing out-of-phase signal deflections, referred to as paradoxical movement[5].

Another method of estimating changes in cavity dimensions is the use of strain gauges, usually consisting of piezoelectric transducers. These measure changes in thoracic and abdominal cavity circumference, rather than cross-sectional area. Surface EMG electrodes placed over the sixth or seventh intercostal spaces may be used to record intercostal and diaphragmatic EMG. In central apneas and during REM sleep, the phasic EMG activity of inspiration will be absent.

*Oxyhemoglobin saturation and CO2 concentration*

Measurement of changes in blood gases provides a measure of the physiological effects of reduced airflow. Pulse oximetry is used to monitor oxyhemoglobin saturation by measuring absorption of red light by different forms of hemoglobin when it is passed through a capillary bed, such as in the ear lobe or the nail bed of a finger. The oximeter displays a continuous digital signal and a list of analog voltages, with accuracy at determining acute changes depending on the sampling frequency. Because of circulation time, the nadir of the oxyhemoglobin saturation graph usually follows the termination of the respiratory event by 7–9 s in the case of ear-lobe placement of the oximeter, and longer when it is placed on the fingertip.

End-tidal partial pressure of $CO_2$ ($p CO_2$, sampled at the end of expiration) is approximately the same as alveolar $p CO_2$, and may be measured to determine $CO_2$ changes with respiration. Transcutaneous $p CO_2$ may also be measured, but is less responsive to rapid changes. These measures are less frequently used in routine clinical practice.

*Upper airway sound*

A microphone should be used to monitor sounds, including snoring, stridor and vocalization. The output may be displayed directly on the polygraph or as an integrated signal. An audiotape may be helpful in distinguishing the actual sounds. The technician may also utilize a semiquantitative scale of snoring intensity (grade 1 audible only by bending over the patient's bed, grade 2 clearly audible in the bedroom but not outside, grade 3 audible outside the bedroom with the door open, grade 4 audible outside the bedroom with the door closed). The appearance of crescendo snoring (progressively increasing amplitude of sounds over several breaths leading to an arousal) may be a helpful marker of subtle upper airway obstruction.

*ECG*

A single ECG derivation is monitored, most frequently lead I from the right and left shoulders. This provides an opportunity to monitor heart rate and any brady- or tachy-arrhythmias that may occur during sleep, especially in relation to respiratory events.

## Staging of sleep

Polysomnographers formally score the absolute time spent in each stage of sleep. The standard scoring system for sleep stages is published in *A Manual of Standardized Terminology, Techniques, and Scoring System for Sleep Stages of Human Subjects*, edited by Allan Rechtschaffen and Anthony Kales in 1968[6]. Some modifications have been suggested, such as in the scoring of arousals and in the elimination of the distinction between stages 3 and 4 NREM sleep, but the manual still remains the basic standard used in scoring sleep. A broad account of sleep staging is discussed here (Table 4.4), but it is essential to read the manual itself before attempting to stage clinical records.

The formal unit used for sleep staging is the epoch. An epoch is one window of sleep recording and is conventionally 30 s in duration, although some laboratories may use slightly shorter or longer windows. Each epoch is given a single sleep stage, according to the activity that constitutes the highest percentage of the epoch. For example, if a 30-s epoch consists of 8 s of stage 2 sleep

Table 4.4 Characteristics of sleep stages. Reproduced with permission from reference 4, copyright 1998, American Academy of Neurology

|  | Stage W | Stage 1 | Stage 2 | Stage 3 | Stage 4 | Stage REM |
|---|---|---|---|---|---|---|
| EEG | alpha or mixed frequency | theta or mixed frequency | K-complexes or spindles | 20–50% delta activity | > 50% delta activity | mixed frequency; sawtooth waves |
| EOG | blinks and voluntary REMs | slow eye movements | none or slow eye movements | none | none | REMs |
| EMG | high | usually lower than in stage W | as in stage 1 | as in stage 2, or lower | as in stage 3 | low or absent; phasic twitches |

EEG, electroencephalography; EOG, electro-oculography; EMG, electromyography; REM, rapid eye movement followed by 8 s of wakefulness and then 14 s of stage 1 sleep, the epoch will be scored as stage 1.

Polysomnograms are usually scored visually by a trained technician, using a computer-assisted technique that allows entry of the stage on a keyboard and later automated calculation of the time spent in each stage. Computer algorithms are available for automated scoring[7], but visual inspection of the raw data is essential. Abnormal sleep architecture, such as may be seen in sleep heavily fragmented by respiratory arousals or in neurodegenerative diseases, may pose especial difficulties for automated scoring systems. Staging of polysomnograms of neonates and infants requires special knowledge, because EEG stages are defined differently from those of older children and adults.

### Stage W (wakefulness)

During wakefulness with the eyes closed, the EEG shows alpha rhythm or occasionally low-voltage, mixed-frequency activity. When the eyes are open, the EOG shows eye blinks and voluntary rapid eye movements. When the eyes are closed, eye blinks continue until drowsiness develops, when slow, rolling eye movements replace them even before alpha rhythm disappears. The EMG tone is relatively high.

### Stage I NREM sleep

The EEG of stage 1 non-rapid eye movement (NREM) sleep (Figure 1.5) shows low-voltage, mixed-frequency activity with prominent theta rhythms. Stage 1 sleep may include the presence of monophasic vertex waves or rudimentary sleep spindles with durations of less than 0.5 s. The EOG shows slow eye movements, and the submental EMG amplitude may be lower than that of wakefulness.

### Stage 2 NREM sleep

The EEG of stage 2 NREM sleep (Figure 1.6) must include either sleep spindles or K-complexes. Sleep spindles are defined as 12–14-Hz central activity with a duration of $\geq 0.5$ s. K-complexes are high-amplitude diphasic wave forms, usually with a relatively sharp initial surface negativity followed by a slower surface positivity, with a duration of $> 0.5$ s. Stage 2 sleep changes back to stage 1 sleep once 3 min have elapsed after the last spindle or K-complex ('3-min rule'). After an arousal, sleep reverts to stage 1 until the next spindle or K-complex. Slow eye movements may sometimes persist into stage 2 sleep. Submental EMG amplitude may remain unchanged or fall further.

### Stage 3 NREM sleep

In stage 3 NREM sleep, the EEG consists of delta activity constituting 20–50% of each epoch. The delta activity is a subset of delta frequencies (all EEG wave forms $< 4$ Hz) and is defined as waves with a frequency of $\leq 2$ Hz and a peak-to-peak amplitude of $> 75\ \mu v$, based on a referential derivation ($C_3$–$A_2$ or $C_4$–$A_1$) and a low-frequency filter setting of $\leq 0.5$ Hz. Sleep spindles may persist into stage 3 sleep. Eye movements are usually absent, and EMG tone is equal to or less than that seen in stage 2 sleep.

*Stage 4 NREM sleep*

Stage 4 sleep is defined identically to stage 3 sleep, but the delta activity must constitute more than 50% of each epoch. Because they really represent a continuum of increasing sleep depth, many laboratories today combine stages 3 and 4 sleep and refer to them as slow-wave sleep (Figure 1.7). With increasing age, the amplitude of the EEG drops. EEG activity in the 0.5–2-Hz range may still occur in older persons, but its amplitude rarely exceeds 75 $\mu$V. Accordingly many laboratories now score stages 3 and 4 sleep in the elderly if the amplitudes of these waves reach at least 50 $\mu$V, but there is no established consensus regarding this practice.

*Stage REM sleep*

The EEG of REM sleep consists of low-voltage, mixed-frequency activity, resembling that of wakefulness with the eyes open (Figure 1.8). Sawtooth waves, especially before bursts of rapid eye movements, may be seen but are not essential for the scoring of REM stage. The EOG shows bursts of conjugate, irregular, rapid eye movements that are most commonly horizontal, but may be vertical or oblique. The submental EMG amplitude is markedly diminished, and should not be higher than that seen during any other sleep stage. Phasic EMG twitches are superimposed on this atonia, often occurring at the same time as bursts of rapid eye movements. Even if rapid eye movements develop only in subsequent epochs, REM sleep is scored from the onset of submental EMG atonia as long as K-complexes and spindles have ceased. At the end of a period of REM sleep, epochs should continue to be scored as REM until EMG tone increases, an arousal occurs or K-complexes or sleep spindles return. REM sleep may be divided into phasic or tonic periods. During phasic REM, eye movements become more frequent, many chin EMG twitches occur, and there is increased variability in ECG and respiration. Tonic REM epochs are relatively devoid of these phasic features.

*Movement time*

The term 'movement time' is used when movement artifact obscures the recording for more than 50% of an epoch, as long as the preceding and subsequent epochs are scored as sleep. The term is used because of uncertainty about whether the patient awakened during the movement or whether it occurred during ongoing sleep.

*Alpha intrusion into NREM sleep*

Alpha intrusion into NREM sleep, also called alpha–delta sleep, is described when alpha activity is superimposed on the normal activity of NREM (usually slow-wave) sleep[8] (Figure 4.5). This phenomenon is of uncertain clinical significance, but is common in patients with chronic musculoskeletal pain such as caused by fibromyalgia or rheumatoid arthritis, and has been described in chronic fatigue syndrome. It has been linked to a complaint of non-restorative sleep, but is neither a specific nor a sensitive finding in any disorder, and may be observed in normal polysomnograms[9].

*Cyclic alternating pattern*

Within long periods of a specific stage of sleep, a subpattern can often be discerned. For example, in stage 2 NREM sleep, minutes of relatively monotonous EEG activity can be flanked by periods with a high frequency of K-complexes. In REM sleep, periods with few rapid eye movements or phasic twitches (tonic REM) can alternate with periods with a high frequency of phasic activity (phasic REM). This sequence of alternating periods of continuous and paroxysmal physiological activity has been called the cyclic alternating pattern (CAP). A CAP scoring system has been devised[10], and various abnormalities of CAP sequences have been noted in a number of sleep disorders. The exact physiological or clinical significance of the phenomenon remains to be determined.

## Scoring of arousals

The identification of arousals from sleep is essential to understand the physiological consequences of events such as obstructive apneas and periodic limb movements. The current American Sleep Disorders Association (ASDA) definition of arousals

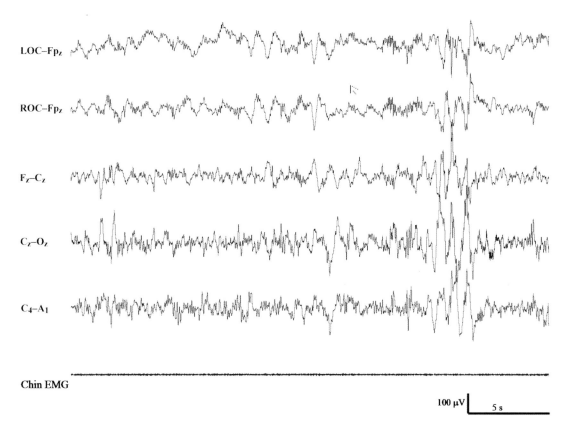

Figure 4.5 Alpha intrusion into non-rapid eye movement (NREM) sleep. This polysomnogram (PSG) fragment shows alpha activity superimposed on the slower frequencies of stage 3 NREM sleep. EMG, electromyogram

differs from the definition in the 1968 Rechtschaffen and Kales manual. An EEG arousal is now defined as an abrupt shift in EEG frequency to the alpha, beta (greater than 16 Hz) or theta frequency bands. The EEG frequency shift must be greater or equal to 3 s in duration and must follow at least 10 s of continuous sleep[11]. During NREM sleep, the scoring of an arousal is not dependent on increased EMG activity, but during REM sleep, arousals are scored only if the submental EMG amplitude increases at the same time as the change in EEG frequency. If the arousal lasts for more than 15 s, it is considered to be an awakening.

Shifts to beta frequencies of 14–16 Hz are excluded, to avoid confusion with sleep spindles. K-complexes alone are not considered evidence of arousal, as they may occur spontaneously in stage 2 sleep as well as in response to an external stimulus. However, a K-complex followed by 3 s of alpha activity ('K–alpha-complex') would qualify as an arousal (Figure 4.6). A burst of delta activity may sometimes indicate an arousal from sleep, especially in children, but is not included in formal criteria for an EEG arousal, to avoid confusion with delta waves of slow-wave sleep. The vast majority of arousals are characterized by a shift to alpha

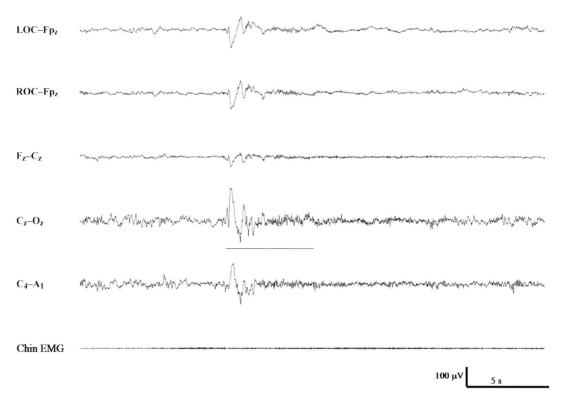

**Figure 4.6** K–alpha-complex. This polysomnogram (PSG) fragment shows a K-complex followed by about 4 s of alpha rhythm (underlined). EMG, electromyogram

frequencies. The additional criterion of increased submental EMG activity in REM sleep is included, because runs of alpha activity may be a normal finding during REM sleep.

## Scoring of respiratory and movement events

Various criteria have been proposed for scoring of obstructive and central apneas, hypopneas and respiratory-related arousals. These are discussed in detail in Chapter 8. Periodic limb movements of sleep are scored according to the Coleman criteria (Chapter

15). Parasomnias, such as confusional arousals (Chapter 16), are noted but not formally scored. Although a scoring system has been proposed for REM sleep without atonia[12], in clinical practice its presence is usually determined by the subjective judgment of an experienced polysomnographer (Chapter 16).

## The polysomnogram report

After all aspects of the polysomnogram have been scored, a report with summary statistics is generated (Figure 4.7). Various standard terms are employed. Time in bed (TIB) is

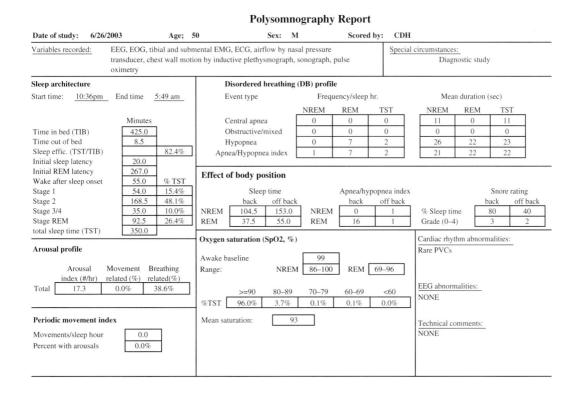

**Figure 4.7** Summary of data from a polysomnogram. See text for explanation of variables

defined as time from lights out in the evening to the end of the study in the morning, excluding time spent out of bed during the night. Total sleep time (TST) is all the time scored as NREM and REM sleep during the study. Sleep efficiency is the ratio TST/TIB expressed as a percentage. The initial sleep latency is the time from lights out to the first epoch of any stage of sleep. Some laboratories also use other indicators of sleep onset, such as the time to either the first epoch of stage 2 sleep or three continuous epochs of stage 1 sleep. Wake after sleep onset (WASO) is the time that the patient was awake from the first epoch of sleep until the end of the study. The initial REM latency is the time from the first epoch of any stage of sleep to the first epoch of REM sleep. This varies with age, being shorter in infants and older subjects than in children and adults (Table 4.5). An initial REM latency shorter than expected for a patient's age raises the possibility of major depression, sleep deprivation, narcolepsy or withdrawal of REM-suppressing medications.

**Table 4.5** Normal lower limits for initial rapid eye movement (REM) latency. Reproduced with permission from reference 13

| Age (years) | Initial REM latency (min) |
| --- | --- |
| 15–24 | 70 |
| 25–34 | 60 |
| 35–44 | 45 |
| 45–60 | 35 |
| > 61 | 30 |

The arousal index is the number of awakenings and arousals per sleep hour. Patients in a sleep laboratory have a high frequency of arousals, presumably related to the attached sensors, the strange bed and anxiety regarding the procedure. The normal range for an arousal index depends on the scoring criteria used, and may vary from laboratory to laboratory. A study of arousals in normal subjects revealed a mean of 4/h using the original Rechtschaffen and Kales definition, and a mean of 20/h using the current ASDA criteria described above[14]. In our laboratory, we consider 15 or fewer arousals per hour to be normal. The arousals should be subdivided into those due to respiratory events, periodic limb movements and unexplained factors.

Surprisingly few normative data are available for the absolute and relative amounts of each stage of sleep at different ages. The most detailed monograph describes values based on a slightly different staging system from the usual Rechtschaffen and Kales method, and a low-frequency filter setting of 1 Hz rather than the currently used 0.5 Hz[15]. Compared with sleep at home, a patient's first night in a sleep laboratory may be more disrupted, with lighter sleep and increased wakefulness[16]. This so-called first-night effect can be obviated by performing two studies on successive nights and using only the data from the second, but this is not feasible in routine clinical practice. Interpretation of sleep stages and indices requires clinical judgment, and a conservative approach should be utilized.

Most laboratories also generate a graphical representation of the night's sleep, sometimes called a hypnogram (Figure 4.8). The patient is also asked to complete a

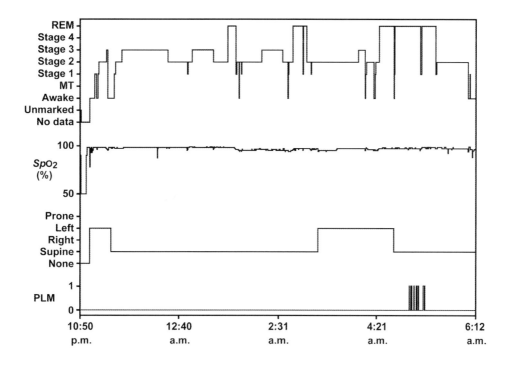

**Figure 4.8** Graphical representation of a night's sleep. This graphical representation of a night's sleep (hypnogram) gives a condensed summary of sleep stages, oxyhemoglobin saturation ($SpO_2$), body position and presence of periodic limb movements (PLM). REM, rapid eye movement; MT, movement time. Reproduced with permission from reference 13

questionnaire the morning after the study. Major discrepancies between the patient's estimation of such variables as initial sleep latency and total sleep time may suggest sleep state misperception (Chapter 10), and can sometimes be diagnostically helpful.

## Partial and unattended monitoring

Because of the inconvenience and cost of full laboratory polysomnograms as well as the inability of many sleep centers to meet demand for testing, many partial and unattended monitoring systems have been devised. These range from overnight pulse oximetry to complex home-based polysomnograms. These modalities have been chiefly used to diagnose obstructive sleep apnea syndrome, and are discussed in Chapter 8.

## MULTIPLE SLEEP LATENCY TESTS

In addition to polysomnography, most sleep laboratories perform daytime sleep studies for the assessment of sleepiness and alertness. The most important of these tests is the multiple sleep latency test, in which a patient is given 4–5 opportunities to sleep in the course of a day and the initial sleep latencies measured. A variant is the maintenance of wakefulness test, in which the patient is asked to keep awake in a sleep-inducing environment. These tests are discussed in detail in Chapter 6.

## ACTIGRAPHY

Actigraphs are small devices the size of a wristwatch that can record movement. They can be worn on the wrist for long periods during both the night and the day, and need only be removed while bathing or swimming. Sampling frequency varies depending on the machine. Computer algorithms allow for display of the data graphically and estimation of times with movements above or below a set threshold (Figure 4.9). Periods of relative absence of movements are interpreted as sleep, and periods of high activity as wakefulness, with adequate validity and reliability

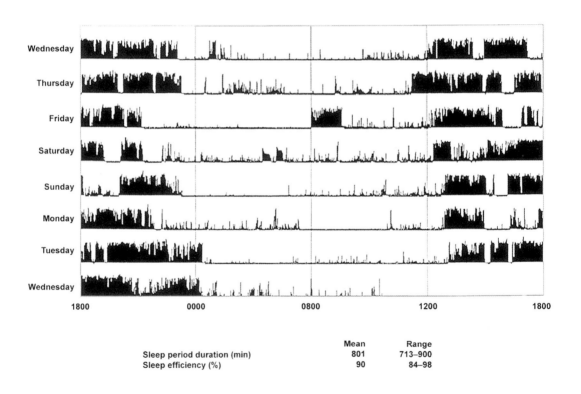

| | Mean | Range |
|---|---|---|
| Sleep period duration (min) | 801 | 713–900 |
| Sleep efficiency (%) | 90 | 84–98 |

**Figure 4.9** Display of actigraphy recording. This 8-day recording of rest–activity cycles shows black as activity (approximately corresponding to wake) and white as rest (approximately corresponding to sleep). This patient has variable bedtimes and a long sleep period of over 12 h. On Friday a period of apparent wakefulness is present between 8 and 9 a.m. Estimated sleep periods and sleep efficiency as calculated by the algorithm are shown

in normal subjects[17]. However, excessive motor activity at night caused by frequent arousals from periodic limb movements or obstructive sleep apnea may result in a falsely low estimate of sleep. Conversely, patients with depression, fatigue or psychophysiological insomnia may lie awake but immobile in bed, resulting in an overestimation of sleep time.

Actigraphy has proved a useful adjunct to the diagnosis of circadian rhythm disorders (Chapter 13), and may provide objective evidence of sleep and wake patterns in some cases of chronic insomnia (Chapter 11). It is increasingly being used to ensure that total sleep time is adequate in the week preceding a multiple sleep latency test (Chapter 6). Ankle actigraphy has been used experimentally to monitor periodic limb movements in drug trials. Evidence-based indications for actigraphy have recently been published[18].

## REFERENCES

1. Polysomnography Task Force. American Sleep Disorders Association Standards of Practice Committee. Practice parameters for the indications for polysomnography and related procedures. *Sleep* 1997;19:152–5

2. American Sleep Disorders Association Standard of Practice Committee. Practice parameters for the use of polysomnography in the evaluation of insomnia. *Sleep* 1995;18:55–7

3. Aldrich MS, Jahnke B. Diagnostic value of video-EEG polysomnography. *Neurology* 1991;41:1060–6

4. Daube JR, Cascino GD, Dotson RM, Silber MH, Westmoreland BF. Clinical neurophysiology. *Continuum* 1998;4:149–72

5. Staats BA, Bonekat HW, Harris CD, Offord KP. Chest wall motion in sleep apnea. *Am Rev Resp Dis* 1984;130:59–63

6. Rechtschaffen A, Kales A. *A Manual of Standardized Terminology, Techniques, and Scoring System for Sleep Stages of Human Subjects*. Bethesda, MD: National Institute of Neurological Disease and Blindness, 1968

7. Hirshkowitz M, Moore CA. Issues in computerized polysomnography. *Sleep* 1994;17:105–12

8. Hauri P, Hawkins DR. Alpha-delta sleep. *Electroencephalogr Clin Neurophysiol* 1973;34:233–7

9. Older SA, Battafarano DF, Danning CL, *et al.* The effects of delta wave sleep interruption on pain thresholds and fibromyalgia-like symptoms in healthy subjects; correlations with insulin-like growth factor I. *J Rheumatol* 1998;25:1180–6

10. Terzano MG, Parrino L, Sherieri A, *et al.* Atlas, rules and recording techniques for the scoring of cyclic alternating pattern (CAP) in human sleep. *Sleep Med* 2001;2:537–53

11. Sleep Disorders Atlas Task Force of the American Sleep Disorders Association. EEG arousals: scoring rules and examples. *Sleep* 1992;15:173–84

12. Lapierre O, Montplaisir J. Polysomnographic features of REM sleep behavior disorder: development of a scoring method. *Neurology* 1992;42:1371–4

13. Hauri PJ, Harris CD, Silber MH. Physiologic assessment of sleep. In Daube JR, ed. *Clinical Neurophysiology*. New York: Oxford University Press, 2002:493–512

14. Mathur R, Douglas NJ. Frequency of EEG arousals from nocturnal sleep in normal subjects. *Sleep* 1995;18:330–3

15. Williams RL, Karacan I, Hursch CJ. *Electroencephalography (EEG) of Human Sleep: Clinical Applications*. New York: John Wiley & Sons, 1974

16. Agnew HWJ, Webb WB, Williams RL. The first night effect: an EEG study of sleep. *Psychophysiology* 1966;2:263–6

17. Sadeh A, Sharkey KM, Carskadon MA. Activity-based sleep–wake identification: an empirical test of methodological issues. *Sleep* 1994;17:201–7

18. Ancoli-Israel S, Cole R, Alessi C, Chambers M, Moorcroft W, Pollack CP. The role of actigraphy in the study of sleep and circadian rhythms. *Sleep* 2003;26:342–92

# Section II
# The sleepy patient

# Chapter 5

# Sleepiness and its causes

*Protect me from unreasonable and immoderate sleep.*

**Samuel Johnson, *Prayers and Meditations***

It has taken a paradigm shift for society to regard sleepiness as a disorder, rather than a moral failing or sin. Patients often take several years to bring a complaint of sleepiness to the attention of a physician, and physicians have only recently started using a medical model to approach the problem. While many diseases causing excessive sleep have probably existed for centuries, sleepiness has become an epidemic in modern times. Since the invention of electric lighting, time spent awake has increased, and social and economic pressures have further reduced the time available for sleep. It was estimated in 1975 that Americans were sleeping one and a half hours less than in 1900[1]. At least 20% of American workers do shift work, a clear contributor to hypersomnolence. Obstructive sleep apnea syndrome, the commonest disease causing sleepiness, has increased in frequency as a result of the increasing prevalence of obesity.

Epidemiological studies of the prevalence of sleepiness in the community are difficult to compare, as many different questionnaires have been used. However, most studies have suggested a prevalence of 5–15%, with higher percentages in men compared with women, and in adolescents and the elderly compared with other age groups[2–4]. Sleepiness has profound public-health implications. Motor vehicle accidents

between 7 p.m. and 7 a.m. account for 30% of the total and 54% of the fatal accidents over a 24-h period, despite the much lower frequency of vehicles on the roads at night[5]. Single-vehicle accidents, more likely to be related to lapses in attention, clearly peak at night[6] (Figure 5.1). Sleep deprivation and night-shift work have been important contributing factors to most of the technological catastrophes of our age, including the nuclear disasters of Three Mile Island in Pennsylvania and Chernobyl in the Ukraine, the chemical industrial catastrophe in Bhopal, India and the explosion of the space shuttle *Challenger*.

The results of a large epidemiological study of 1.1 million subjects aged 30–102 years have suggested that long sleep at night is associated with increased mortality[7]. A self-reported nocturnal sleep time of 8.5 h or more was linked to a 15% increased mortality risk, which increased with increased duration of sleep. In particular, risk of death from cerebrovascular disease increased. The reason for this association is unknown, but sleep-disordered breathing may play a role. There is no direct evidence that the longer sleep duration itself is a causative factor for the increased mortality risk, and it should also be noted that increased nocturnal sleep time does not necessarily translate into daytime sleepiness.

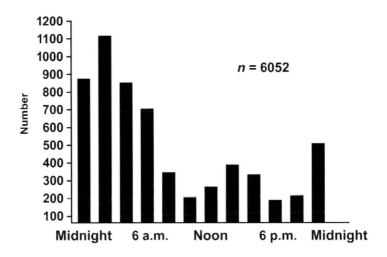

**Figure 5.1** Sleepiness-related motor vehicle accidents. This figure shows pooled data from 6052 motor vehicle accidents in Israel, Texas and New York, believed to be due to falling asleep at the wheel. There is a major peak after midnight and a minor peak between 1 and 4 p.m. Reproduced with permission from reference 6

## TERMINOLOGY OF SLEEPINESS

Patients and physicians use many different terms to express the concepts of tiredness, sleepiness and fatigue. As there are no universally accepted definitions of these and similar expressions, diagnostic confusion can frequently result from varying interpretations of their meaning. This section attempts to provide definitions and explanations of some of these concepts in order to present a structure for accurate clinical diagnosis.

### Tiredness

This is a non-specific term, including sleepiness and fatigue, and should not be used to describe a patient's complaint. When a patient complains of tiredness, physicians should make every effort to establish the more precise meaning of the symptom.

### Sleepiness

Sleepiness is a physiological phenomenon, determined by circadian factors and by the length of time from the last sleep period. However, sleepiness can be excessive owing to a number of extrinsic environmental factors and intrinsic pathologies. Daytime sleepiness usually comprises two components: first, the subjective perception of a need to sleep, and second, the ability to fall asleep. The perception of a need to sleep is usually accompanied by behavioral manifestations, including yawning, transient loss of neck tone, ptosis, pupillary constriction and lapses of attention. The increased ability to fall asleep in circumstances in which alertness is desired is a more objective criterion, implying that physiological, measurable indices of sleep onset have occurred. It is assessed by tests such as the multiple sleep latency test (MSLT) (Chapter 6) that determine whether the patient has commenced sleeping under permissive circumstances more rapidly than would be expected. Occasional patients will experience episodes of sleep commencing without a warning perception of the need to sleep (see 'Sleep attacks'), and this is usually included under the rubric of excessive daytime sleepiness. In contrast, some patients have a strong desire to sleep, but are unable to do so, because of a competing increased state of arousal, such as may be seen in psychophysiological insomnia or caused by symptoms of restless legs syndrome. Whether the latter group should be called sleepy is controversial; in the absence of an accepted term to describe this phenomenon, the symptoms should rather be described as a desire to sleep during the day but the inability to do so.

### Drowsiness

Drowsiness is the state of transition between wakefulness and sleep. Subjectively, it is characterized by a desire to sleep, and is accompanied by observable signs of sleepiness. A drowsy patient is synonymous with a sleepy patient. In the interpretation of the MSLT, sleep onset is arbitrarily defined as the first epoch of any stage of sleep, most commonly stage 1 non-rapid eye movement (NREM) sleep[8]. However, a continuum exists between full alertness and established sleep (Figure 5.2). Many neurophysiological phenomena of impending sleep precede the

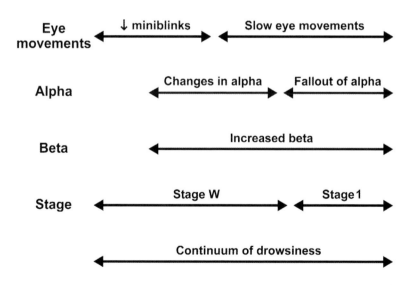

**Figure 5.2** The continuum of drowsiness. Reduction in miniblink rate, slow eye movements, frontotemporal spread of alpha rhythm with interspersed theta waves and beta rhythms all precede the loss of alpha rhythm which constitutes the formal start of stage 1 non-rapid eye movement (NREM) sleep. Reproduced with permission of the American Academy of Neurology from reference 9

loss of alpha rhythm and development of slower rhythms that characterize stage 1 NREM sleep. One of the earliest changes is a slowing of the rate of miniblinks, which are present at a frequency of 1–2 Hz during full alertness with the eyes closed. As drowsiness deepens, slow, rolling, predominantly horizontal eye movements replace them. Before alpha rhythm attenuates, it often spreads frontocentrally and may either increase or decrease in amplitude. Theta transients appear while alpha rhythm still predominates, and frontocentral beta rhythms develop. The descent into sleep is not always a smooth process, with several returns to full wakefulness often interrupting drowsiness before full sleep is established. The degree of drowsiness can also be assessed by psychophysiological responses, and these do not always correlate with sleep onset as defined by neurophysiological measures. Subjects are asked to tap a switch in response to auditory or visual stimuli of varying intensity. Different subjects will cease responding at variable times; many will continue to tap the switch into stage 1 and some even into stage 2 sleep[10].

## Microsleeps

For a 30-s epoch on a polysomnogram (PSG) or MSLT to be scored as sleep, scoring rules dictate that more than 15 s should show sleep activity[8]. A microsleep is defined as less than 15 s of polysomnographic phenomena which would have allowed the epoch to be classified as sleep if they had been present for more than 15 s. These include theta rhythm with slow eye movements, K-complexes or sleep spindles. They may or may not be accompanied by behavioral changes of drowsiness. Despite their brief duration, microsleeps may result in sufficient loss of environmental awareness to be inconvenient to workers or students and hazardous to drivers. The term microsleeps has also been used to describe brief subjective periods of drowsiness of unspecified duration, especially in drivers or experimentally sleep-deprived subjects, but this imprecise use of the word should be avoided.

## Sleep attacks

Sleep attacks are sudden descents into sleep without any preceding subjective awareness that it is about to occur. Originally they were felt to be typical of narcolepsy, and are certainly common in that condition. More recently, sleep attacks have been described in patients using the non-ergot dopamine agonists pramipexole and ropinirole for the treatment of Parkinson's disease. However, sleep attacks are entirely non-specific. Most people are aware of impending sleep, but a small minority may at times experience no warning of sleep onset. This phenomenon can occur with any cause of excessive daytime sleepiness, including sleep deprivation, medication-induced sleepiness, obstructive sleep apnea syndrome and narcolepsy. It can be confusing to physicians, and many patients have been investigated for a seizure disorder or cardiac rhythm abnormality before the correct diagnosis has been reached. Sleep attacks can be especially dangerous when driving, and it can be very difficult to assess whether treatment of the underlying disorder has produced adequate alertness. A maintenance of wakefulness test (Chapter 6) is often necessary in deciding whether such a patient can resume driving a motor vehicle.

## Fatigue

In the practice of sleep medicine, the term fatigue is used to describe a type of tiredness very different from excessive daytime sleepiness. Fatigue is a sense of exhaustion, an inability to perform physical activity at the intensity or for the duration that one might expect. It is often associated with a sense of mental fatigue with poor concentration and memory. When patients with fatigue lie down to rest, they may sleep, but this differs from the inappropriate, irresistible sleep of excessive sleepiness. The MSLT is normal in patients with fatigue, demonstrating normal duration sleep latencies. There are many causes of chronic fatigue (Table 5.1), but primary sleep disorders do not usually cause

**Table 5.1** Causes of chronic fatigue

*Medical causes*
Chronic infections
Malignancies
Autoimmune disorders
Endocrinopathies, including hypothyroidism
and Addison's disease

*Neurological causes*
Myasthenia gravis
Myopathies and neuropathies
Multiple sclerosis
Parkinson's disease

*Psychiatric causes*
Depression
Somatoform disorders
Personality disorders

*Miscellaneous*
Chronic fatigue syndrome

this symptom. The differentiation of sleepiness and fatigue is a fundamental step in understanding the tired patient.

## MECHANISMS OF SLEEPINESS

The neurophysiological and neurochemical mechanisms that result in sleepiness are uncertain. Sleepiness can be conceptualized as being the result of a balance between drives towards sleep and drives towards wakefulness. As discussed in Chapter 2, sleep and alertness are both active processes involving networks of neurons in the brainstem, thalamus, hypothalamus, basal forebrain and cortex. Two biological processes encourage sleep: a homeostatic sleep factor (process S) which increases proportionally to the degree of sleep debt, and a circadian factor (process C) which produces a major trough of alertness between 2 and 6 a.m. and a minor trough 12 h earlier.

Disorders increasing factors S and C will produce sleepiness, as will disorders reducing the drive towards wakefulness (Table 5.2) (Figure 5.3). Sleep deprivation and sleep fragmentation will increase sleep debt. While it seems obvious that insufficient sleep will result in a compensatory drive towards sleep, the effects of sleep fragmentation are less intuitive. However, many studies have demonstrated that brief interruptions in sleep continuity, often lasting only seconds, will result in increased daytime somnolence and that treatment of the causes restores alertness. Experimental fragmentation of sleep by the presentation of audible tones causes subjective daytime sleepiness, decreased sleep latencies on the MSLT and deterioration of performance on psychomotor tasks[11,12]. Even when the tones presented

**Table 5.2** Putative mechanisms of sleepiness

*Increased sleep drive*
Increased sleep debt (process S)
  sleep deprivation
  sleep fragmentation (e.g. obstructive sleep apnea syndrome)
Circadian dysrhythmias (process C)
  extrinsic circadian factors (e.g. shift work)
  disorders of the biological clock (e.g. delayed sleep phase syndrome)

*Decreased wakefulness drive*
Reduction of monoaminergic activity by hypocretin deficiency  (e.g. narcolepsy)
Inhibition by GABA-A of wake-active neurons (e.g. benzodiazepines)
Inhibition of histamine-1 receptors (e.g. histamine-1 antagonists)

GABA-A, $\gamma$-aminobutyric acid-A

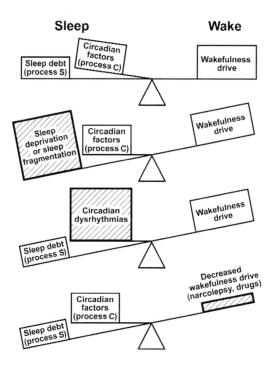

**Figure 5.3** Mechanisms of sleepiness. This figure illustrates sleep and wake as a seesaw. The wakefulness drive is normally balanced by sleep debt and circadian factors causing the drive towards sleep. The seesaw tilts towards excessive sleepiness if sleep debt increases (due to sleep deprivation or fragmentation), circadian dysrhythmias occur or if the wakefulness drive diminishes

cause only transient increases in blood pressure or heart rate without changes in the scalp electroencephalogram (EEG), sleep latencies on the MSLT shorten[13]. Thus, disorders such as obstructive sleep apnea syndrome can cause significant sleepiness without the patient even being aware that sleep has been disrupted. External factors disrupting circadian rhythm, such as shift work or travel across multiple time zones can cause sleepiness, as can intrinsic disorders of the biological clock, such as delayed sleep phase syndrome (Chapter 13).

Decreased waking drive as a cause for sleepiness is more speculative, but may play a role in somnolence caused by narcolepsy and some sedating medications. The exact mechanism of sleepiness in narcolepsy and related conditions is uncertain. However, hypocretin-containing neurons have excitatory effects on brainstem dopaminergic and noradrenergic pathways comprising parts of the reticular activating system. Thus, loss of hypocretin-containing neurons as appears to occur in most cases of narcolepsy (Chapter 7) most probably results in sleepiness by reducing the drive towards wakefulness[14]. The anatomical sites mediating drug-induced sleep have not been fully established. The classic hypnotics, barbiturates and benzodiazepines, activate the γ-aminobutyric acid-A (GABA-A) receptor, which results in an intracellular chloride flux causing postsynaptic neuronal inhibition. It has been suggested that they may act in the anterior hypothalamus and basal forebrain area, perhaps by inhibiting populations of wake-active neurons[15]. Similarly, histamine activity peaks during wakefulness and results in cortical activation[16], while histamine-1 antagonists decrease alertness.

## CAUSES OF SLEEPINESS

### Classification

Causes of sleepiness can best be considered as intrinsic or extrinsic. Extrinsic causes are due to environmental or motivational factors, while intrinsic causes consist of diseases resulting in somnolence (Table 5.3).

### Extrinsic causes

Extrinsic causes are discussed here, with the exception of shift work sleep disorder and jet lag syndrome (see Chapter 13).

#### Sleep deprivation

Sleep deprivation has been studied in animals and humans for over a century. The

**Table 5.3** Causes of excessive daytime sleepiness

| |
| --- |
| *Extrinsic causes* |
| Sleep deprivation (insufficient sleep syndrome) |
| Drug-related hypersomnia |
| Shift work sleep disorder |
| Jet lag syndrome |
| Environmental sleep disorder |
| |
| *Intrinsic causes* |
| Sleep-disordered breathing |
| Narcolepsy |
| Idiopathic hypersomnia |
| Restless legs syndrome and periodic limb movement disorder |
| Circadian rhythm sleep disorders (including delayed sleep phase syndrome) |
| Periodic hypersomnia (including Kleine–Levin syndrome) |

classic experiments conducted by Allan Rechtschaffen and his team at the University of Chicago in the 1980s demonstrated the effects of sleep deprivation in the rat[17]. An experimental and a control animal with implanted EEG electrodes were housed on either side of a rotating horizontal disk suspended over a shallow bath of water (Figure 5.4). When the experimental rat slept, the disc rotated, and both rats were forced to walk in the opposite direction to avoid falling into the water. Conversely, when the control rat slept, the disk remained stationary. This experimental design resulted in a mean of 72% sleep loss in the experimental animals and only 9% sleep loss in the controls. The sleep-deprived rats all

died after a mean of 21 days if the experiment was allowed to continue. Death was preceded by loss of weight, ulcerative skin lesions, hypothermia and a hypercatabolic state. When the experiment was stopped prior to death, most rats survived, with recovery sleep characterized by large amounts of paradoxical (rapid eye movement, REM) sleep. Selective deprivation of paradoxical sleep produced similar results, but with longer survival (mean of 37 days). Autopsy studies did not yield a definite cause of death. However, subsequent experiments have suggested that the sleep-deprived rats were bacteremic, and that death may have resulted from overwhelming sepsis[19]. The hypothesis that sleep loss may impair the

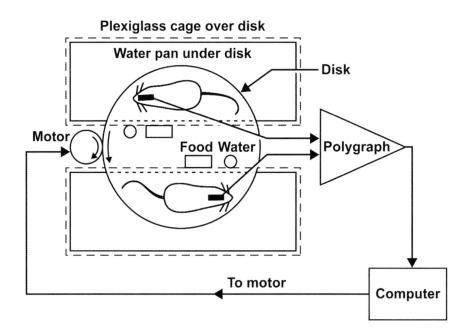

**Figure 5.4** Diagram of the experimental model used to study sleep deprivation in rats. The disk rotates when the experimental rat sleeps but remains still when the control rat sleeps. See text for details. Modified with permission from reference 18

immune system is an attractive explanation but remains unproven, as the subsequent administration of antibiotics did not prevent progression towards death[20].

It is hard to produce sustained total sleep deprivation in humans. Short periods of sleep start intruding, and experiments usually terminate after a maximum of 5–10 days. The principal effect of such sleep deprivation is an intense desire for sleep. EEG studies show intrusion of slow rhythms and failure of alpha activity to develop with eye closure. Psychomotor test performance declines and mood changes are noted. Visual distortions or hallucinations may occur. The effects of partial sleep deprivation have been thoroughly studied. As little as 2 h sleep deprivation per night may result in measurable increases in sleepiness[21]. Chronic partial sleep deprivation results in sleepiness, impaired cognitive and psychomotor skills, and feelings of anxiety, sadness and hostility. Experimental sleep deprivation over 14 days led to cumulative deficits in cognitive performance, demonstrating that adaptation to chronic sleep loss does not occur. However, subjective measurements of sleepiness on the Stanford sleepiness scale (Chapter 6) showed that the subjects did not perceive themselves as becoming progressively more impaired[22] (Figure 5.5). Thus, the potentially dangerous situation may arise

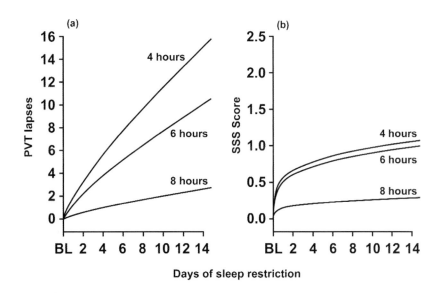

**Figure 5.5** Effects of cumulative partial sleep deprivation on performance testing and subjective sleepiness. This figure illustrates progressive difficulties with a psychomotor vigilance task (PVT) as partial sleep deprivation continued over 14 days (a). The three graphs show subjects restricted to 4, 6 and 8 h sleep per night. In contrast, subjects did not perceive themselves as experiencing increasing sleepiness, as indicated by Stanford sleepiness scale (SSS) self-reports not worsening with time (b). BL, baseline. Modified with permission from reference 22

when a chronically sleep-deprived person may perceive adequate adaptation to loss of sleep while, objectively, performance progressively worsens. The amount of sleep needed to recuperate following complete or partial sleep deprivation is less than the amount of sleep debt incurred. The subject usually sleeps 12–15 h on the first recovery night, with marked rebound of slow-wave sleep and high sleep efficiency. The second recovery night demonstrates REM sleep rebound, but by the third night, sleep architecture has usually returned to normal.

Sleep deprivation in medical residents has attracted much attention, and serves as an example of the effects of chronic partial sleep deprivation due to life-style or occupational factors. It has long been traditional for physicians in training to work long hours, with night call sometimes required as frequently as twice a week with little or no compensatory time off during the day. This results in weekly work hours far in excess of those permitted by almost any other profession. Various explanations have been suggested for this situation, including the unproven belief that it offers residents increased learning opportunities and the means to develop a sense of professional responsibility, while providing better continuity of care for patients. It has been compared to a rite of passage that must be undergone before the young physician can formally join the profession. However, economic factors are probably most important, as the cost of providing additional medical coverage can be high. Studies of surgical residents have shown more surgical errors, a longer time to complete procedures and a higher complication rate after sleep deprivation[23]. Impairment of electrocardio-

gram interpretation and the performance of other psychomotor tests deteriorated after medical residents spent a night on call[23]. The risk of falling asleep while driving increased in sleep-deprived residents, with descriptions of traffic citations and accidents[24]. Stress and depression have also been related to sleep loss in residents. The Libby Zion case in New York highlighted the problem, bringing the stresses of graduate medical training to the attention of the public. Libby Zion was an 18-year-old woman who died of bronchopneumonia at a New York teaching hospital in 1984, while under the care of junior residents who had been on duty for 18 h. A grand jury later found that, among other factors, the physicians' sleep deprivation contributed to her demise[25]. Although the state of New York subsequently placed restrictions on the work hours of junior physicians, it was only in July 2003 that a nationwide 80-h work week was mandated by the Accreditation Council for Graduate Medical Education.

## Case 5.1

A first-year surgical resident admitted 12 patients to a busy acute-care service over the course of a night, during which he obtained only 1 h of sleep. One of the patients, admitted by the resident at 8 p.m., was an elderly diabetic woman with gangrene of the leg. On rounds the following morning, the attending surgeon decided that the leg needed to be amputated and told the resident to prescribe the usual antibiotic regimen, including intravenous penicillin. Without checking his notes written 12 h earlier, in which he had recorded that the patient was allergic to penicillin, he prescribed the medications, which were duly administered. Twenty minutes later the patient died of anaphylaxis. A judge later determined that sleep deprivation in the resident had played a major role in the event.

This case occurred 25 years ago. Today, most hospitals have instituted checks in the system involving nursing staff and pharmacists, which should prevent similar occurrences. Nevertheless, it illustrates how a combination of short-term memory impairment and poor judgment from severely reduced sleep can contribute to serious medical errors.

### Drug-related hypersomnia

Excessive daytime sleepiness may result from prescribed, over-the-counter and recreational drugs. Benzodiazepines used as hypnotics, especially those with a long half-life such as clonazepam, can cause daytime sleepiness, as can sedating antihistamines. Most antidepressants can cause sedation in a minority of patients, and hypersomnia can complicate the use of antiepileptic drugs, dopaminergic agents and α-adrenergic agonists. The role of alcohol and drugs of abuse should always be considered.

### Environmental sleep disorder

Environmental causes of hypersomnia include any disturbing environmental factors that fragment sleep, including excessive heat, cold, noise or light. It is a special problem in a hospital, especially in an intensive care unit, where multimodal sensory input can cause severe sleep loss. Parents of infants or companions of invalids may have sufficient nocturnal sleep deprivation to cause sleepiness during the day. Pets sleep-

ing on their owners' beds may also cause sleep disruption through movement or snoring. In a study of 300 patients seen at a sleep disorders center, 41% reported having pets sleep on their bed. A similar percentage felt that their pets caused them some sleep loss[26].

The spousal arousal syndrome refers specifically to sleepiness caused by frequent arousals from the sound of a bed partner's snoring. A study of the wives of ten men with obstructive sleep apnea syndrome[27] showed poor sleep efficiency with frequent arousals, often temporarily related to their husbands' snores. After the husbands received continuous positive airway pressure therapy halfway through the night, their wives' sleep parameters improved significantly. This syndrome can be extended to any abnormal sleep behavior that causes sleep disruption in a bed partner, including high-amplitude periodic limb movements, the dream enactment behavior of REM sleep behavior disorder and the restless sleep of chronic insomnia.

## Intrinsic causes

Intrinsic causes are discussed in subsequent chapters (see Chapters 7 and 8).

## REFERENCES

1. Webb WB, Agnew HW. Are we chronically sleep-deprived? *Bull Psychonomic Soc* 1975;6:47

2. Lavie P. Sleep habits and sleep disturbances in industrial workers in Israel: main findings and some characteristics of workers complaining of excessive daytime sleepiness. *Sleep* 1981;4:147–58

3. Hublin C, Kaprio J, Partinen M, Heikkila K, Koskenvuo M. Daytime sleepiness in an adult, Finnish population. *J Int Med* 1996; 239:417–23

4. Martikainen K, Urponen H, Partinen M, Hasan J, Vuori I. Daytime sleepiness: a risk factor in community life. *Acta Neurol Scand* 1992;86:337–41

5. Webb WB. The cost of sleep-related accidents: a reanalysis. *Sleep* 1995;18:276–80

6. Mitler MM, Carskadon MA, Czeisler CA, Dement WC, Dinges DF, Graeber RC. Catastrophes, sleep and public policy: consensus report. *Sleep* 1988;11:100–9

7. Kripke DF, Garfinkel L, Wingard DL, Klauber MR, Marler MR. Mortality associated with sleep duration and insomnia. *Arch Gen Psychiatry* 2002;59:131–6

8. Carskadon MA, Dement WC, Mitler MM, *et al.* Guidelines for the multiple sleep latency test (MSLT): a standard measure of sleepiness. *Sleep* 1986;9:519–24

9. Daube JR, Cascino GD, Dotson RM, Silber MH, Westmoreland BF. Clinical neurophysiology. *Continuum* 1998;4:149–72

10. Ogilvie RD, Wilkinson RT. The detection of sleep onset: behavioral and physiological convergence. *Psychophysiology* 1984;21:510–20

11. Bonnet MH. Performance and sleepiness as a function of frequency and placement of sleep disruption. *Psychophysiology* 1986;23:263–71

12. Bonnet MH. Effect of sleep disruption on sleep, performance, and mood. *Sleep* 1985;8:11–19

13. Martin SE, Wraith PK, Deary IJ, Douglas NJ. The effect of nonvisible sleep fragmentation on daytime function. *Am J Respir Crit Care Med* 1997;155:1596–601

14. Mignot E, Taheri S, Nishino S. Sleeping with the hypothalamus: emerging therapeutic targets for sleep disorders. *Nature Neurosci* 2002;5:1071–5

15. Mendelson WB, Martin JV. Characterization of the hypnotic effects of triazolam microinjections into the medial preoptic area. *Life Sci* 1992;50:1117–28

16. Orr E, Quay WB. Hypothalamic 24-hour rhythms in histamine, histidine decarboxylase, and histamine-*N*-methyltransferase. *Endocrinology* 1975;96:941–5

17. Rechtschaffen A, Bergmann BM, Everson CA, Kushida CA, Gilliland MA. Sleep deprivation in the rat: X. Integration and discussion of the findings. *Sleep* 1989;12:68–87

18. Bergmann BM, Kushida CA, Everson CA, Gilliland MA, Obermeyer W, Rechtschaffen A. Sleep deprivation in the rat: II. Methodology. *Sleep* 1989;12:5–12

19. Everson CA. Sustained sleep deprivation impairs host defense. *Am J Physiol* 1993;265:R1148–54

20. Bergmann BM, Gilliland MA, Feng P, *et al.* Are physiological effects of sleep deprivation in the rat mediated by bacterial invasion? *Sleep* 1996;19:554–62

21. Rosenthal L, Roehrs TA, Rosen A, Roth T. Level of sleepiness and total sleep time following various time in bed conditions. *Sleep* 1993;16:226–32

22. Van Dongen HPA, Maislin G, Mullington JM, Dinges DF. The cumulative cost of additional wakefulness: dose–response effects on neurobehavioral functions and sleep physiology from chronic sleep restriction and sleep deprivation. *Sleep* 2003;26:117–26

23. Veasey S, Rosen R, Barzansky B, Rosen I, Owens J. Sleep loss and fatigue in residency training: a reappraisal. *J Am Med Assoc* 2002;288:1116–24

24. Marcus CL, Loughlin GM. Effect of sleep deprivation on driving safety in housestaff. *Sleep* 1996;19:763–6

25. Asch DA, Parker RM. The Libby Zion case. *N Engl J Med* 1988;318:771–5

26. Shepard JW. Pets and sleep. *Sleep* 2002; 25:A520

27. Beninati W, Harris C, Herold DL, Shepard JW. The effect of snoring and obstructive sleep apnea on the sleep quality of bed partners. *Mayo Clin Proc* 1999;74:955–8

# Chapter 6

# Approach to the sleepy patient

*To sleep: perchance to dream....*

**William Shakespeare,** *Hamlet*

## CLINICAL APPROACH

An assessment of the sleepy patient commences with a comprehensive sleep history and relevant examination as discussed in Chapter 3. The physician must then determine whether a clear diagnosis has emerged, allowing a management plan to be developed, or whether further investigations are needed. A starting point in this decision-making process is to decide whether the patient is describing sleepiness or fatigue (Chapter 5). It is essential to provide patients with an understandable definition of these symptoms, as they are often used interchangeably in everyday language. In a study of 190 patients with sleep apnea, 57% described themselves as fatigued and 47% as sleepy, when no definitions were provided for these terms[1]. Sleepiness should be described in terms of the eyelids drooping, the head sagging and short periods of sleep occurring inappropriately under sedentary circumstances when it is undesired. Fatigue, on the other hand, should be defined as a lack of physical energy and a sense of muscular exhaustion. When daytime sleep occurs with fatigue, it usually follows a period of rest, and does not have the same irresistible quality as with hypersomnolence.

Many patients are able to distinguish the two symptoms fairly easily when they are defined, but others cannot make the distinction or may perceive that they suffer from both. If the problem is clearly fatigue, an attempt should be made to elucidate the cause (Table 5.1). Primary sleep disorders are rarely the primary etiology. If the patient is sleepy, the cause may be determined by the history, especially if it is due to extrinsic factors. However, sleep studies are often needed, including polysomnography and the multiple sleep latency test (MSLT). Objective tests of sleepiness are helpful, especially in patients who cannot easily distinguish between sleepiness and fatigue, and the MSLT is especially valuable in determining the presence of premature intrusion of rapid eye movement (REM) sleep in patients with narcolepsy. Table 6.1 lists the quantitative tests of sleepiness and alertness that are discussed in detail in the remainder of this chapter. Figure 6.1 provides an algorithm for the diagnosis of sleepiness. However, each patient should be assessed individually, and it should be kept in mind that many patients have more than one contributing factor.

## SLEEPINESS SCALES

### Epworth sleepiness scale

The Epworth sleepiness scale (ESS) is the commonest scale used to assess sleepiness.

**Table 6.1** Quantitative measures of sleepiness and alertness

Sleepiness scales
    Epworth sleepiness scale
    Stanford sleepiness scale
    visual analog scale

Multiple sleep latency test

Maintenance of wakefulness test

Pupillometry

Performance tests

The patient is presented with eight situations and, for each, is asked to rate the chance of dozing on a scale of 0–3, with a maximum score of 24 points[2] (Table 3.1). The upper limit of normality derived from two studies of 72[3] and 182[4] subjects is generally accepted as 10–11 points. The scale shows acceptable test–retest reliability[5]. Studies have shown little or no correlation between ESS scores and MSLT results, suggesting that the two tests measure different aspects of sleepiness[6,7]. The ESS correlates with the intensity of psychological symptoms[8], and is consistently higher in

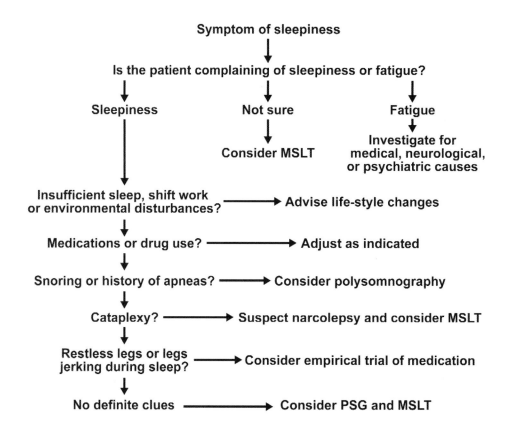

**Figure 6.1** Algorithmic approach to the sleepy patient. PSG, polysomnogram; MSLT, multiple sleep latency test

women compared with men[1]. Proponents of the ESS emphasize that it reflects sleepiness under a variety of real-life situations, but others have argued that its subjectivity reduces its usefulness as a quantitative tool. Many clinicians consider it a useful diagnostic supplement to the MSLT, and also helpful in monitoring the response of sleepy patients to treatment.

### Stanford sleepiness scale

This scale assesses a patient's sleepiness at a specific moment, using seven descriptions thought to indicate increasing depths of drowsiness (Table 6.2). It is often administered before each nap opportunity of an MSLT, to assess whether the patient's perception of sleepiness correlates with the objective results.

### Visual analog scale

A simple visual analog scale, similar to a scale of pain intensity, can provide a quan-

tifiable measure of a patient's sleepiness. This may be especially useful in comparing the efficacy of various doses of stimulant medication at different times of the day.

## THE MULTIPLE SLEEP LATENCY TEST

### Performance of the MSLT

The MSLT is the most widely used objective measure of sleepiness. In broad outline, the test consists of four or five nap opportunities offered at 2-h intervals over the course of a day. The time taken to fall asleep is measured for each nap and the average sleep latency is calculated. Any sleep-onset REM periods (SOREMPs) within 15 min of the start of sleep are noted. Test–retest reliability over several months has been demonstrated for both the mean latency[10] and the number of SOREMPs[11]. The essential simplicity of the concept masks the many details that need to be addressed for the results to be meaningful.

Table 6.2 Stanford sleepiness scale. Reproduced with permission from reference 9

| | |
|---|---|
| (1) | Feeling active and vital; alert; wide awake |
| (2) | Functioning at a high level, but not at peak; able to concentrate |
| (3) | Relaxed; awake; not at full alertness; responsive |
| (4) | A little foggy; clearly not at peak; let down |
| (5) | Fogginess; beginning to lose interest in remaining awake; slowed down |
| (6) | Sleepiness; prefer to be lying down; fighting sleep; woozy |
| (7) | Almost in reverie; sleep onset soon; lost struggle to remain awake |

The test is sensitive to sleep deprivation, and thus attention must be paid to ensuring an adequate total sleep time for at least a week before the study. If necessary, patients should be urged either to go to bed earlier or to rise later than usual, and to keep a sleep log while doing so. When available, wrist actigraphy for 1–2 weeks before the MSLT provides extremely useful objective confirmation of times awake and asleep. In almost all situations, a polysomnogram (PSG) should be performed the night before an MSLT. This allows a formal check on time spent asleep as well as ruling out causes of sleep fragmentation, such as unexpected sleep-disordered breathing. Every effort should be made to achieve adequate total sleep time the night before the test, preferably at least 7 h, even if patients need to remain in bed until 7 a.m. or later.

A range of psychotropic drugs influences both the MSLT sleep latency and the presence of SOREMPs, and the commonest error in performing the test is to ignore this confounding factor. All stimulants, hypnotics, sedatives, antidepressants, major tranquillizers and opioids should be discontinued at least 2 weeks before the study. Pharmacological agents with lengthy half-lives, such as fluoxetine, should be stopped even earlier. This step may pose inconveniences to patients, such as the worsening of sleepiness with the need for temporary driving restrictions, but cannot be avoided if interpretable MSLT results are to be obtained. It may not be possible to withdraw safely some medications such as antidepressants in patients with partially treated major depression, or antiseizure medications in patients with epilepsy. Rather than obtain uninterpretable data, it is often better in these situations not to perform the test at all, and to rely on clinical judgment in deciding diagnosis and therapy. In patients with heavy caffeine use, caffeinated beverages should be slowly weaned before the study and kept to a minimum for a week before the test. A urine drug screen should be obtained the day of the test, both to ensure that the patient is not continuing to take medications that could influence the test results, and to rule out the presence of illicit drugs.

On the day of the test, the patient should remain in the laboratory and not perform physical exercise, as this has been shown to delay significantly MSLT sleep latency[12]. Between nap opportunities, the patient should be out of bed, dressed in street clothes, and every effort should be made to prevent unscheduled naps. The patient should not smoke for 30 min before each test, and should not drink caffeinated beverages. The nap opportunities should be offered at 2-h intervals, commencing approximately 2 h after the patient wakes in the morning. At the start of each test, the patient should lie in bed in a dark, quiet room with a comfortable ambient temperature, wearing non-constricting clothing and no shoes. After calibration of the system, the technician should switch off the lights and instruct the patient to lie still and try to sleep. The time from lights out to the first epoch of any stage of sleep is defined as the sleep latency. Once sleep has been achieved, the study should continue for 15 min to determine whether a SOREMP has occurred. Once unequivocal REM sleep is recorded, many laboratories terminate the study even if 15 min of sleep have not elapsed. If no sleep occurs, the study is stopped after 20 min and an arbitrary figure of 20 min is assigned as the sleep latency. Either four or five nap opportunities can be offered, but in practice the only situation when a fifth test is generally performed is when a single SOREMP has been recorded during one of the first four naps.

Usually, the arithmetic mean is used as a measure of the average sleep latency, but ooccasionally one latency is an outlier, usually longer than the others. This results in a skewed distribution, and use of the mean will result in an inappropriately high average latency. In these circumstances, the median sleep latency is a more accurate measure of central tendency[13]. In addition to the average sleep latency, the number of naps with SOREMPs should be recorded.

## Interpretation of the MSLT

Despite the MSLT being used clinically for 25 years, there is still considerable controversy about its interpretation. The original two studies of 14 controls and 27 narcoleptics demonstrated a significant difference between the mean sleep latencies of the two groups (10.7 vs. 3.0 min)[14]. Despite standard deviations of greater than 5 min in the control samples, the authors suggested a 'preliminary guideline' of less than 5 min as the minimum cut-off point for documentation of pathological sleepiness. This was later enshrined as a 'generally accepted rule of thumb' in a widely cited 1986 guideline paper of the American Association of Sleep Disorders Centers[15]. Mean latencies of less than 5 min were interpreted as indicating definite excessive somnolence, latencies of greater than 10 min were considered indicative of normal alertness and the range of 5–10 min was defined as a 'diagnostic gray area' of uncertain significance. Mean laten-

cies of under 5 min have been associated with impaired performance on psychometric tests in sleep-deprived subjects[16], providing some measure of validity for considering very short latencies to be pathological. More recently, there has been a tendency to consider less than 8 min as indicating definite pathological sleepiness, but this figure seems to be based on clinical experience rather than normative data.

Several other studies have examined MSLT mean latencies in control populations, but this was not the primary goal in any of them. Interpretation of these data is also affected by concerns about possible sleep deprivation in some of the subjects, small numbers of participants and differences in methodology from that employed in the standard clinical MSLT. Table 6.3 summarizes the results of those studies utilizing a single epoch of any stage of sleep to indicate sleep onset. The mean latencies range between 10.0 and 15.1 min with standard deviations varying between 3.9 and 4.6 min. Two standard deviations below the mean represents the traditional statistical cut-off point separating the lower 5% from the upper 95% in a normally distributed population. For the first two studies, this point was 5.6 and 7.1 min, while for the latter two, the equivalent figures were considerably lower at 1.6 and 2.2 min, respectively. There is a strong possibility that sleep deprivation may have affected the latter results, as self-reported sleep times are not always accurate. In another study of 34 healthy volunteers who reported sleeping 6–9 h a night, 23 had unexpectedly short mean latencies on an MSLT[20]. Extending their time in bed to 10 h for 2 weeks resulted in normalization of their latencies (Figure 6.2).

With these imperfect data, how should the clinician judge the clinical significance of mean sleep latency on an MSLT? The MSLT results must be interpreted in the overall setting of the patient's problem, and should not be considered an absolute diagnostic test, overriding other considerations. The range of latencies should be regarded as representing a continuum of sleepiness, with lower values reflecting greater somnolence than higher values. While some ostensibly normal subjects in research studies may have mean latencies of less than 5 min, this range generally indicates pathological somnolence, due either to disease or to extrinsic causes such as sleep deprivation. The nearer the mean latency approaches 10 min, the more overlap there will be with a normal population, but some patients with abnormally excessive sleepiness will fall into this range. Other diagnostic tools, such as the use of clinical judgment or a quantitative sleepiness scale, should be used to supplement the MSLT in these patients. Mean latencies of above 10 min clearly fall within the statistically normal range, and probably do not indicate a degree of objective sleepiness very different from that of a control population.

The presence of a SOREMP is defined as at least one epoch of REM sleep occurring within 15 min of sleep onset. Most normative studies have confirmed that, at most, a single SOREMP is found during MSLT naps in normal subjects, and two or more SOREMPs are generally considered to be

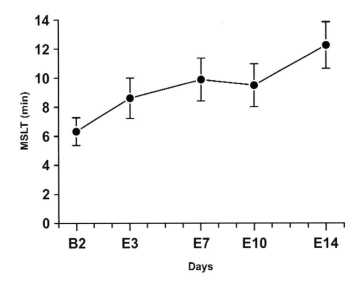

**Figure 6.2** Effect on the multiple sleep latency test (MSLT) of extending sleep time in sleepy subjects. This figure shows the effect on the MSLT of extending time in bed from 8 to 10 h over 2 weeks in 11 subjects. Mean sleep latencies increased from about 6 to 12 min. B2, baseline night 2, E3–E14, extended sleep nights 3–14. Modified with permission from reference 20

**Table 6.3** Normative multiple sleep latency test (MSLT) data. Sleep latency values are expressed as mean ± SD

| Reference | Number of subjects | Sleep latency (mins) | Comments |
|---|---|---|---|
| Zwyghuizen-Doorenbos et al. (1988)[10] | 14 | 13.4 ± 3.9 | all men; age 21–40 years; no preceding PSG |
| Kronholm et al. (1995)[17] | 77 | 15.1 ± 4.0 | age 35–55 years; no preceding PSG |
| Bishop et al. (1996)[18] | 139 | 10.0 ± 4.2 | about 15% reported usual sleep time as < 6 h; 17% with two or more SOREMPS |
| Carskadon et al. (1998)[19] | 25 | 11.4 ± 4.6 | age 14–16 years; preceding sleep time by actigraphy < 7 h in approximately 50% of subjects |

PSG, polysomnogram; SOREMP, sleep-onset rapid eye movement period

abnormal. The one exception is the study of 139 subjects[18] (Table 6.3), in which 17% had two or more SOREMPs. However, the SOREMP group had shorter mean sleep latencies than the group without SOREMPs, and this may indicate that the group with early REM sleep intrusion was sleep-deprived. Although SOREMPs are considered a neurophysiological marker for narcolepsy, they are not specific, and can result from many disturbances of sleep (Table 6.4). Seven per cent of patients with sleep apnea will have SOREMPs[21], and their presence in the setting of untreated sleep-disordered breathing cannot be accepted as providing evidence for narcolepsy. If both sleep apnea and narcolepsy are suspected in the same patient, sleep apnea must be treated for several weeks before the MSLT can be accurately interpreted. In general,

**Table 6.4** Causes of sleep-onset rapid eye movement periods (SOREMPs) on a multiple sleep latency test (MSLT)

Narcolepsy

Moderate or severe obstructive sleep apnea syndrome

Withdrawal of REM suppressant medication

REM sleep deprivation

Sleep–wake schedule disorders

Major depression

Prader–Willi syndrome[22]

meticulous attention to performing the MSLT correctly can result in the exclusion of most other causes, and thus, in the correct setting, two or more SOREMPs may be both sensitive and specific for a diagnosis of narcolepsy.

## Case 6.1

A 23-year-old woman presented with a history of daytime tiredness, starting rather abruptly at age 15 years at the time of an influenza-like febrile illness. It was extremely difficult to determine whether she was describing sleepiness or fatigue. She endorsed both symptoms, but thought that fatigue predominated. She described feeling exhausted after a day's work and would often doze while lying down to watch TV in the late afternoon. She did not fall asleep in conversations, nor in meetings at work. However, when driving in the evenings she had felt the car beginning to drift towards the side of the road after about 40 min. Her Epworth sleepiness scale score was 9. She was a receptionist in a physician's office, working from 7 a.m. to 3:30 p.m. She felt too tired to exercise. She reported sleeping well at night with few awakenings from 10 p.m. to 5 a.m., but felt exhausted on waking with an alarm in the morning. She did not snore, had not experienced cataplexy and denied symptoms of depression or systemic illness. She wore an actigraph for a week. This suggested that she was actually going to bed at about 11 p.m. and confirmed a waking time of 5 a.m. She was encouraged to extend her time in bed, and repeat actigraphy showed that she had achieved an average of about 7 h of sleep at night. Despite this, she reported feeling as tired as before. She had difficulty sleeping in the laboratory during the PSG and felt that her sleep quality was less good than at home. Her sleep efficiency was 73%, and she had achieved only 6 h 40 min of sleep by 7:30 a.m. No disordered breathing events or periodic limb movements of sleep were noted, but her sleep was fragmented by 17 non-specific arousals per hour. Despite the suboptimal sleep, an MSLT was performed the following day. This revealed sleep latencies of 15.5, 12.5 and 14.5 min on the first, third and fourth naps, with the patient being unable to sleep at all on the second nap opportunity. The mean latency was 15.6 min. No REM sleep was recorded. The mean sleep latencies, clearly within the normal range despite a marginal previous night's sleep, suggested that the problem was fatigue rather than sleepiness. No obvious medical cause was detected, and a psychiatric examination did not reveal evidence for depression. She was diagnosed with chronic fatigue syndrome and was encouraged to pursue a graded exercise program and a course of cognitive-behavioral therapy.

This case illustrates how some patients find it difficult to distinguish sleepiness from fatigue, and how these can be differentiated by means of a properly performed MSLT. It also shows how the use of actigraphy before an MSLT may demonstrate a degree of sleep deprivation not predicted by the patient's history. It also demonstrates how in practice it may sometimes be difficult to achieve an optimal amount of sleep the night before an MSLT. If the mean sleep latency is then clearly normal, as in this patient, useful conclusions can be reached. However, if a borderline short latency is obtained after a curtailed night's sleep, interpretation may be very difficult.

## THE MAINTENANCE OF WAKEFULNESS TEST

### Performance of the MWT

The maintenance of wakefulness test (MWT) is a variant of the MSLT in which, rather than attempt to sleep, the patient is asked to remain awake as long as possible. The MWT is not a diagnostic test for degree of sleepiness but rather a test of the ability to remain awake. It is used to assess efficacy of treatment once a diagnosis has been reached, and thus is performed under real-life conditions while the patient is taking stimulant medication or being treated for sleep-disordered breathing. A PSG is not usually performed the night before the test. It is used to assess a patient's fitness to fly a plane or drive a truck or bus, and is mandated by the United States Federal Aviation Administration before pilots treated for sleep apnea are permitted to regain their licenses. It is also useful for assessing narcoleptic patients who complain of continued tiredness, despite the use of high quantities of stimulant medication. The MWT is more subject to motivational factors than the MSLT.

As in the MSLT, four trials are performed at 2-h intervals. The patient is positioned sitting up in bed, with the back and head supported by a bed rest cushion. Alternatively, the patient can be seated in a recliner, with the trunk at a 45–90° angle with respect to the legs. A night-light (about 7.5 W) is positioned behind the patient's head. The patient is asked to try to remain awake with eyes open, but is not allowed to use extraordinary measures such as singing or slapping the face. The latency to the first epoch of sleep is measured for each trial and the mean sleep latency calculated. Two variants of the test have been described: in the first, a trial is terminated after 20 min if no sleep occurs, while in the second, each trial can last up to 40 min.

### Interpretation of the MWT

A multicenter normative study of the MWT involving 64 subjects aged 30–70 years has been reported[23]. The mean total sleep time on PSG the night before the MWT was $417 \pm 63$ min. The mean MWT latencies did not correlate with total sleep time, suggesting that sleep deprivation did not significantly affect the results. The study showed that the mean latencies followed a truncated distribution, with full wakefulness preserved for 40 min in over 75% of the trials. The mean latency for the test based on 40-min trials was 32.6 min; with 20-min trials this fell to 18.1 min due to accentuation of the ceiling effect. The authors recommend that the 20-min version be used, and suggest that an impairment of wake tendency be diagnosed if the mean latency is below 11 min, corresponding to the 8th centile and two standard deviations below the mean.

These recommendations raise philosophical issues regarding the degree of alertness that is acceptable for the performance of potentially hazardous tasks that put others at risk. As the MWT is not designed as a diagnostic test, a cut-off point that defines acceptable alertness as equivalent to that of the lowest 8% of the normal population may be inappropriately low. We have chosen to use 22.5 min, a mean latency one standard deviation below the mean (approximately the 15th centile) on the less truncated 40 min version, as a slightly more stringent guideline to societally acceptable alertness. However, this measure is not validated, and it can be argued that there is little evidence that the MWT correlates with lack of alertness in practical situations such as driving or piloting a plane.

### Case 6.2

An unmarried 42-year-old rural mail delivery man was driving down a hill into a small town one winter afternoon when he abruptly and without warning lost awareness. He rear-ended a truck in front of him at the bottom of the hill and immediately recovered consciousness. He denied feeling sleepy before the event. A few weeks later he was involved in a single-vehicle accident when his car rolled off the road into a ditch. His last recollection was driving near the site of the accident, but he recovered immediately the car came to a halt. He was uncertain whether or not the episodes were those of sleep. On questioning he admitted to falling asleep easily while watching television. He recalled dozing in the cab of his postal truck while doing paperwork at the end of a shift but denied sleepiness driving. His Epworth sleepiness scale score was 4. He estimated his usual total sleep time as 7 h, and this was confirmed with a week's actigraphy. He did not snore and did not experience cataplexy. He was on no medications. Extensive investigations for a seizure disorder or cardiac arrhythmia were negative. A polysomnogram was normal. An MSLT showed a mean initial sleep latency of 2.1 min, with no REM sleep recorded during any of the four naps. The patient misperceived the latencies of his naps, believing that he had fallen asleep in about 10 min on each occasion. A diagnosis of idiopathic hypersomnia was made and the patient treated with modafinil. At a daily dose of 400 mg, he did not perceive any change in his alertness. A 40-min MWT while taking modafinil revealed a mean sleep latency of 9.1 min. His medication was changed to methylphenidate, in increasing doses. At a dose of 20 mg three times a day, he still did not perceive a change in alertness. An MWT was repeated and this showed a mean latency of 28 min. He returned to driving and has not experienced any further motor vehicle accidents.

This case illustrates the unusual situation of severe objective sleepiness on an MSLT in association with sleep attacks, but little or no subjective perception of sleepiness. The MWT was essential in assessing the patient's response to medication. On modafinil his mean latency was below the 5th centile, but on a daily dose of 60 mg methylphenidate, it was within one standard deviation of the mean.

### PUPILLOMETRY

During drowsiness, the pupils constrict and become unstable. Electronic pupillometry was used as a measure of sleepiness many years before the development of the MSLT. Various algorithms have been used and most measures correlate with mean MSLT latencies. While abnormal pupillometry is predictive of short mean MSLT latencies, normal results may sometimes be seen in patients with MSLT latencies of less than 5 min[24]. Although experimental work with the technique still continues, it is rarely used clinically today.

## PERFORMANCE TESTING

Decrements in the performance of repetitive tasks involving attention and sensory processing may be used as indirect measures of alertness. Various tasks have been used, including standard psychometric tests and motor responses to sounds of varying intensity. Driving simulators can test vigilance in both sensory tracking and motor tasks, and may provide a more realistic measure of alertness in real-life situations. None of these tests have been used widely in clinical settings.

## REFERENCES

1. Chervin RD. Sleepiness, fatigue, tiredness, and lack of energy in obstructive sleep apnea syndrome. *Chest* 2000;118:372–9

2. Johns MW. A new method for measuring daytime sleepiness: the Epworth sleepiness scale. *Sleep* 1991;14:540–5

3. Johns MW, Hocking B. Daytime sleepiness and sleep habits of Australian workers. *Sleep* 1997;20:844–9

4. Parkes JD, Chen SY, Clift SJ, Dahlitz MJ, Dunn G. The clinical diagnosis of the narcoleptic syndrome. *J Sleep Res* 1998; 7:41–52

5. Johns MW. Sleepiness in different situations measured by the Epworth sleepiness scale. *Sleep* 1994;17:703–10

6. Benbadis S, Mascha E, Perry MC, Wolgamuth BR, Smolley L, Dinner D. Association between the Epworth sleepiness scale and the multiple sleep latency test in a clinical population. *Ann Intern Med* 1999;130:289–92

7. Chervin RD, Aldrich MS. The Epworth sleepiness scale may not reflect objective measures of sleepiness or sleep apnea. *Neurology* 1999;52:125–31

8. Olson LG, Cole MF, Ambrogetti A. Correlations among Epworth sleepiness scale scores, multiple sleep latency tests and psychological symptoms. *J Sleep Res* 1998; 7:248–53

9. Hoddes E, Dement WC, Zarcone V. The development and use of the Stanford Sleepiness Scale [Abstract]. *Psychophysiology* 1972;9:150

10. Zwyghuizen-Doorenbos A, Roehrs T, Schaefer M, Roth T. Test–retest reliability of the MSLT. *Sleep* 1988;11:562–5

11. Folkerts M, Rosenthal L, Roehrs T, *et al.* The reliability of the diagnostic features in patients with narcolepsy. *Biol Psychiatry* 1996;40:208–14

12. Bonnet MH, Arand DL. Sleepiness as measured by modified multiple sleep latency testing as a function of preceding activity. *Sleep* 1998;21:477–83

13. Benbadis SR, Perry MC, Wolgamuth BR, Turnbull J, Mendelson WB. Mean versus median for the multiple sleep latency test. *Sleep* 1995;18:342–5

14. Richardson GS, Carskadon MA, Flagg W, Van den Hoed J, Dement WC, Mitler MM. Excessive daytime sleepiness in man: multiple sleep latency measurement in narcoleptic and control subjects. *Electroencephalogr Clin Neurophysiol* 1978;45:621–7

15. Carskadon MA, Dement WC, Mitler MM, Roth T, Westbrook PR, Keenan S. Guidelines for the multiple sleep latency test (MSLT): a standard measure of sleepiness. *Sleep* 1986;9:519–24

16. Carskadon MA, Dement WC. Effects of total sleep loss on sleep tendency. *Percept Mot Skills* 1979;48:495–506

17. Kronholm E, Hyyppa MT, Alanen E, Halonen J, Partinen M. What does the multiple sleep latency test measure in a community sample? *Sleep* 1995;18:827–35

18. Bishop C, Rosenthal L, Helmus T, Roehrs T, Roth T. The frequency of multiple sleep onset REM periods among subjects with no excessive daytime sleepiness. *Sleep* 1996;19:727–30

19. Carskadon MA, Wolfson AR, Acebo C, Tzischinsky O, Seifer R. Adolescent sleep patterns, circadian timimg, and sleepiness at a transition to early school days. *Sleep* 1998;21:871–81

20. Roehrs T, Shore E, Papineau K, Rosenthal L, Roth T. A two-week sleep extension in sleepy normals. *Sleep* 1996;19:576–82

21. Aldrich MS, Chervin RD, Malow BA. Value of the multiple sleep latency test (MSLT) for the diagnosis of narcolepsy. *Sleep* 1997;20:620–9

22. Hertz G, Cataletto M, Feinsilver SH, Angulo M. Sleep and breathing patterns in patients with Prader Willi Syndrome (PWS): effects of age and gender. *Sleep* 1993;16:366–71

23. Doghramji K, Mitler MM, Sangal RB, *et al.* A normative study of the maintenance of wakefulness test (MWT). *Electroencephalogr Clin Neurophysiol* 1997;103:554–62

24. McLaren JW, Hauri PJ, Lin S, Harris CD. Pupillometry in clinically sleepy patients. *Sleep Med* 2002;3:347–52

# Chapter 7

# Narcolepsy and related conditions

*Thy sweet child Sleep, the filmy-eyed,*
*Murmured like a noontide bee,*
*Shall I nestle near thy side?*
*Wouldst thou me? – And I replied,*
*No, Not thee!*

**Percy Bysshe Shelley,** *To Night*

## NARCOLEPSY

Narcolepsy is the classic example of a true sleeping sickness. First described in 1877, the disorder was given its name by the French neuropsychiatrist Jean Baptiste Gelineau. Understanding of narcolepsy has slowly developed over the past 50 years, culminating in a flood of knowledge since 1999. Diagnostic techniques have evolved and new drugs have provided increasing relief for patients. However, much remains to be understood, especially about the disorder's pathogenesis and the borderlands where it merges with other conditions such as idiopathic hypersomnia.

### Clinical features

In 1957, Yoss and Daly suggested that there was a core tetrad of narcoleptic symptoms comprising excessive daytime sleepiness, cataplexy, hypnagogic hallucinations and sleep paralysis. However, many patients do not have all four of these symptoms, leading to controversies regarding minimal diagnostic criteria. Diagnostic considerations are explored later in this chapter.

### Excessive daytime sleepiness

Most patients with narcolepsy are initially identified because of inappropriate, severe daytime sleepiness that interferes with their functioning. Essentially all patients with narcolepsy experience this potentially disabling symptom, which can lead to motor vehicle accidents, occupational difficulties and social problems. It occurs most commonly in circumstances that induce drowsiness such as boredom and inactivity, but may also occur at strikingly inappropriate times. Narcoleptic patients may experience sleep attacks (see Chapter 5) in which periods of sleep occur without preceding drowsiness, but at other times a pervasive sense of impending sleep precedes loss of awareness. Patients often feel refreshed after a nap, but drowsiness soon returns. Daytime drowsiness may lead to episodes of automatic behavior without recall, such as typing or driving, as well as diplopia, blurred vision and ptosis. The sleepiness of narcolepsy is non-specific, and other causes such as sleep deprivation and sleep apnea syndromes must be considered. However, it is often extremely severe and persistent, with onset usually in adolescence or early adulthood.

*Cataplexy*

Cataplexy is the most specific symptom of narcolepsy, and its occurrence in the setting of excessive daytime sleepiness is virtually pathognomonic for the disorder. Isolated cataplexy is very rare, but can be found in conditions such as Niemann–Pick disease type C[1] and occasional pontomedullary lesions[2]. The percentage of narcoleptic patients with cataplexy is usually quoted as 75–80%[3,4], but in a population-based study in which narcolepsy was defined as excessive sleepiness with either cataplexy or more than two sleep-onset rapid eye movement periods (SOREMPs) on a multiple sleep latency test (MSLT), it was present in only 64%[5].

Cataplexy is a sudden episode of transient loss of muscle strength precipitated by emotion. It should be bilateral and involve more than just a subjective sensation of internal weakness. In complete attacks, only the respiratory and extraocular muscles are spared, but partial attacks are more common, with symptoms such as buckling of the knees, sagging of the face or weakness of the jaw or neck. Sensory input and memory are intact, and patients can describe what transpired after the episode has resolved. The ability to observe and recall events during most cataplectic episodes is a helpful feature in discriminating between cataplexy and other states of immobility, such as syncope, seizures and sleep. Most episodes resolve within seconds to minutes, but during occasional prolonged attacks, dream-like hallucinations may occur and the patient may actually enter rapid eye movement (REM) sleep.

Cataplexy is most frequently precipitated by laughter, while the patient is either telling a joke or hearing one told by others. The response is extremely dependent on the individual patient's particular sense of humor, and many patients can describe the exact type of joke that will result in muscle atonia. Cataplexy can also be induced by other strong emotions, including anger, excitement, surprise, sadness or fear, but it is very rare for true cataplexy never to be caused by laughter. It can reduce the enjoyment of recreational activities by occurring at critical moments while hunting, fishing or playing ball games. Cataplexy can be subdivided into a typical form, in which joking or laughing triggers events, and an atypical form triggered only by other emotions[6].

During an episode of cataplexy, deep tendon reflexes are transiently lost, and this usually occurs even if the attack is a partial one[7]. The patient is otherwise medically stable, without cardiovascular or respiratory compromise. The electroencephalogram (EEG) does not usually change, and limited surface electromyogram (EMG) recordings are rarely helpful unless the attack is complete. The H-reflex, a neurophysiological correlate of the deep tendon reflex, is inhibited in REM sleep and during cataplectic attacks. Unless a physician observes transient areflexia during a spell of unresponsiveness, cataplexy can be difficult to diagnose with complete certainty. Table 7.1 indicates the percentages of patients with narcolepsy and controls who answered affirmatively to questions regarding muscle weakness precipitated by different emotions[8]. While all the positive responses were more frequent in narcoleptic patients, a sizeable minority of control subjects also perceived experiencing weakness with emotion. Algorithms have been suggested to help make the diagnosis[8,9] (Figure 7.1), but

**Table 7.1** Muscle weakness precipitated by emotion. Modified with permission from reference 8

| Question | Cataplexy, yes (n = 55) | Control, yes (n = 47) | Sensitivity (95% CI) | Specificity (95% CI) |
|---|---|---|---|---|
| Laugh | 53 (96%) | 7 (15%) | 0.96 (0.87–1.00) | 0.85 (0.72–0.94) |
| Hear or tell a joke | 47 (85%) | 8 (17%) | 0.85 (0.73–0.94) | 0.83 (0.69–0.92) |
| Surprised | 48 (87%) | 10 (21%) | 0.87 (0.76–0.95) | 0.79 (0.64–0.89) |
| Excited | 45 (82%) | 8 (17%) | 0.82 (0.69–0.91) | 0.83 (0.69–0.92) |
| Elated | 40 (73%) | 7 (15%) | 0.73 (0.59–0.84) | 0.85 (0.72–0.94) |
| Angry | 40 (73%) | 8 (17%) | 0.73 (0.59–0.84) | 0.83 (0.69–0.92) |
| Remember a happy moment | 35 (64%) | 4 (9%) | 0.64 (0.50–0.76) | 0.91 (0.80–0.98) |
| Remember an emotional event | 40 (73%) | 10 (21%) | 0.73 (0.59–0.84) | 0.79 (0.64–0.89) |

CI, confidence interval

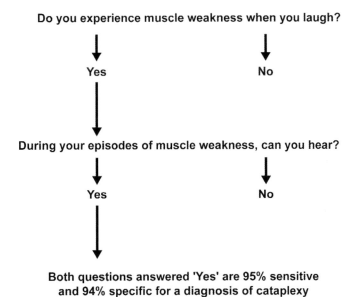

**Figure 7.1** An algorithm for the diagnosis of cataplexy[8]

generally one relies on the clinical judgment of experienced physicians.

Cataplexy usually develops after the onset of daytime sleepiness, most often within 4 years, but occasionally 10 or more years later (Figure 7.2)[10]. With increasing age, cataplexy is often said to become less frequent, but this may be due to patients learning to control the emotional responses that precipitate the events. In some older patients, cataplexy may actually become more frequent, and may be less clearly precipitated by emotions alone.

*Sleep paralysis and hypnagogic hallucinations*

Sleep paralysis refers to the transient inability to move at the onset of sleep, or upon wakening, with retained consciousness. The spell always resolves spontaneously within seconds or minutes, but touching the patient often aborts the paralysis. Hypnagogic hallucinations occur at the transition between wakefulness and sleep, and many patients report difficulty in distinguishing them from dreams at sleep onset or termination. They are usually visual, but can occasionally be auditory, tactile or vestibular. The frequency of hypnagogic hallucinations and sleep paralysis in a community-based study of narcoleptic patients with and without cataplexy is indicated in Table 7.2[11]. They commence before, simultaneously with or after the onset of excessive daytime sleepiness[10]. However, these phenomena are not specific:

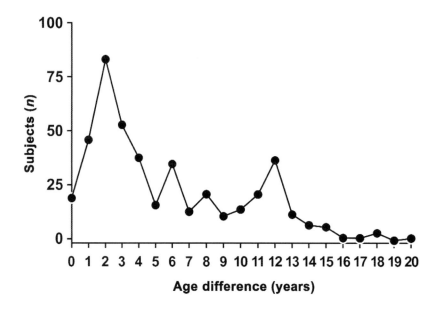

**Figure 7.2** Age of onset of cataplexy in relation to age of onset of sleepiness. Most patients experienced cataplexy onset within 4 years of onset of sleepiness, but onset of cataplexy was occasionally delayed for up to two decades. Reproduced with permission from reference 10

25% of a community sample of 13 057 subjects reported hallucinations on falling asleep and 7% on wakening[12]. A similar study of 8085 subjects revealed that the lifetime prevalence of sleep paralysis was 6%[13]. These phenomena may be more prevalent in normal adolescents than in older subjects. They probably occur with greater frequency over a longer period of time in patients with narcolepsy, compared with a normal population (see Chapter 16).

*Disturbed nocturnal sleep*

Patients with narcolepsy often develop fragmented nocturnal sleep with multiple awakenings (Figure 7.3). Total sleep time over 24 h is often not prolonged, with sleep distributed during the night and the day. REM sleep may occur earlier than usual during the night, and may be more evenly distributed through the different sleep cycles. Patients with narcolepsy may develop REM sleep behavior disorder in which muscle tone is retained during REM sleep (see Chapter 16). Arousal parasomnias (sleepwalking and sleep terrors) may also occur, but the frequency has not been established. Periodic limb movements of sleep are common in patients with narcolepsy, but rarely contribute significantly to patients' hypersomnia.

**Table 7.2** Hypnagogic hallucinations and sleep paralysis in narcolepsy

|  | *Hypnagogic hallucinations* (%) | *Sleep paralysis* (%) |
|---|---|---|
| Narcolepsy with cataplexy | 59 | 66 |
| Narcolepsy without cataplexy | 32 | 11 |

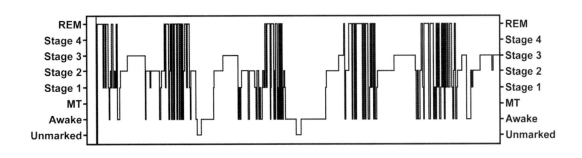

**Figure 7.3** A typical hypnogram of a patient with narcolepsy. This hypnogram shows early onset of rapid eye movement (REM) sleep. REM sleep is highly fragmented and is distributed through all sleep cycles rather than clustered in cycles towards the end of the night. Sleep efficiency is poor with periods of wakefulness during the night. MT, movement time. Reproduced with permission from reference 14

*Increased body mass*

A number of studies have shown that the body mass index of a population of patients with narcolepsy is higher than in age- and gender-matched controls[15–17]. Occasionally, a sudden increase in body mass seems to accompany the onset of the disorder. The mechanism of increased mass is uncertain; it is possible that reduced physical activity due to sleepiness plays a role, but low cerebrospinal fluid (CSF) hypocretin and alterations in serum[15] and CSF[16] leptin concentrations may indicate a state of altered energy homeostasis.

## Case 7.1

A 28-year-old man presented with a 9-year history of paralysis accompanying orgasm. He was unable to move, his eyelids closed involuntarily and he could only talk in a slurred mumble. He was able to retain his erection and achieve a full orgasm with complete retention of consciousness. The spell occurred during about every second orgasm, and lasted for about 15 s. He denied similar episodes with any other emotion, including with laughter. He also reported waking once a week from dreams, unable to move, with the dream imagery continuing for a few moments. The paralysis could be overcome by his wife touching him. On rare occasions he would act out his dreams, and recalled kicking his wife during sleep. He was only mildly sleepy, and did not believe this was a significant problem. An overnight polysomnogram (PSG) revealed an initial REM sleep latency of 2.5 min, with 480 min of total sleep time recorded. No significant disordered breathing

events were recorded. Muscle tone during REM sleep was increased. A multiple sleep latency test the following day showed a mean sleep latency of 7.5 min, with REM sleep being recorded on three of the four nap opportunities. A diagnosis of narcolepsy with cataplexy was made, and treatment commenced with protriptyline. At a dose of 15 mg before bed, cataplexy ceased and episodes of sleep paralysis became less frequent. After about a year, he became more conscious of daytime sleepiness and modafinil was prescribed. At a dose of 200 mg in the morning, his alertness returned to normal.

This case illustrates how cataplexy can occur with emotions highly specific to individual patients. Even with laughter, the special type of humor may be vitally important in determining whether or not the spell occurs. The patient also experienced sleep paralysis, hypnopompic hallucinations and REM sleep behavior disorder, but surprisingly little sleepiness. It is extremely unusual for cataplexy to antecede the onset of hypersomnolence. The case report also illustrates how the premature intrusion of REM sleep in both the PSG and the MSLT may provide helpful confirmation of the diagnosis, even when the MSLT mean sleep latency is greater than 5 min.

### Epidemiology

A community-based study in Olmsted County, Minnesota[5] demonstrated that the incidence rate of narcolepsy was 1.4/100 000 population per year, implying that one would expect 14 new narcoleptics to be diagnosed every year in an area with 1 million population. The prevalence was 56/100 000, indicating that one would expect to find at any one time about 560 narcoleptics in an area of 1 million population. This is very similar to the prevalence of 26–67/100 000 found in other American and European studies[18–22]. Narcolepsy commences most frequently in adolescence, with second-decade incidence rates more than twice that seen in the third decade, and more than three times that seen in the first and fourth decades (Figure 7.4). It is extremely unusual for idiopathic narcolepsy to commence after the age of 40 years. Narcolepsy appears to be slightly commoner in men than in women (approximately 1.5 : 1)[5].

## Etiology and pathogenesis

### A disorder of REM sleep

The first step in understanding the pathogenesis of narcolepsy was the recognition in 1960 that REM sleep occurred close to sleep onset[23]. This premature intrusion of REM sleep has been utilized diagnostically in the MSLT. In addition, inappropriate dissociation of the phenomena of REM sleep is also characteristic of the condition. Cataplexy and sleep paralysis represent REM sleep muscle atonia occurring during wakefulness, and hypnagogic hallucinations are the dreams of REM sleep occurring before sleep

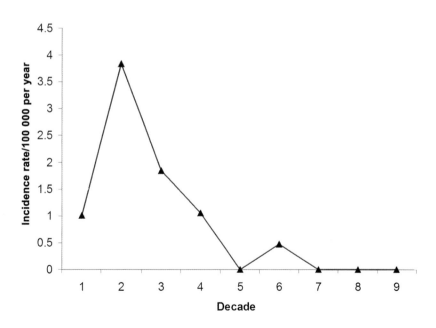

**Figure 7.4** Age of onset of narcolepsy. This graph demonstrates that narcolepsy most commonly commences in the second decade followed by the third and then the first and fourth decades

onset or after sleep termination. REM sleep behavior disorder in narcolepsy also represents abnormal REM sleep, with loss of skeletal muscle atonia providing the substrate for acting out of dreams.

### HLA and narcolepsy

The next phase in unraveling narcolepsy was triggered by the observation in 1984 that Japanese narcoleptic patients were highly likely to carry the human leukocyte antigen (HLA) haplotype DR2[24], a finding later confirmed in American Caucasians. A lower frequency of HLA DR2 in African-American narcoleptic patients led to the conclusion that the actual predisposing antigen was DQ1 rather than DR2. Finally, the responsible subtype was identified as HLA DQB1*0602. The region on chromosome 4 surrounding the HLA DQB1*0602 locus has been fully sequenced, and this seems to be the actual predisposing gene. Of narcoleptics with clear-cut cataplexy, 85–93% are positive for HLA DQB1*0602, compared with 35–56% of narcoleptics without cataplexy and about 20% of the control Caucasian population[4,6,25]. The relationship of narcolepsy to a specific HLA antigen highlights the issue of a genetic component to the disorder. However, only 1–2% of first-degree relatives of narcoleptics develop the disease[26], and 70–75% of monozygotic twins are discordant for the disorder, suggesting strong environmental influences[27]. In addition, patients with familial narcolepsy are less likely to be HLA DQB1*0602-positive than sporadic cases, suggesting that a mechanism separate from the HLA system may underlie these familial cases. Diseases associated with a specific HLA subtype are generally autoimmune in nature, and this remains the most likely mechanism in sporadic narcolepsy. However, searches for general serum autoimmune markers in narcolepsy have been negative[28], and there are no reported magnetic resonance imaging (MRI) or CSF changes to suggest an inflammatory disorder.

### Secondary (symptomatic) narcolepsy

Occasional cases of narcolepsy apparently caused by other disorders of the brain have been reported since the early 20th century. Most patients have had pathology of the hypothalamic–pituitary region[29], including suprasellar pituitary tumors, hypothalamic sarcoidosis and an arteriovenous malformation. Rare cases of brainstem pathology have also been reported, but the relationship is less clear. The onset of narcolepsy has also been reported to follow head injuries, brain radiation and hypoxic–ischemic insults, but the anatomical areas involved have not been determined. Despite the primary REM sleep generator being in the pons, these data support the possibility that the hypothalamus has a role in pathogenesis of the disease.

### Monoamines and narcolepsy

A number of lines of evidence from studies of narcolepsy in humans and dogs suggest that the disorder may be associated with decreased brainstem catecholamine activity. Autopsy studies of patients with narcolepsy suggest that altered $\alpha_1$-adrenergic receptor functioning is associated with the disease[30]. The anticataplectic effects of antidepressants in human and canine narcolepsy appear to be mediated via inhibition of norepinephrine uptake at the synaptic cleft. The effect of stimulant therapy in controlling the sleepiness of narcolepsy is predominantly mediated via dopamine. The firing rate of adrenergic locus ceruleus cells in the brainstem tegmentum falls during canine cataplexy.

*Hypocretins (orexins) and narcolepsy*

The dramatic breakthrough in the understanding of narcolepsy came following the discovery of the hypocretin (Hcrt) neurotransmitter system (Chapter 1). Narcolepsy in dogs is transmitted as an autosomal recessive trait. In 2000, Emmanuel Mignot and colleagues discovered that the disorder was caused by a deletion in the Hcrt receptor-2 gene[31]. Another group of investigators, working with a Hcrt knock-out mouse model, serendipitously recognized that the mutant mice developed episodes of either REM sleep or cataplexy while awake[32]. The observation that different abnormalities in the Hcrt system caused a narcolepsy-like syndrome in two animal species led to a search for evidence that Hcrt was involved in narcolepsy in humans. It was soon noted that Hcrt-1 could be measured in the CSF, and that narcoleptics had absent or markedly

**Table 7.3** Normal and abnormal ranges for cerebrospinal fluid (CSF) hypocretin-1 (Hcrt-1) concentration[6]

| Normal | > 200 pg/ml |
| --- | --- |
| Borderline low | 111–200 pg/ml |
| Low | ≤ 110 pg/ml |
| Undetectable | depends on sensitivity of assay, often < 40 pg/ml |

reduced Hcrt-1 concentrations. Table 7.3 summarizes normal and abnormal ranges for CSF Hcrt-1 concentration. In the largest published study of 101 narcoleptics with typical cataplexy and the HLA DQB1*0602 antigen, 87% had low or undetectable levels of CSF Hcrt-1[6]. This was in contrast with 29% of seven narcoleptics with cataplexy but negative for HLA DQB1*0602, and 14% of 21 narcoleptics without cataplexy (all three positive for HLA DQB1*0602). Only four of 228 non-narcoleptic neurological controls had low or undetectable levels of CSF Hcrt-1: three had Guillain–Barré syndrome and one Hashimoto's encephalitis. Levels may be borderline low in a range of other disorders, including acute leukemia, head injuries, central nervous system (CNS) infections, seizure disorders and CNS tumors[33].

Eight of 21 patients from nine families with familial narcolepsy had low or undetectable CSF Hcrt-1 levels[6]. However, the search for human mutations in the Hcrt system as a cause for narcolepsy has been disappointing. A point mutation in the Hcrt signal peptide has been described in a single patient, resulting in unusually early-onset disease[34]. However, a screen of 74 patients, including 27 with a family history of the disorder and 29 who were HLA DQB1*0602-negative, failed to reveal any pathogenic mutations in the genes for Hcrt or its receptors[34], suggesting that abnormalities in other neurotransmitter systems may be responsible for most cases of familial narcolepsy.

Autopsy studies of the brains of narcoleptics have shown absent Hcrt in the hypothalamus, cortex and pons. Hcrt neurons are reduced by 90% compared with controls, while melanin-concentrating hormone neurons, which are intermixed with Hcrt neurons in the hypothalamus, are preserved[34]. Conflicting findings regarding the presence or absence of hypothalamic gliosis have been reported[34,35]. Low levels of CSF Hcrt-1 have also been described in some patients with narcolepsy related to hypothalamic tumors[36,37], and in a patient with Prader–Willi syndrome[6].

How do abnormalities in the Hcrt system cause the symptoms of narcolepsy? Hcrt neurons project widely to the brainstem, and especially the ascending reticular activating system. Hcrt may facilitate arousal mechanisms by an excitatory influence on dopaminergic, histaminergic and cholinergic neurons, and its absence may thus cause hypersomnolence. Similarly, Hcrt may activate pontine noradrenergic pathways that prevent REM sleep intruding into wakefulness, and its absence may promote dissociated states such as cataplexy.

### Summary (Table 7.4)

*Narcolepsy with cataplexy (sporadic)* Approximately 90% of these patients are positive for the HLA DQB1*0602 antigen, and 90% have low or absent CSF Hcrt-1 levels. The disorder in these patients is most probably caused by loss of Hcrt-synthesizing cells in the hypothalamus. The mechanism for the cell loss is unknown, but the very tight association with a specific HLA antigen suggests that it may be autoimmune-mediated.

*Narcolepsy without cataplexy (sporadic)* These patients with multiple SOREMPS have a frequency of HLA DQB1*0602 positivity intermediate between narcoleptics with cataplexy

**Table 7.4** Subtypes of narcolepsy

|  | Narcolepsy with cataplexy (sporadic) | Narcolepsy without cataplexy (sporadic) | Familial narcolepsy | Symptomatic narcolepsy |
|---|---|---|---|---|
| ≥ 1 SOREMP on MSLT | 84%[3] | 100% (by definition) | uncertain | 75% (total 18 cases)[29] |
| HLA DQB1*0602 | 85–93% | 35–56% | 65–79%[38] | uncertain |
| Low or undetectable CSF Hcrt-1 levels | 87%[6] | 14% (total 21 cases)[6] | 38% (total 21 cases)[6] | uncertain, some low |
| Proposed pathogenesis | autoimmune destruction of Hcrt synthesizing neurons | partial Hcrt deficiency in some; unknown mechanism in others | multiple genotypes; some, but not all, involving Hcrt system | damage to hypothalamic Hcrt synthesizing neurons |

SOREMP, sleep-onset rapid eye movement period; MSLT, multiple sleep latency test; HLA, human leukocyte antigen; CSF, cerebrospinal fluid; Hcrt, hypocretin and a control population. The majority have normal CSF Hcrt-1 levels but some, especially those who are HLA-positive, have low or absent levels. This group may be heterogeneous, with some patients having a partial Hcrt deficiency sufficient to cause sleepiness, but insufficient to cause cataplexy or to reduce the CSF concentration of Hcrt-1 below the normal range. Others may have a different condition altogether, unrelated to dysfunction of the Hcrt system and not associated with an immune mechanism.

*Familial narcolepsy* This appears to be a heterogeneous group of conditions, with probably a variety of underlying genotypes. Some families have low CSF Hcrt-1 levels, but the underlying genetic defect has only been established in a single patient. In other families, the Hcrt system may not be involved at all.

*Symptomatic narcolepsy* Secondary narcolepsy is largely associated with hypothalamic–pituitary pathology, and limited studies have found low CSF Hcrt-1 levels. The available data suggest that it is most often due to damage to Hcrt-synthesizing cells in the hypothalamus.

## Case 7.2

A 45-year-old woman had no sleep complaints until she underwent a hysterectomy. She was later told that she 'stopped breathing in the recovery room'. Notes obtained from the surgical admission were scanty, but indicated that she was reintubated. Arterial blood gases measured soon after she was placed back on a ventilator showed a pH of 7.25 and a carbon dioxide partial pressure ($p$CO$_2$) of 55 mmHg, sug-

gesting that she was in acute respiratory failure. Before discharge from hospital 2 days later, she noticed profound sleepiness. On the day she returned home, she laughed while sitting at a meal and noted that her head fell forward. Multiple similar brief episodes of neck weakness and slurring of speech with laughter, excitement and later on attempting to enter a conversation occurred daily. Severe sleepiness persisted and she was unable to return to work. Occasional episodes of sleep paralysis associated with hypnagogic hallucinations occurred, and she began acting out her dreams, with flailing arms and vocalizations. Polysomnography showed a total sleep time of 443 min without significant disordered breathing events. Muscle tone in REM sleep was abnormally increased. An MSLT the following day showed a mean sleep latency of 1.1 min with SOREMPs on all four naps. HLA testing revealed positivity for DR2 and DQ1. An MRI scan of the head was normal. A diagnosis of narcolepsy with cataplexy was made and she was commenced on stimulant and antidepressant therapy. Despite high doses of methylphenidate, some sleepiness persisted, but cataplexy was better controlled.

This case illustrates some of the difficulties in deciding whether narcolepsy is primary or secondary. The vast majority of cases are not associated with another CNS disorder, but the close temporal relationship here to a postoperative hypoxic event suggests a probable relationship. The age of onset is very unusual for sporadic narcolepsy. On the other hand, the event was not well documented, and an MRI scan did not reveal evidence for an infarct of the hypothalamus or brainstem. The patient was also positive for HLA antigens known to be associated with sporadic narcolepsy, but these are also seen in normal subjects, and might have predisposed her to secondary narcolepsy following a hypoxic insult. On the balance of probabilities, the patient was classified as having symptomatic narcolepsy.

**Diagnosis**

The minimum criteria required for the diagnosis of narcolepsy are controversial. The criteria of the 1997 International Classification of Sleep Disorders (ICSD) are complex and have not been validated. The presence of unequivocal cataplexy in the setting of hypersomnia is diagnostic of the disorder, even without laboratory confirmation. The problem is that cataplexy with transient areflexia is rarely observed by physicians, and the diagnosis is usually made on history alone. Even experienced sleep specialists may sometimes be uncertain, and the symptoms can be feigned by intelligent drug-seeking impostors. Thus, it is optimal for the diagnosis to be confirmed by a correctly performed MSLT, seeking both reasonably short mean sleep latency and the presence of SOREMPs. When cataplexy is not present, then an MSLT is essential, as the presence of SOREMPs with other causes excluded defines the condition.

There is very little role for HLA-typing in clinical practice. Although the presence of HLA DQB1*0602 is 90% sensitive for the diagnosis of narcolepsy with cataplexy, its frequency in the general population of 20% makes its specificity low. Thus, considering a prevalence of 1 : 2000 for the disease, its positive predictive value is only about 10%. Currently, CSF Hcrt-1 determination should be considered a research tool, but the test may soon be available clinically. While the sensitivity of a low or undetectable level for the diagnosis of narcolepsy with cataplexy is about the same as the presence of HLA DQB1*0602, its specificity is far higher, and may reach close to 100% in the absence of a few easily distinguishable neurological disorders. However, in the absence of cataplexy, the test will not provide useful diagnostic information. CSF Hcrt-1 measurement requires a spinal tap, but not the often-cumbersome preparations needed for an MSLT. It may be especially useful in the diagnosis of sleepy patients with suspected cataplexy who are taking REM suppressant medications, when withdrawal of these drugs may be inconvenient or potentially harmful.

**Treatment**

*Non-pharmacological management*

Non-pharmacological approaches to narcolepsy management include avoidance of sleep deprivation, regular sleep and wake times, work in a stimulating environment and avoidance of shift work. Patients with narcolepsy should be educated about the risks of driving when sleepiness is inadequately treated. It is commonly believed that naps of even brief duration are restorative, but objective data are contradictory. A study of 2-h duration naps ending at noon showed some objective decrease in sleepiness on an MSLT up to 2-h later, while a 15-min nap showed no effect[39]. Similarly, long naps caused improvement in reaction times, whereas short naps did not[40]. In contrast, another study showed that a 15-min nap at 4 p.m. resulted in increased latency on a further nap opportunity offered 15, but not 30, min later[41].

### Stimulant therapy

The mainstay of treatment of excessive daytime sleepiness in narcolepsy or idiopathic hypersomnia is the use of stimulant medication. Ephedrine and amphetamines were first used in the 1930s and methylphenidate in 1956. With the possible exception of modafinil, whose mechanism of action is uncertain, all stimulants are centrally acting sympathomimetic agents that enhance the release of monoamines in the synaptic cleft and block their reuptake. Stimulants can be divided into short-acting agents, needing several doses a day to maintain sustained alertness, and long-acting agents (including controlled-release forms of some of the short-acting drugs) that can often be taken once daily (Table 7.5). Rigorous assessment of the stimulants is difficult because few double-blind trials of the agents have been undertaken with the exception of modafinil, and there have been no head-to-head comparisons of different drugs. However,

**Table 7.5** Commonly used short- and long-acting stimulants

|  | Common daily starting dose (mg) | Recommended maximum daily dose (mg) |
|---|---|---|
| *Short-acting stimulants* | | |
| Methylphenidate | 30 | 100* |
| Dextroamphetamine | 15 | 100* |
| Mixed dextro- and levo-amphetamine (Adderall®) | 20 | 60† |
| Methamphetamine | 15 | 80* |
| | | |
| *Long-acting stimulants* | | |
| Extended-release methylphenidate | 20 | 60† |
| Extended-release methylphenidate (Concerta®) | 18 | 54 (attention deficit and hyperactivity disorder)† |
| Extended-release dextroamphetamine (Dexedrine spansules®) | — | 60† |
| Extended-release mixed dextro- and levo-amphetamine (Adderall XR®) | 20 | 60‡ |
| Modafinil | 100 | 400† |
| Pemoline | 18.75 | 150* |

*American Academy of Sleep Medicine recommendations[42] (note that some of these maximum doses exceed manufacturer's recommendations); †manufacturer's recommendations; ‡derived from recommended maximum dose of short-acting Adderrall

considerable information is available from clinical experience and reported case series.

The goal of stimulant therapy should be to produce as near normal alertness as possible with a minimum of side-effects. Stimulant dosage should commence low and be increased as required and tolerated. Occasional patients need higher doses than recommended, but careful monitoring for toxicity, including psychiatric symptoms and hypertension, is needed. The short-acting drugs have durations of action ranging between 3 and 5 h, often resulting in peak and trough effects with the patient oscillating between states of heightened alertness and distressing sleepiness. These drugs are usually administered 3–4 times a day, initially at 4-h intervals. Long-acting drugs can be administered once or twice daily. The timing of the last dose of stimulants should be regulated to prevent nocturnal insomnia. Physicians are often cautious about increasing doses of stimulants because of fear of inducing tolerance, dependence or toxicity, or concern over possible audit by governmental bodies. Tolerance does occur in some patients, with 31 of a series of 100 narcoleptics requiring doubling of the dose of amphetamines to achieve the same degree of control over 1 year[43]. However, abuse of the drugs is very rare in narcoleptic patients, who do not have a previous problem of chemical dependency. A study of the discontinuation of modafinil after 9 weeks' therapy showed no evidence for the development of withdrawal symptoms, suggesting that dependence did not develop[44]. There is inadequate evidence that drug holidays reduce the development of tolerance, and discontinuing stimulants for even a day every week results in considerable patient distress.

Sympathomimetic side-effects are dose-related, and the dose at which they occur varies from drug to drug and from patient to patient. They include anxiety, irritability, palpitations, tremor, anorexia, headache and insomnia. The risk of inducing psychoses at recommended doses is low (0.3–0.6%)[45,46], but may be considerably higher when maximum suggested doses are exceeded. There is little evidence that moderate-dose stimulants induce hypertension, although high-dose amphetamines may cause a modest rise in blood pressure. Stimulants are not contraindicated in patients with underlying hypertension, but careful attention should be paid to blood pressure control. A relationship to stroke or other vascular disease has not been established. Conventional stimulants have been reported to cause impairment of growth in children, but the long-term effect seems small. Pemoline has been associated with a 4–17 times greater than expected risk of acute hepatic failure, and as a result, the manufacturers now recommend that serum alanine aminotransferase concentration be measured every 2 weeks[47]. Modafinil does not usually produce sympathomimetic toxicity, but headache, nausea, nervousness and rhinitis occurred more frequently than with placebo in controlled trials[44,48,49]. Modafinil may reduce the efficacy of certain drugs metabolized via the cytochrome P450 system, including oral contraceptives. The potential for stimulants to cause teratogenicity is unknown, and therefore it may be advisable to discontinue medications during pregnancy.

How effective are conventional stimulants? In the only reported placebo-controlled trial, doses of 40–60 mg methamphetamine daily in eight patients with narcolepsy produced mean initial sleep latencies on an MSLT, statistically indistinguishable from those of eight normal control subjects[50]. In large case series, 73–92% of patients have shown moderate to excellent responses to a variety of stimulants[51,52]. In contrast to the conventional stimulants, extensive data are available from controlled and open trials regarding the efficacy of modafinil[48]. A series of controlled studies have demonstrated that the drug produces significant increases in mean maintenance of wakefulness test (MWT) latencies and reductions in Epworth sleepiness scale (ESS) scores, although these values did not

return to normal. Quality-of-life measures improved with modafinil, compared with placebo[53]. Long-term studies have shown that 62–71% of patients initially treated with modafinil continue to use it[54,55]. Despite controlled trials showing no apparent difference between the effects of 200 mg and 400 mg daily doses, 75% of patients in one study requested the initial dose to be increased with time to 400 mg daily. Patients changed from high-dose conventional stimulants to modafinil often perceive the new drug as less effective. In the absence of any direct studies comparing different stimulants, an indirect analysis has been performed, comparing MWT and MSLT data with published norms (Figure 7.5). This

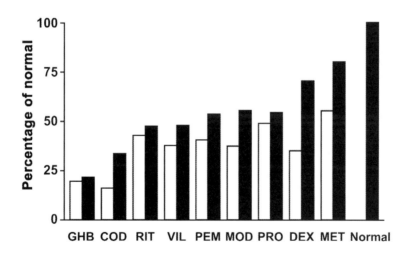

**Figure 7.5** Relative efficacy of drugs for the treatment of narcolepsy. The information in this figure was derived from different studies and is presented in terms of percentage of normal levels of alertness, using multiple sleep latency test (MSLT) and maintenance of wakefulness test (MWT) data. White bar, baseline level; black bar, post-treatment level; direct comparisons of the different drugs have not been performed.  GHB, γ-hydroxybutyrate; COD, codeine; RIT, ritanserin; VIL, viloxazine; PEM, pemoline; MOD, modafinil; PRO, protriptyline; DEX, (+)-amphetamine; MET, methylphenidate. Reproduced with permission from reference 56

suggests that methylphenidate, metham-phetamine and dextroamphetamine all result in alertness levels 65–75% of normal, while pemoline and modafinil result in alertness of about 50% of normal[56,57].

Modafinil is the usual first choice for patients newly diagnosed with narcolepsy, in view of its long duration of action, its relative lack of adverse effects and apparent low potential for the development of dependence. However, its cost as a new medication and its potential for interaction with other drugs such as oral contraceptives result in the use of conventional stimulants for some patients. For patients with severe narcolepsy, modafinil may not produce adequate alertness, and drugs such as methylphenidate may be needed. The decision to increase the dose of a stimulant is primarily based on

careful clinical assessment. Patients should be asked the time from taking the medication to onset of action and the duration of action. Peak and trough alertness can be estimated using a 10-point scale, with 10 being maximal alertness and 0 maximal sleepiness (Figure 7.6). The ESS may also be useful in monitoring progress. The physician must then decide whether to increase the dose or frequency of the medication, or whether to convert to a longer-acting drug. Sometimes a combination of long- and short-acting medications may be best, if there are times of the day when maximum alertness is essential. In complex situations when the dose is escalating and it is unclear whether the patient's symptoms of fatigue actually represent sleepiness, performing an MWT on medication may be helpful.

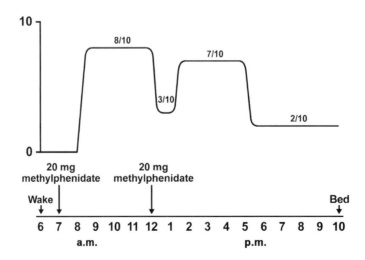

**Figure 7.6** Example of a chart documenting a patient's response to stimulant therapy. This is an example of a useful schema for considering the response of a patient to stimulants. The time the drug is taken, the time to onset of action, the duration of action and a simple rating of effectiveness at different times of the day (scale of 1–10) may be very useful in determining whether doses should be increased or the drug administered more frequently

**Case 7.3**

A 23-year-old woman had noted sleepiness from the age of 8 years. She did not experience cataplexy, was not on any medications and had an adequate nocturnal sleep time. An MSLT following a normal PSG showed a mean sleep latency of 4.5 min, with SOREMPs on the second and fourth naps. A diagnosis of narcolepsy without cataplexy had been made, and she was commenced on therapy with modafinil. Despite increasing the dose from 200 mg in the morning to 600 mg, she perceived no improvement in alertness. Methylphenidate was substituted in a dose of 20 mg three times a day, and resulted in an increase in alertness for about 3.5 h after each dose. While the drug was working, she rated her alertness as increasing from 2/10 to 5/10 on a 10-point scale, with 0 being the worst sleepiness she could imagine and 10 being complete alertness. Modafinil was reintroduced to supplement the methylphenidate in a dose of 400 mg in the morning, and her alertness improved by a further point. She remained especially troubled by sudden surges in sleepiness after each dose of methylphenidate wore off, and by a feeling of anxiety while it was working. Modafinil and methylphenidate were discontinued, and she was prescribed extended-release methylphenidate in the form of Concerta®, commencing at 18 mg at 7 a.m. and increasing to 36 mg. At this dose, she described increased alertness (score of 7/10) for about 11 h without the peak and trough effects she had experienced on the short-acting drug. A further

18 mg was added at 9 a.m., which resulted in alertness of 8/10 until about 9 p.m.

This case illustrates how modafinil may not be strong enough for some patients with severe narcolepsy, and how short-acting agents can produce distressing fluctuations in alertness and mood. It also shows how a quantitative scale can be used to assess the effects of drugs and how extended-release agents can be beneficial.

*Management of cataplexy and other symptoms*

Stimulant therapy alone often improves control of cataplexy, by alleviating drowsiness. Tricyclic antidepressants have been used to treat cataplexy since 1960, and are still commonly used today. Although there is little evidence that any specific drug is more effective, imipramine, clomipramine and protriptyline have been generally favored. In a study of 33 patients taking one of these agents, 64% reported a moderate or good response[43]. Imipramine and clomipramine are used in single daily doses of 10–200 mg at night, while protriptyline is prescribed in doses of 5–15 mg three times a day. Common side-effects include dry mouth, weight gain, postural hypotension and sedation. Rarer, more serious, complications include arrhythmias, seizures and acute urinary retention. Selective serotonin reuptake inhibitors, such as fluoxetine and paroxetine, and newer antidepressants, such as venlafaxine, are alternative agents with fewer side-effects.

Sodium oxybate (γ-hydroxybutyrate) is the first drug to be specifically approved by the US Food and Drug Administration (FDA) for the treatment of cataplexy. The frequency of cataplexy was reduced by 69% at maximal dose in a controlled trial, compared with a 28% reduction with placebo[58]. The drug also increased delta sleep, and may reduce daytime sleepiness. It should be administered in two doses, the first before sleep and the second 2.5–4 h later. The initial total daily dose is 4.5 g, with the possibility of increasing to 9 g daily by increases of 1.5 g at 2-week intervals. Sodium oxybate is metabolized in the liver and excreted as carbon dioxide. It is potentially dependence-producing, and side-effects include headache, dizziness, nausea, constipation, sleepwalking and nocturnal confusion. It can produce CNS and respiratory depression, and should never be used with alcohol or other CNS depressants. It is contraindicated in untreated sleep apnea, obesity–hypoventilation syndrome and chronic obstructive pulmonary disease. Its mechanism of action is unknown.

Hypnagogic hallucinations and sleep paralysis rarely need treatment, but tricyclic antidepressants are often effective. It is appropriate to prescribe short-acting hypnotics for insomnia in narcolepsy, and triazolam has been shown to increase total sleep time and sleep efficiency without effecting alertness the following day[59]. Drug therapy is not always needed for REM sleep behavior disorder in narcolepsy. The standard treatment is clonazepam (Chapter 16), but its long duration of action may result in increased sleepiness, and shorter-acting benzodiazepines can be tried.

## IDIOPATHIC HYPERSOMNIA

### Definition and diagnosis

As understanding of narcolepsy increased, it became evident that not all patients with excessive sleepiness of uncertain cause had cataplexy or evidence of premature occurrence of REM sleep. Various terms have been suggested to describe these patients, including non-rapid eye movement (NREM) narcolepsy, primary central nervous system hypersomnolence, primary hypersomnia, essential hypersomnia, subwakefulness syndrome and hypersomnia with sleep drunkenness, but the most accepted current term is idiopathic hypersomnia (IH). The disorder is variably defined, with little consensus regarding required laboratory findings.

Sleep center-based studies suggest that IH is 3–12 times less common than narcolepsy[60]. At the Stanford Sleep Disorders Clinic, for example, 71 patients with IH were seen at the same time as 266 with narcolepsy and cataplexy and 73 with narcolepsy without cataplexy[3,60]. The little information available about age of onset suggests that it is similar to narcolepsy, commencing most frequently in childhood, adolescence or early adulthood. A consistent relationship with a HLA type has not been found. CSF Hcrt-1 concentrations have been normal in most patients studied[6,61].

The broadest criteria for IH include patients with a history of excessive daytime somnolence not explainable by other extrinsic or intrinsic causes, no cataplexy and fewer than two SOREMPs on an MSLT. Comparing such patients with those with narcolepsy, IH patients describe their nocturnal sleep as having fewer awakenings and their naps as being less refreshing[62]. PSG data confirm that sleep efficiency is higher in IH[63], with more slow-wave sleep and less stage 1 NREM sleep. MSLT mean latencies are slightly longer[64]. There appear to be at least two subtypes of IH, IH without long sleep time (also called narcolepsy-like IH or monosynaptic IH) and IH with long sleep time (also called classic IH, or polysynaptic IH). IH without long sleep time has only excessive sleepiness, which may resemble that of narcolepsy with short refreshing naps and perhaps a higher than normal frequency of associated hypnagogic hallucinations and sleep paralysis[63]. IH with long sleep time presents with prolonged deep nocturnal sleep with difficulty rousing in the morning and sometimes early-morning confusion and disorientation (sleep drunkenness). Naps are long, often lasting several hours, and are unrefreshing. It is not clear whether these two subtypes are separate disorders, or whether they represent a spectrum of disease. The relative frequency of the two types varies between different series[60,63]. To diagnose either type, a PSG is essential to rule out other causes of sleepiness, such as sleep-disordered breathing. An MSLT is necessary to be certain that SOREMPs are not present and to provide objective confirmation of excessive somnolence. As with narcolepsy, no definite cut-off of mean MSLT latency can be defined, although ICSD criteria suggest a figure of less than 8 min. French authorities believe that the MSLT may not always be the most appropriate test for the classic form of IH, suggesting instead a 24-h PSG with the diagnosis based on a long nocturnal total sleep time with high sleep efficiency and one or more prolonged naps during the day[60] (Table 7.6).

## Differential diagnosis

Care must be taken to rule out other causes of sleepiness before concluding that IH is present (Table 7.7). Apart from narcolepsy, subtle forms of sleep-disordered breathing (upper airway resistance syndrome)

**Table 7.6** Practical diagnostic criteria for idiopathic hypersomnia (IH)

---

*IH without long sleep time (monosynaptic IH or narcolepsy-like IH)*
A complaint of excessive daytime sleepiness present for at least 6 months
No history of cataplexy
No other principal cause of sleepiness by clinical assessment and PSG
An MSLT shows a mean initial sleep latency of < 8 min and fewer than two SOREMPs

*IH with long sleep time (polysynaptic IH or classic IH)*
A complaint of excessive daytime sleepiness present for at least 6 months
No history of cataplexy
No other principal cause of sleepiness by clinical assessment and PSG
History of long, deep nocturnal sleep with difficulty rousing in the morning
Prolonged, unrefreshing naps
Either an MSLT showing a mean initial sleep latency of < 8 min and fewer than two SOREMPs, or a 24-h sleep recording showing a long nocturnal sleep time and one or more naps lasting > 1 h and without SOREMPs

---

PSG, polysomnogram; MSLT, multiple sleep latency test; SOREMP, sleep-onset rapid eye movement period

109

**Table 7.7** Differential diagnosis of idiopathic hypersomnia

Insufficient sleep syndrome

Delayed sleep phase syndrome

Narcolepsy with or without cataplexy

Sleep-disordered breathing, including upper airway resistance syndrome

Drug-induced sleepiness

Sleep fragmentation from pain

Hypersomnia following head injury

Hypersomnia following viral infections

Sleepiness associated with psychiatric disorders

(Chapter 8), insufficient sleep syndrome, delayed sleep phase syndrome, hypersomnia due to sleep fragmentation from pain and the effects of sedating medications may all mimic IH. The controversial entity of the long sleeper may also be confusing. Long sleepers have a need for a longer total nocturnal sleep time than the average person, and do not feel refreshed unless they achieve it. However, once the required amount of sleep is present, daytime somnolence resolves, in contrast with patients with IH who continue to feel sleepy despite lengthy nocturnal sleep.

Less well-defined entities are chronic sleepiness commencing soon after head injury or a viral infection. Both these entities have been described, but no case–control studies have been reported. Another condition is that of persistent sleepiness documented by an MSLT following apparently adequate treatment of obstructive sleep apnea with nasal continuous positive airway pressure (CPAP). These patients are often diagnosed with IH and respond to stimulant therapy, but the pathogenesis is probably different from the true idiopathic form of the disorder.

The lifetime prevalence of psychiatric disorders in IH is high (57% in one study[63]), especially in the classic form. An entity of hypersomnia related to psychiatric disorders has been postulated, and may be easily confused with IH. In one study[65–67], an attempt has been made to compare these two conditions in untreated patients, by having experienced psychiatrists determine whether the associated psychiatric disorders were the primary cause of the sleepiness (23 patients) or a secondary diagnosis (59 patients). The psychiatric hypersomnia group had longer sleep latency on PSG, lower sleep efficiency and a lower percentage of REM sleep. An unconventional nap study (two 60-min nap opportunities) showed mean latencies for the psychiatric group to be no shorter than in normal controls. These results suggest that the sleepiness described by the patients in the psychiatric group was really fatigue associated with insomnia, and easily distinguishable from IH on objective testing.

## Management

Treatment of IH is the same as treatment of narcolepsy, and involves the use of stimulant medication. Anecdotal reports suggest that IH, especially the classic form, is more difficult to treat than narcolepsy, but this has not been confirmed in large studies.

## RECURRENT HYPERSOMNIA

Recurrent (periodic) hypersomnia is a rare disorder, characterized by recurrent episodes of hypersomnolence lasting days to weeks and occurring months apart. It is essentially synonymous with Kleine–Levin syndrome (KLS), although the minimum criteria for this eponymic disorder remain controversial.

The illness occurs predominantly in men (76–83%), with age of onset averaging 15–16 years[68,69]. Patients average four attacks a year[68], with each attack lasting a mean of 12 days[68,69]. Most patients seem to recover within about 4 years[68], although the course appears to be more prolonged in a minority.

The recurrent episodes of sleep constitute the essential clinical criterion for a diagnosis of periodic hypersomnia. However, three other symptoms are often present in KLS (Table 7.8). The first is the presence of varied cognitive and mood disturbances only during the episodes, including irritability, confusion, mutism, aggressiveness, hallucinations and depression. One set of investigators requires at least one of these disturbances as a minimum criterion for the diagnosis[69]. The second additional symptom, reported to be present in 57–66% of patients[68,69], is that of hyperphagia, with compulsive and often binge eating during episodes. Third, 44–47% of patients experience hypersexuality with inappropriate sexual acts and language[68,69]. Most patients return to normal psychosocial functioning between episodes.

**Table 7.8** Practical diagnostic criteria for recurrent hypersomnia (Kleine–Levin syndrome)

| | |
|---|---|
| A | Recurrent episodes of hypersomnia lasting days to weeks, recurring at intervals of weeks to months |
| B | Cognitive or mood disturbances during the episodes only |
| C | Hyperphagia during the episodes |
| D | Hypersexuality during the episodes |
| E | Onset commonest in the second decade |

A is essential for the diagnosis, B is almost always present, C–E are confirmatory, but may be absent

Polysomnography during attacks reveals increased total sleep time with reduced sleep efficiency, reduced percentage slow-wave sleep and increased percentage stage 1 NREM sleep[68–70]. MSLTs have generally shown reduced mean sleep latencies, occasionally with SOREMPs[70]. Polysomnography returns to normal between attacks, apart from showing reduced sleep efficiency. MRI scans and CSF examinations are normal. Endocrine studies have revealed inconsistent results, but growth hormone secretion appears to dissociate from slow-wave sleep, and 24-h mean plasma melatonin concentration is raised[71].

The pathogenesis of KLS is uncertain, but hypothalamic dysfunction has been suggested. An autoimmune hypothesis has been postulated based on the age of onset, preceding viral infections in 32–53% of patients[68,69], and an association with HLA DQB1*0201[69]. A few autopsies, mostly of atypical patients, have shown inflammatory infiltrates in the thalamus, midbrain amygdala or hypothalamus.

Interpretation of reports of treatment is difficult because of small numbers of patients and the natural history of the disorder. However, stimulants during attacks seem to be of little benefit to most patients. Lithium is the most promising prophylactic agent, and carbamazepine has also been used with varying success.

## Case 7.4

A 13-year-old boy presented during the third of three episodes of hypersomnia and altered behavior that had occurred over the preceding year. The first episode lasted 8 and the second 10 days. The patient was reported to sleep 20 h a day during the events. He had a voracious appetite when awakened, and inappropriate behavior characterized by confusion, restlessness and disinhibited hypersexual behavior. Between attacks, he was described as a normally achieving, popular 13-year-old with no evidence of psychiatric disease. On examination 8 days after the start of the episode, the patient did not speak spontaneously, but answered questions with little emotional tone. He was disoriented for the day of the week and the date. He could learn four words and accurately recall them after 5 min. General knowledge, arithmetic and constructional abilities were normal. He was interviewed at the termination of his PSG and spent most of the time ripping off the electrodes that had been used during the study. A PSG showed a total sleep time of 649 min with 78% sleep efficiency. Sleep stages were normal, but the REM latency was short at 31 min. The patient was given methylphenidate at a dose of 5 mg three times a day and recovered after a further 48 h. Further follow-up information was not available.

This case illustrates the typical clinical and PSG features of KLS. A slightly short REM latency has been reported, but is of uncertain significance. Judging the effects of stimulant therapy can be difficult in a disorder characterized by spontaneously terminating episodes.

## REFERENCES

1. Boor R, Reitter B. Cataplexy in Niemann–Pick disease type C. *Klin Padiatr* 1997;209:88–90

2. D'Cruz OF, Vaughn BV, Gold SH, Greenwood RS. Symptomatic cataplexy in pontomedullary lesions. *Neurology* 1994;44: 2189–91

3. Guilleminault C, Mignot E, Partinen M. Controversies in the diagnosis of narcolepsy. *Sleep* 1994;17:S1–6

4. Mignot E, Hayduk R, Black J, Grumet FC, Guilleminault C. HLA DQB1*0602 is associated with cataplexy in 509 narcoleptic patients. *Sleep* 1997;20:1012–20

5. Silber MH, Krahn LE, Olson EJ, Pankratz VS. The epidemiology of narcolepsy in Olmsted County, Minnesota: a population based study. *Sleep* 2002;25:197–202

6. Mignot E, Lammers GJ, Ripley B, *et al*. The role of cerebrospinal fluid hypocretin measurement in the diagnosis of narcolepsy and other hypersomnias. *Arch Neurol* 2002;59: 1553–62

7. Krahn LE, Boeve BF, Olson EJ, Herold DL, Silber MH. A standardized test for cataplexy. *Sleep Med* 2000;1:125–30

8. Krahn LE, Lymp J, Moore WR, Slocumb N, Silber MH. Characterizing cataplexy: exploring the mind–body interface. *J Neuropsychiatr Clin Neurosci* 2004;in press

9. Anic-Labat S, Guilleminault C, Kraemer HC, Meehan J, Arrigoni J, Mignot E. Validation of a catplexy questionnaire in 983 sleep-disorders patients. *Sleep* 1999;22: 77–87

10. Okun ML, Lin L, Pelin Z, Hong S, Mignot E. Clinical aspects of narcolepsy–cataplexy across ethnic groups. *Sleep* 2002;25:27–35

11. Silber MH, Krahn LE, Slocumb N. Clinical and polysomnographic findings of narcolepsy with and without cataplexy: a population-based study [Abstract]. *Sleep* 2003;26: A282–3

12. Ohayon MM. Prevalence of hallucinations and their pathological associations in the general population. *Psychiatr Res* 2000;97: 153–64

13. Ohayon MM, Zulley J, Guilleminault C, Smirne S. Prevalence and pathologic associations of sleep paralysis in the general population. *Neurology* 1999;52:1194–200

14. Krahn LE, Black JL, Silber MH. Narcolepsy: new understanding of irresistible sleep. *Mayo Clin Proc* 2001;76: 185–94

15. Schuld A, Blum WF, Uhr M, *et al*. Reduced leptin levels in human narcolepsy. *Neuroendocrinology* 2000;72:195–8

16. Nishino S, Ripley B, Overeem S, *et al*. Low cerebrospinal fluid hypocretin (orexin) and altered energy homeostasis in human narcolepsy. *Ann Neurol* 2001;50:381–8

17. Dahmen N, Bierbrauer J, Kasten M. Increased prevalence of obesity in narcoleptic patients and relatives. *Eur Arch Psychiatr Clin Neurosci* 2001;251:85–9

18. Ohayon MM, Priest RG, Caulet M, Guilleminault C. Hypnagogic and hypnopompic hallucinations: pathological phenomena? *Br J Psychiatry* 1996;169: 459–67

19. Hublin C, Kaprio J, Partinen M, *et al*. The prevalence of narcolepsy: an epidemiologic study of the Finnish twin cohort. *Ann Neurol* 1994;35:709–16

20. Dement WC, Carskadon MA, Ley R. The prevalence of narcolepsy II [Abstract]. *Sleep Res* 1973;2:147

21. Dement WC, Zarcone V, Varner V, *et al*. The prevalence of narcolepsy [Abstract]. *Sleep Res* 1972;1:148

22. Ohayon MM, Priest RG, Zulley J, Smirne S, Paiva T. Prevalence of narcolepsy sympto-

matology and diagnosis in the European general population. *Neurology* 2002;58: 1826–33

23. Vogel G. Studies in the psychophysiology of dreams, III: the dream of narcolepsy. *Arch Gen Psychiatry* 1960;3:421–8

24. Juji T, Satake M, Honda Y, Doi Y. HLA antigens in Japanese patients with narcolepsy: all the patients were DR2 positive. *Tissue Antigens* 1984;24:316–19

25. Rogers AE, Meehan J, Guillamcnault C, Grumet FC, Mignot E. HLA DR15 (DR2) and DQB1*0602 typing studies in 188 narcoleptic patients with cataplexy. *Neurology* 1997;48:1550–6

26. Guilleminault C, Mignot E, Grumet FC. Familial patterns of narcolepsy. *Lancet* 1989;2:1376–9

27. Mignot E. Genetic and familial aspects of narcolepsy. *Neurology* 1998;50:S16–22

28. Black JL, Krahn LE, Pankratz VS, Silber MH. Search for neuronal-specific and non-neuronally-specific antibodies in the sera of patients with HLA DQB1*0602 positive and negative narcolepsy. *Sleep* 2002;25: 719–23

29. Malik S, Boeve BF, Krahn LE, Silber MH. Narcolepsy associated with other central nervous system disorders. *Neurology* 2001; 57:539–41

30. Aldrich M, Propokowicz G, Ockert K, Hollingsworth Z, Penney JB, Albin RL. Neurochemical studies of human narcolepsy: α-adrenergic receptor autoradiography of human narcoleptic brain and brainstem. *Sleep* 1994;17:598–608

31. Lin L, Faraco J, Li R, *et al*. The sleep disorder canine narcolepsy is caused by a mutation in the hypocretin (orexin) receptor 2 gene. *Cell* 1999;98:365–76

32. Chemelli RM, Willie JT, Sinton CM, *et al*. Narcolepsy in orexin knockout mice: molecular genetics of sleep regulation. *Cell* 1999;98:437–51

33. Ripley B, Overeem S, Fujiki N, *et al*. CSF hypocretin/orexin levels in narcolepsy and other neurological conditions. *Neurology* 2001;57:2253–8

34. Peyron C, Faraco J, Rogers W, *et al*. A mutation in a case of early onset narcolepsy and a generalized absence of hypocretin peptides in human narcoleptic brain. *Nat Med* 2000;6:991–7

35. Thannickal TC, Moore RY, Nienhuis R, *et al*. Reduced number of hypocretin neurons in human narcolepsy. *Neuron* 2000;27: 469–74

36. Scammell TE, Nishino S, Mignot E, Saper CB. Narcolepsy and low CSF orexin (hypocretin) concentration after a diencephalic stroke. *Neurology* 2001;56:1751–3

37. Arii J, Kanbayashi T, Tanabe Y, Ono J, Nishino S, Kohno Y. A hypersomnolent girl with decreased CSF hypocretin level after removal of a hypothalamic tumor. *Neurology* 2001;56:1775–6

38. Mignot E, Meehan J, Grumet FC. HLA class II and narcolepsy in thirty-three multiplex families [Abstract]. *Sleep Res* 1996;25: 303

39. Helmus T, Rosenthal L, Bishop C, Roehrs T, Syron ML, Roth T. The alerting effects of short and long naps in narcoleptic, sleep deprived, and alert individuals. *Sleep* 1997; 20:251–7

40. Mullington J, Broughton R. Scheduled naps in the management of daytime sleepiness in narcolepsy–cataplexy. *Sleep* 1993;16:444–56

41. Roehrs T, Zorick F, Wittig R, Lamphere J, Sticklesteel J, Roth T. Alerting effects of naps in narcolepsy. *Sleep* 1986;9:194–9

42. American Academy of Sleep Medicine Standards of Practice Committee. Practice parameters for the treatment of narcolepsy: an update for 2000. *Sleep* 2001;24:451–66

43. Parkes JD, Baraitser M, Marsden CD, Asselman P. Natural history, symptoms and treatment of the narcoleptic syndrome. *Acta Neurol Scand* 1975;52:337–53

44. US Modafinil in Narcolepsy Multicenter Study Group. Randomized trial of modafinil as a treatment for excessive daytime somnolence in narcolepsy. *Neurology* 2000;54:1166–75

45. Parkes D. Introduction to the mechanism of action of different treatments of narcolepsy. *Sleep* 1994;17:S93–6

46. Guilleminault C. Amphetamines and narcolepsy: use of the Stanford database. *Sleep* 1993;16:199–201

47. Littner M. Sleep practitioners need to be aware of new changes in the labeling of pemoline (CYLERT) [Letter]. *Sleep* 1999;22:833

48. Broughton RJ, Fleming JA, George CF, *et al*. Randomized, double-blind, placebo-controlled crossover trial of modafinil in the treatment of excessive daytime sleepiness in narcolepsy. *Neurology* 1997;49:444–51

49. US Modafinil in Narcolepsy Multicenter Study Group. Randomized trial of modafinil for the treatment of pathological somnolence in narcolepsy. *Ann Neurol* 1998;43:88–97

50. Mitler MM, Hajdukovic R, Erman MK. Treatment of narcolepsy with methamphetamine. *Sleep* 1993;16:306–17

51. Honda Y, Hishikawa Y, Takahashi Y. Long-term treatment of narcolepsy with methylphenidate (Ritalin). *Curr Ther Res* 1979;25:288–98

52. Yoss RE, Daly D. Treatment of narcolepsy with Ritalin. *Neurology* 1959;9:171–3

53. Beusterien KM, Rogers AE, Walsleben JA, *et al*. Health-related quality of life effects of modafinil for treatment of narcolepsy. *Sleep* 1999;22:757–65

54. Besset A, Chetrit M, Carlander B, Billiard M. Use of modafinil in the treatment of narcolepsy: a long term follow-up study. *Neurophysiol Clin* 1996; 26:60–6

55. Mitler MM, Harsh J, Hirshkowitz M, Guilleminault C, for the US Modafinil in Narcolepsy Multicenter Study Group. Long-term efficacy and safety of modafinil (Provigil) for the treatment of excessive daily sleepiness associated with narcolepsy. *Sleep Med* 2000;1:231–43

56. Mitler MM, Hajdukovic R. Relative efficacy of drugs for the treatment of sleepiness in narcolepsy. *Sleep* 1991;14:218–20

57. Mitler MM, Aldrich MS, Koob GF, Zarcone VP. Narcolepsy and its treatment with stimulants. ASDA standards of practice. *Sleep* 1994;17:352–71

58. The US Xyrem Multicenter Study Group. A randomized, double blind, placebo-controlled multicenter trial comparing the effects of three doses of orally administered sodium oxybate with placebo for the treatment of narcolepsy. *Sleep* 2002;25:42–9

59. Thorpy MJ, Snyder M, Aloe FS, Ledereich PS, Starz KE. Short-term triazolam use improves nocturnal sleep of narcoleptics. *Sleep* 1992;15:212–16

60. Billiard M. Idiopathic hypersomnia. *Neurol Clin* 1996;14:573–82

61. Takashi K, Inoue Y, Chiba S, *et al*. CSF hypocretin-1 (orexin-A) concentrations in narcolepsy with and without cataplexy and idiopathic hypersomnia. *J Sleep Res* 2002; 11:91–3

62. Bruck D, Parkes JD. A comparison of idiopathic hypersomnia and narcolepsy–cataplexy using self report measures and sleep diary data. *J Neurol Neurosurg Psychiatry* 1996;60:576–8

63. Bassetti C, Aldrich MS. Idiopathic hypersomnia. A series of 42 patients. *Brain* 1997; 120:1423–35

64. Aldrich MS. The clinical spectrum of narcolepsy and idiopathic hypersomnia. *Neurology* 1996;46:393–401

65. Vgontzas AN, Bixler EO, Kales A, Criley C, Vela-Bueno A. Differences in nocturnal and daytime sleep between primary and psychiatric hypersomnia: diagnostic and treatment implications. *Psychosom Med* 2000;62: 220–6

66. Guilleminault C, Mondini S. Infectious mononucleosis and excessive daytime sleepiness: a long term follow-up study. *Arch Intern Med* 1986;146:1333–5

67. Guilleminault C, Faull KF, Miles L, van den Hoed J. Posttraumatic excessive daytime sleepiness: a review of 20 patients. *Neurology* 1983;33:1584–9

68. Gadoth N, Kesler A, Vainstein G, Peled R, Lavie P. Clinical and polysomnographic characteristics of 34 patients with Kleine–Levin syndrome. *J Sleep Res* 2001;10:337–41

69. Dauvilliers Y, Mayer G, Lecendreux M, *et al.* Kleine–Levin syndrome. An autoimmune hypothesis based on clinical and genetic analysis. *Neurology* 2002;59.1739–45

70. Rosenow F, Kotagal P, Cohen BH, Green C, Wyllie E. Multiple sleep latency test and polysomnography in diagnosing Kleine–Levin syndrome and periodic hypersomnia. *J Clin Neurophysiol* 2000;17: 519–22

71. Mayer G, Leonhard E, Krieg J, Meier-Ewert K. Endocrinological and polysomnographic findings in Kleine–Levin syndrome: no evidence for hypothalamic and circadian dysfunction. *Sleep* 1998;21:278–84

# Chapter 8

# Sleep apnea syndromes

*"Sounds like – like hogs grunting.*
*No – it's somebody snoring, Tom."*
*"That IS it! Where 'bouts is it, Huck?"*
*"I b'leeve it's down at t'other end. Sounds so, anyway.*
*Pap used to sleep there, sometimes,*
*'long with the hogs, but laws bless you,*
*he just lifts things when HE snores."*

**Mark Twain,** *The Adventures of Tom Sawyer*

Respiration is a highly regulated physiological function designed primarily to maintain homeostasis of arterial oxygen and carbon dioxide tension, $PaO_2$ and $PaCO_2$, and pH over a wide range of human activities. Physical exertion, infection and other physiological stresses require increased metabolism, and the respiratory system must respond with great precision to prevent hypoxia, acidosis, tissue injury and even death. In addition to homeostatic functions, more specialized intermittent tasks requiring respiratory control include speech and activities needing breath-holding or forceful ventilatory efforts, such as micturition, defecation, emesis, coughing, parturition, inflation of a balloon or playing a brass instrument. Sleep substantially influences respiratory control, and some of the most common sleep disorders involve abnormal breathing patterns, often termed 'sleep-disordered breathing' (Table 8.1)[1]. To understand these disorders, a review of key concepts in respiratory physiology and the effects of sleep on pulmonary function is necessary.

## PHYSIOLOGY OF RESPIRATION DURING WAKEFULNESS AND SLEEP

Rhythmicity of breathing begins during fetal development and continues until death. The origin of this rhythmicity lies in the central nervous system, and is the result of integrated neural networking of at least six different nuclei located primarily in the medulla. The unique breathing patterns experienced during health and disease are influenced by two general regulatory systems, the automatic and the voluntary control systems. During sleep, the voluntary control system becomes inactive. The clinical significance of this is most striking in patients with 'Ondine's curse', an extreme form of selective failure of the automatic

**Table 8.1** Sleep-disordered breathing

| Syndrome | Characteristics |
| --- | --- |
| Obstructive sleep apnea syndrome (OSAS)/ obstructive sleep apnea–hypopnea syndrome* | recurrent episodes of partial or complete upper airway obstruction during sleep; breathing events noted include obstructive apneas, obstructive hypopneas, mixed apneas and respiratory effort-related arousals |
| Central sleep apnea syndrome (CSAS)/ central sleep apnea–hypopnea syndrome* | recurrent apneic episodes during sleep in the absence of upper airway obstruction or hypercapnia (hypercapnic patients are considered to have alveolar hypoventilation syndrome) |
| Cheyne–Stokes respiration (CSR) (Cheyne–Stokes breathing syndrome)* | cyclic fluctuation in ventilatory pattern during sleep with periods of central apnea or hypopnea alternating with hyperpnea in a crescendo and decrescendo manner |
| Alveolar hypoventilation syndrome (AHS) (sleep hypoventilation syndrome, SHVS)* | hypercapnia and hypoxemia during sleep due to inappropriate central hypoventilation and not due exclusively to obstructive apneas and hypopneas; diurnal hypercapnia is often present |

*Adapted from an American Academy of Sleep Medicine Task Force report[1]

respiratory control system. Afflicted patients cannot generate involuntary rhythmic breathing movements even when awake, but are able to breathe voluntarily. With sleep or pharmacological sedation, when the voluntary respiratory system is suppressed, such patients require mechanical ventilation to survive.

Automatic control is best visualized as a classic feedback system, with the central controller located in the medulla (Figure 8.1). The efferents from the central controller provide output to an array of respiratory muscles that effect ventilation.

Afferents (influencing inputs to the controller) include signals from chemoreceptors that detect levels of $CO_2$ and $O_2$ and $H^+$ ions in various body fluids, and mechanoreceptors that detect physical changes in the lungs, respiratory muscles, chest wall and upper airway. There is also input to this center from the cerebral cortex, especially for voluntary respiratory control. The components of the feedback system are listed in Table 8.2.

Sleep inactivates the voluntary control system and also substantially affects the automatic control system. The automatic control system maintains homeostatic set points over a wide range of activities, with one of the primary set points being maintenance of a target $PaCO_2$ (typically 40 mmHg in non-pregnant awake adults at sea level). The ventilatory response to deviation from the target $PaCO_2$ can be depicted graphically (Figure 8.2). The ventilatory response to $PaCO_2$ is blunted in sleep compared with wakefulness, resulting in a 3–7-mmHg rise in

**Table 8.2**  Components influencing respiratory control

| | | |
|---|---|---|
| *I* | *Automatic respiratory control system* | |
| A | Medullary respiratory center | |
| B | Afferents to the medullary respiratory center | |
| | *chemoreceptors* | |
| | central chemoreceptors | medullary chemoreceptors: influenced predominantly by $PaCO_2$ via changes in CSF pH; to lesser extent influenced by $PaO_2$, oxygen consumption |
| | peripheral chemoreceptors | carotid bodies, aortic bodies: influenced predominantly by $PaO_2$ |
| | *mechanoreceptors* | |
| | receptors in the upper respiratory tract | influenced by temperature, pressure, contact/touch, humidity and various chemical substances |
| | receptors in lower respiratory tract and lungs (irritant, stretch and J receptors) | irritant receptors: respond to mechanical as well as non-specific chemical irritation<br>stretch receptors: responsible for the Hering–Breuer reflex<br>J receptors: stimulate ventilation in response to a variety of stimuli, including microembolization of the pulmonary circulation, pulmonary edema |
| | muscle spindles and tendon organs in respiratory muscles | monitor effectiveness of the peripheral effector system |
| C. | Efferents from the medullary respiratory center to respiratory organs | |
| | phrenic nerves | innervate the diaphragm |
| | spinal nerves to intercostal and abdominal muscles | innervate intercostal and abdominal muscles |
| | cranial and spinal nerves to upper airway | innervate numerous muscles of the pharynx, hypopharynx, larynx and tongue, including the genioglossals, tensor palatini, medial pterygoids, cricothyroid and posterior cricoarytenoids |
| *II* | *Voluntary respiratory control system* | |
| | cortex | directs variability in respiratory processes, such as breath-holding, coughing, singing, etc., while awake |

$PaCO_2$, arterial $CO_2$ tension; CSF, cerebrospinal fluid; $PaO_2$, arterial $O_2$ tension

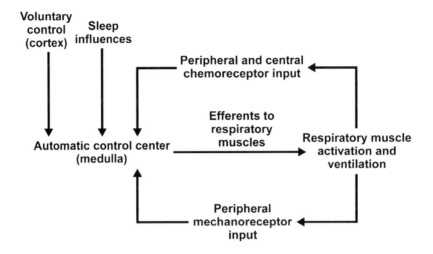

**Figure 8.1**   Respiratory control system

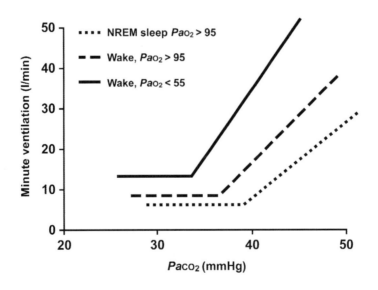

**Figure 8.2**   Ventilatory response to $CO_2$. Schematic depiction of ventilatory response to arterial $CO_2$ tension $PaCO_2$ in the wake state at two different levels of $PaO_2$, and in non-rapid eye movement (NREM) sleep. Hypoxemia increases the ventilatory drive at any given $PaCO_2$. Sleep lowers the ventilatory drive at any particular $PaCO_2$ as well as the sensitivity to increases in $PaCO_2$

$PaCO_2$ with the onset of non-rapid eye movement (NREM) sleep. During rapid eye movement (REM) sleep, ventilation and $CO_2$ sensitivity are further reduced. Reduced ventilation occurs mostly by decreases in tidal volume with deepening levels of NREM sleep, and finds a nadir in phasic REM sleep of only about 75% of that found in the wake state. Frequency of ventilation falls only slightly during NREM sleep compared with wakefulness at rest, but is variable during REM sleep (Figures 8.3 and 8.4).

Changes in $PaCO_2$ are predominantly controlled by chemoreceptors located on the surface of the medulla which respond to changes in cerebrospinal fluid (CSF) hydrogen ion concentration. Surgical or traumatic section of the peripheral arterial chemoreceptors causes only a slight reduction in ventilatory response to $CO_2$. Conversely, Ondine's curse was originally described following surgery involving the brainstem and high cervical spinal cord[3]. In such patients, $CO_2$ responsiveness is markedly reduced.

The automatic control system also increases ventilation when challenged with hypoxia. In contrast to the dominant role of the medullary chemoreceptor in the maintenance of eucapnia, the peripheral arterial chemoreceptors play the major role in regulation of $PaO_2$. The carotid bodies are located close to the bifurcation of the common carotid arteries. Usually only about 6 mm$^3$ in volume, they undergo hypertrophy and hyperplasia under conditions of chronic hypoxia (for example, the high-altitude residents of the Andes). Their afferent pathway is via the carotid sinus nerve and ultimately the ninth cranial nerve. The less vigorous aortic bodies send their inputs via the tenth cranial nerve. Sleep also blunts the ventilatory response to hypoxemia, and again, the degree of blunting increases progressively from stage 1 to stage 4 NREM sleep, and further still in REM sleep (Figure 8.5).

When considering the ventilatory response curves, it is important to recall that the graphs depicted in Figures 8.2 and 8.5 appear linear, but in the case of $CO_2$ response the ordinate is $PaCO_2$, while in the case of $O_2$ response the ordinate is $SaO_2$ (arterial oxygen saturation). Ventilatory responses to $PaO_2$ are not linear, owing to the curvilinear relationship between $PaO_2$ and $SaO_2$ dictated by the oxyhemoglobin dissociation curve. Thus, a fall in initial $PaO_2$ from 80 to 60 mmHg (20 mmHg change) may mean a fall in $SaO_2$ only from 96 to 91%, or a 5% change. Given the linear relationship between $SaO_2$ and ventilation, we would expect a 5% increase in ventilation for this 20-mmHg decline in $PaO_2$. In contrast, if one starts at 60 mmHg, and falls to 40 mmHg (an equivalent fall in $PaO_2$), the $SaO_2$ will fall from 91 to 74%, a dangerously low value, and one would expect a 17% increase in ventilation (Figure 8.6).

Both hypoxia and hypercapnia cause arousals from sleep. Within individuals, there appears to be a threshold that triggers arousal with a given degree of hypoxia or hypercapnia. For $CO_2$, the arousal threshold is fairly constant between sleep states, and in healthy individuals $PaCO_2$ ranges between 55 and 60 mmHg[5]. The arousal threshold for hypoxia varies according to sleep stage, and is lower in REM than NREM sleep. The hypoxic arousal signal is mediated via the

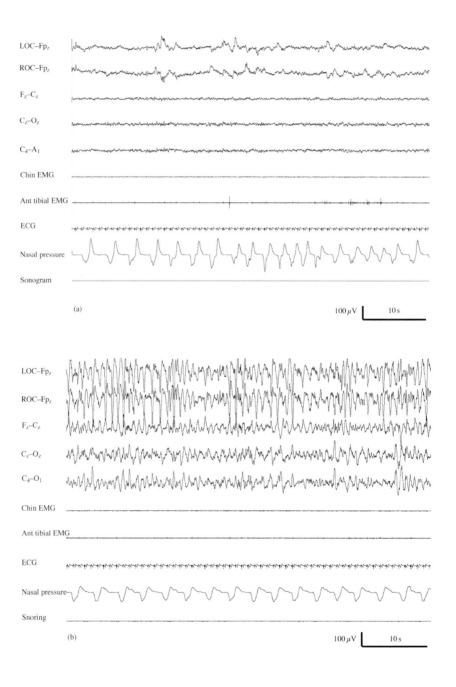

**Figure 8.3** Ventilatory patterns in sleep. Epoch of rapid eye movement (REM) sleep (a) shows variation in both respiratory rate and amplitude in the nasal pressure tracing, a marker of airflow. In contrast, the ventilatory channel in the non-rapid eye movement (NREM) epoch (b) shows regular respiration rate and airflow. Channel labels as in Figure 4.1

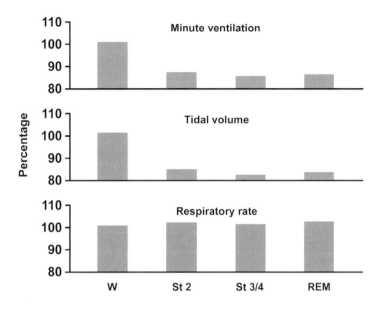

**Figure 8.4** Ventilation and sleep. Minute ventilation decreases with all sleep stages compared with wakefulness. The decrease in ventilation is mostly related to decreases in tidal volume, rather than changes in ventilatory rate. W, wake; St 2, stage 2 non-rapid eye movement (NREM) sleep; St 3/4, stages 3 and 4 NREM sleep. Modified with permission from reference 2

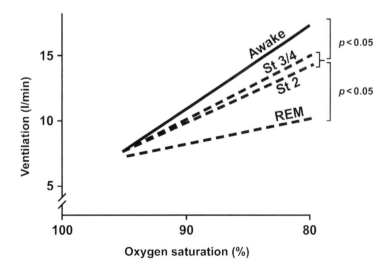

**Figure 8.5** Hypoxic ventilatory drive in wakefulness and sleep. Decreasing oxygen saturation results in increased ventilatory drive. Ventilatory drive at any given oxygen saturation or arterial oxygen tension ($PaO_2$) is less in non-rapid eye movement (NREM) sleep and less still in rapid eye movement (REM) sleep. Reproduced with permission from reference 4

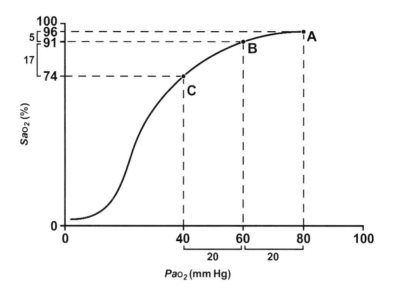

**Figure 8.6** Oxyhemoglobin dissociation curve. The shape of the oxyhemoglobin dissociation curve dictates the relationship of changes in arterial oxygen tension ($PaO_2$) to changes in oxygen saturation ($SaO_2$). At high $PaO_2$, a drop from 80 to 60 mmHg may only mean a fall in $SaO_2$ from 96 to 91% (point A to point B). In contrast, if one starts at 60 mmHg, and falls to 40 mmHg (an equivalent fall in $PaO_2$, B to C), the $SaO_2$ will fall from 91 to 74%, a dangerously low value

carotid bodies, and surgical injury or removal of these organs may significantly lower or eliminate this defense mechanism[6]. Other factors that influence hypoxic arousal thresholds include adaptation to chronic hypoxia, genetic influences and medications, such as nicotine, sedatives and narcotics. In practice, some patients appear very sensitive to even mild hypoxia, while others will seemingly permit alarmingly severe hypoxemia ($SaO_2 < 60\%$) without apparent arousal. When arousals are noted during clinical polysomnography, it is difficult to know whether the stimuli are chemical (hypoxia or hypercapnia) or mechanical.

**Case 8.1**

A 74-year-old woman was diagnosed with bilateral carotid body (glomus) tumors. After radiation of the left glomus tumor, she underwent resection of the right carotid body and vagotomy. Postoperatively she was found to be hypoxic and hypercapnic. She had snored loudly, had been hypersomnolent for years and had developed a well-compensated mild respiratory acidosis sometime in the preceding 6 months. Although she had a remote brief smoking history, her pulmonary function tests were unremarkable and she had never comp-lained of dyspnea. On examination, she had an oxyhemoglobin saturation of 84% on room air and was resting comfortably in no distress. Her respirations were slow and unlabored. She had a mildly crowded pharynx, clear lung sounds with normal diaphragmatic excursion and a normal cardiac examination. Arterial blood gases at rest on 3 l/min $O_2$ via nasal cannula showed a $PaCO_2$ of 50.0 mmHg, with a pH measuring 7.36 and a $PaO_2$ equal to 56 mmHg. Polysomnography showed her to have mild obstructive sleep apnea controlled well with continuous positive airway pressure (CPAP), but ongoing stable mild hypoxemia with hypoventilation shown by an elevated $PaCO_2$ on arterial blood gas measurement. Non-invasive positive pressure ventilation im-proved both sleep quality and hypercapnia.

This case illustrates how carotid body dysfunction following surgical and radiation treatment of bilateral tumors can be sufficient to blunt ventilatory and arousal response to hypoxemia, and, coupled with obstructive sleep apnea syndrome (OSAS), cause compensated respiratory failure.

In addition to the medullary and peripheral chemoreceptors, there are different types of receptors in the lungs, sensitive to the effects of mechanical and chemical stimulation (Table 8.2). The vagus nerves are the predominant afferent pathways to the controller from these receptors. Signals from other respiratory mechanoreceptors present in the chest wall muscles, diaphragm and thoracic skeleton travel via spinal nerves. Stretch receptors in the lungs respond to lung inflation by inhibiting inspiration and promoting expiration. This reflex (the Hering–Breuer reflex) may produce apnea, particularly under conditions when the chemical drive for ventilation is low, such as in hypocapnia. This reflex, as discussed below, may partially explain some elements of abnormal breathing patterns encountered when positive airway pressure is first applied to patients with sleep-related breathing disorders.

## The upper airway during respiration in wakefulness and sleep

The upper airway is also regulated by the control system. Upper airway muscles (genioglossus, tensor palatini, sternohyoid and others) stiffen and dilate the airway during inspiration to prevent collapse. During wakefulness, hypoxia and hypercapnia lead to an increase in upper airway muscle tone proportional to ventilatory stimulation. However, upper airway tone regulation is damped in NREM sleep, with decreases in tone that are generally greater than declines in ventilatory drive. The generalized muscle atonia of REM sleep is reflected in further reductions of upper airway muscle tone, particularly during phasic REM sleep.

Upper airway dimension and muscle tone determine airway resistance and the tendency for airway collapse. The oronasal pressure required to produce airway collapse is termed the critical closing pressure or $P_{crit}$ (Figure 8.7). $P_{crit}$ has been measured during sleep in normal individuals at about −12 to −15 cmH$_2$O[7-9]. Thus, even during sleep when pharyngeal muscle tone is very

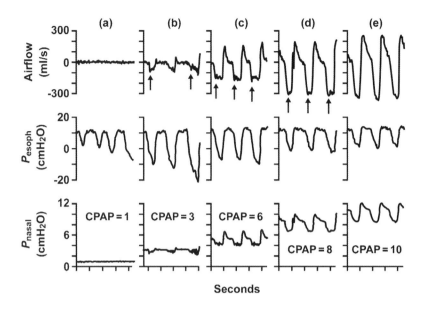

**Figure 8.7** Airway closure pressure ($P_{crit}$) in a patient with obstructive sleep apnea syndrome. In the figure, airflow, esophageal pressure $P_{esoph}$ and nasal pressure $P_{nasal}$ are measured during sleep at different applied nasal continuous positive airway pressures (CPAPs). Efforts to breathe at all CPAP levels are shown by the negative deflection of esophageal pressure. At CPAP=1 cmH$_2$O (a), there is no flow. At CPAP=3, there is minimal flow (b). $P_{crit}$, or the critical closing pressure, is therefore between 1 and 3 cmH$_2$O. As nasal airway pressure is increased, flow normalizes. The shape of the inspiratory flow curve at CPAP $\leq$ 8 (b, c, d) is flattened (arrows) during inspiration, indicating flow limitation. This is confirmed by the large inspiratory pressures (shown by esophageal pressure) required to generate the flows. The inspiratory pressure requirement declines with loss of flow limitation at CPAP=10 (e). This would be a reasonable treatment pressure for the patient. Modified with permission from reference 7

relaxed, there is no tendency for airway collapse, and a negative suction pressure must be applied to close the airway. In contrast, the $P_{crit}$ in patients with OSAS measured while asleep is typically greater than 5–6 cmH$_2$O. This means that pharyngeal muscles are usually applying a distending force to maintain airway patency. When such a patient falls asleep and pharyngeal muscle tone is deeply relaxed, obstruction occurs. Reopening the airway would require that the patient actively distend the airway by pharyngeal muscle contraction, or that an external pressure be applied to the airway to open it. Specifically, applying a CPAP of at least 5–6 cmH$_2$O would be required to keep the airway open. CPAP can be thought of as a pneumatic splint, keeping open an airway that has a tendency to collapse when muscle tone is lost during sleep.

## DEFINITIONS OF SLEEP-RELATED BREATHING EVENTS

### Snoring

Snoring is an acoustic event produced by vibrations of the air column and soft tissue structures due to turbulent flow through a narrowed upper airway. Although snoring is the target of many public jests, it is a highly prevalent problem, affecting both patients and their bed partners (Figure 8.8). Most commonly, snoring occurs after sleep onset, although in some persons it is present even during drowsiness. Thirty to fifty per cent of adults over the age of 50 years snore, and snoring is loud enough to be heard in an adjacent room in 5–10% of adults. In one recent study of patients referred for sleep evaluations, snoring produced sound intensity levels that averaged 46.2 dB, and that exceeded regulatory outdoor noise limits in 12.3% of patients[11]. Snoring is more common in patients with nasal congestion, as measured by rhinometry[12]. Because snoring results from muscle tone-related

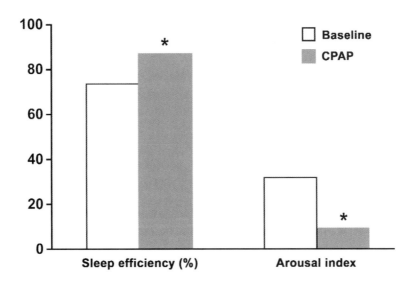

**Figure 8.8** Spousal arousal syndrome[10]. In this study, married couples with one spouse with obstructive sleep apnea syndrome (OSAS) were studied simultaneously by polysomnography with and without nasal continuous positive airway pressure (CPAP) applied to the partner with OSAS. The data illustrated are for the non-apneic spouse, and show significant improvements in sleep quality when the snoring partner used CPAP therapy (*p = <0.01). Sleep efficiency rose and arousals fell

**Table 8.3** Definition of apneas, hypopneas and respiratory effort-related arousals (RERAs)

| | |
|---|---|
| Obstructive apnea | a cessation of airflow for at least 10 s, during which there is effort to breathe |
| Central apnea | a cessation of airflow for at least 10 s, during which there is no effort to breathe |
| Mixed apnea | a cessation of airflow for at least 10 s with the event commencing as a central apnea, but terminating as an obstructive apnea |
| Hypopnea | an abnormal respiratory event lasting at least 10 s with at least a 30% reduction in thoracoabdominal movement or airflow compared with baseline, and with at least a 4% oxyhemoglobin desaturation; a hypopnea can be proved obstructive only with an esophageal balloon that shows increasing effort with reduced airflow, but can often be inferred from the shape of the airflow signal or when snoring intensity increases during the event |
| RERA | sequence of breaths with increasing respiratory effort leading to an arousal from sleep; this is best demonstrated by progressively more negative esophageal pressure efforts for at least 10 s preceding an arousal with resumption of more normal pressures, but often RERAs are inferred from other measured signals (see Figure 8.11) |

reductions in airway dimension, it is frequently also present in patients with apneas and hypopneas.

**Apneas and hypopneas**

The word apnea, derived from the Greek apnoia meaning 'no breath', describes a temporary cessation of breathing. Physiologically, an apnea can arise from two main causes, lack of the central controller signal (central apnea), or an obstruction to breathing despite an adequate central signal and its transmission via efferents to the respiratory muscles (obstructive apnea). Combinations of central and obstructive apneas are called mixed apneas. When a patient experiences a transient reduction in ventilation, the term hypopnea applies. Because there is some normal variance in respiratory pattern from breath to breath, by convention, apneas or hypopneas must last at least 10 s in adults, a period that ordinarily would encompass 2–3 breaths. During the development of our understanding of breathing patterns during sleep, there have been varied specific criteria applied to define apnea or hypopnea. Current definitions are outlined in Table 8.3.

The measurement of respiratory parameters during sleep is covered in Chapter 4. The frequency of apneic and hypopneic events per minute of sleep is expressed as the 'apnea–hypopnea index' (AHI). Using airflow and esophageal pressure measurements as references, Figure 8.9 depicts central, obstructive and mixed apneas.

*Central apneas*

During a central apnea, there is no signal sent from the central respiratory controller, and without effort, there is no airflow (Figure 8.9). Central apneas are most frequent during lighter stages of sleep, particularly with transition from wake to sleep (Figure 8.10). Isolated sleep-onset central apneas are not infrequent in normal sleepers, as the

central controller may interpret the normal $PaCO_2$ of wakefulness as too low when measured against the higher $CO_2$ set point of sleep. Sometimes periodic breathing patterns develop, consisting of series of repetitive central apneic events. Risk factors for this pattern include a low $PaCO_2$ often due to a heightened baseline respiratory drive, such as occurs in congestive heart failure or breathing at high altitude. When this periodic breathing pattern is accompanied by other clinical associations, central sleep apnea syndrome (CSAS) results (see below).

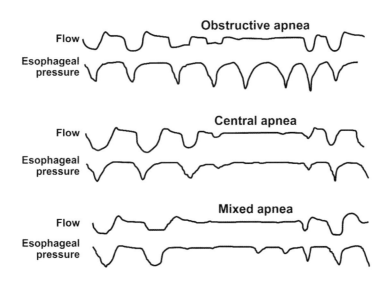

**Figure 8.9** Obstructive, central and mixed apneas. In this figure, airflow signal deflects downwards with inspiration in response to inspiratory efforts that are reflected in negative esophageal pressures. In the top panel an obstructive apnea is illustrated. Apnea occurs despite ongoing inspiratory effort. Flow restarts when the airway opens. The middle panel demonstrates a central apnea. Flow stops in response to an absence of inspiratory effort and begins again as inspiratory efforts recommence. A mixed apnea, seen in the lower panel, begins with a central apnea, but when inspiratory efforts begin, there is upper airway obstruction, and several efforts do not result in airflow. When the upper airway is opened, usually by arousal, airflow begins again

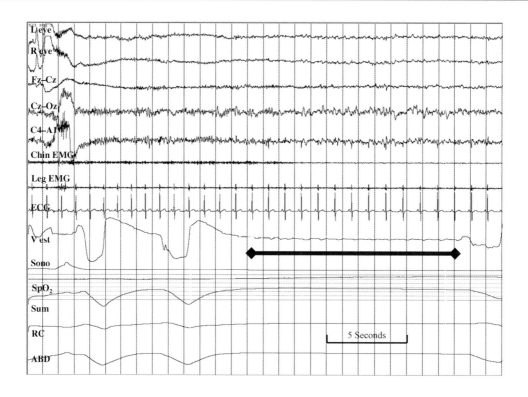

**Figure 8.10** Sleep-onset central apnea. A sleep-onset central apnea is demonstrated in the polysomnogram fragment (apnea between the arrows). As arterial $CO_2$ tension $PaCO_2$ rises and $PaO_2$ falls (changes not evident in this tracing), the ventilatory center is stimulated with resumption of breathing. When $PaCO_2$ rises and $PaO_2$ changes are substantial, hyperpnea and arousal results, setting the patient up for repetitive sleep-onset central apneas alternating with arousals. Channel labels as in Figure 4.1

### Obstructive apneas and hypopneas

When relaxation of the upper airway muscle tone results in an intraluminal pressure less than $P_{crit}$, airway collapse occurs. An obstructive apnea occurs when efforts to breathe continue for at least 10 s against a completely collapsed airway (Figure 8.9). An obstructive hypopnea occurs when efforts to breathe continue for at least 10 s against a partially collapsed airway that restricts ventilation. After either event, normal breathing can resume only after an increase in upper airway muscle tone, which often requires arousal from sleep. Once sleep is resumed, the upper airway muscle tone again decreases, and the tendency for upper airway collapse may cause a repeat of the sequence. Laboratory measurements show increases in sympathetic activation with apneas and arousals, independent from but augmented by any resultant hypoxia. Such increases in sympathetic activation and other humoral responses to this physiological stress are hypothesized to play a role in the development of hypertension, myocardial hypertrophy, impaired glucose tolerance and cerebrovascular and ischemic heart disease. Obstructive apneic and hypopneic events during sleep occur occasionally in asymptomatic individuals.

### Mixed apneas

Occasionally, at the end of an otherwise predominantly central apnea, the resumption of the central signal occurs, but upper airway obstruction interferes with restoration of ventilation. This situation is termed a mixed apnea, and is depicted in Figure 8.9. Such events are similar to obstructive events in their associations with arousals and sleep fragmentation. However, mixed apneas may be more prevalent in patients with risk factors for central sleep apnea syndromes, such as congestive heart failure.

## Respiratory effort-related arousals

The degree of upper airway obstruction and the ventilatory response to such increased upper airway resistance occur over a spectrum of severity ranging from snoring to obstructive apnea. Mild flow limitation and intraluminal narrowing result in snoring, while more severe narrowing may result in hypopneas or apneas despite increased efforts to breathe. When increased upper airway resistance results in increased respiratory efforts sufficient to maintain adequate ventilation but significant enough to trigger an alerting response, the event is called a 'respiratory effort-related arousal' (RERA). Polysomnography (Figure 8.11) reveals a sequence of breaths with increasing respiratory effort leading to an arousal from sleep, but not meeting the criteria for apneas or hypopneas (Table 8.3).

## Periodic breathing

Periodic breathing is a descriptive, not a diagnostic, term referring to a waxing and waning of ventilation as a result of cyclic varying central respiratory drive. It therefore encompasses idiopathic central sleep apnea syndrome, Cheyne–Stokes respiration and high-altitude sleep apnea. High-altitude sleep apnea is periodic breathing that occurs when persons exposed to acute environmental hypoxia experience respiratory control-related instability, with resultant periods of sleep-onset hypoventilation alternating with hyperpnea and arousal. At altitude, inspiratory oxygen content is lower, and the relative hypoxemia drives ventilation during wakefulness. This results in mild hypocapnia. With sleep onset, the $PaCO_2$ level may be below the apneic threshold and a brief central apnea or hypopnea ensues. The repetitive arousals account for insomnia and the poorly restorative quality of sleep often experienced by travelers during their first days at high altitude (Figure 8.12).

## EPIDEMIOLOGY OF SLEEP APNEA SYNDROMES

## Definition and epidemiology of obstructive sleep apnea syndrome

OSAS, first described over 30 years ago, is characterized by repetitive obstructive apneas and hypopneas that disrupt sleep and cause sleepiness[14]. Initial interest focused on severely sleepy patients and on patients in respiratory failure with cor pulmonale. Subsequently, it was discovered that OSAS is common, contributing to impaired quality of life, motor vehicle

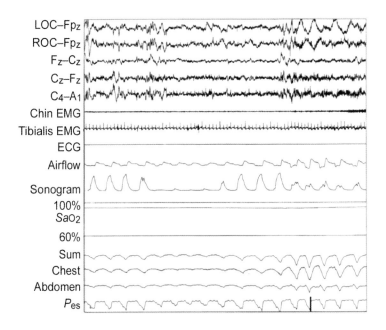

**Figure 8.11** Respiratory effort-related arousal. This 60-s polysomnogram fragment illustrates a series of four crescendo snores terminating in an arousal. There are only minimal changes in airflow, oxyhemoglobin saturation and thoracoabdominal plethysmography preceding the arousal, and these are insufficient to fulfill criteria for a hypopnea. An esophageal pressure recording ($P_{es}$) shows increasing negative pressure preceding the arousal, confirming that respiratory effort has increased. Channel labels as in Figure 4.1

accidents and excessive use of health-care assets. How common is OSAS? The prevalence of any disease depends upon the choice of definition that separates normality from disease.

An initial problem is choosing which variables to measure. For OSAS, the chief components to consider are apneas, hypopneas, RERAs and sleepiness. Apneas, hypopneas and RERAs occur on occasion even in normal sleepers. The AHI is one of the measures used most to quantify the 'severity'

of OSAS. Although the AHI and related arousals are among the strongest variables associated with sleepiness in patients with OSAS, the relationship is far from perfect. In patients with OSAS, some estimate that less than 20% of the variance in daytime sleepiness is explained by AHI or respiratory arousal parameters[15,16]. Thus, some patients complain of severe sleepiness and have relatively low AHI, while others have high AHI and few sleep-related complaints.

Since there is no threshold AHI that predicts sleepiness, what AHI is abnormal? The Wisconsin Sleep Cohort study investigated a random sample of 602 middle-aged men and women[17]. Twenty four per cent of men and 9% of women had an AHI > 5/h, while 9% of men and 4% of women had an AHI > 15/h. Many studies have found the AHI to be an independent risk factor for increases in cardiovascular morbidity and mortality. In the Sleep Heart Health Study, 6424 participants underwent in-home polysomnography. Those with an AHI frequency in the upper quartile (AHI ≥ 11/h) had 42%

greater odds of cardiovascular disease than those in the lowest quartile (< 1.3/h)[18]. Disturbingly, the majority of the increase in cardiovascular risk across the continuum of obstructive sleep apnea developed as the AHI increased between 0 and 10.

These factors challenge our ability to decide rationally what threshold of AHI defines abnormality. Mostly by convention, an AHI of 5 or less is considered normal in adults. For the present, an AHI ≥ 5/h with symptoms of sleepiness, cognitive difficulties or fatigue or documented cardiovascular disease or hypertension, or an AHI ≥ 15/h

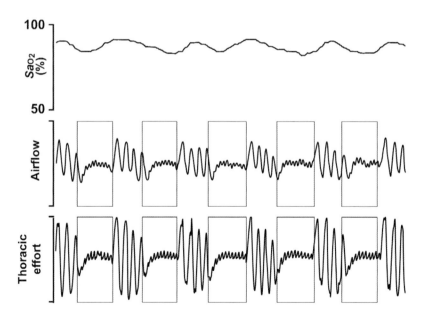

**Figure 8.12** High-altitude sleep apnea. The panel is obtained from a physically fit cyclist, sleeping in a normobaric, hypoxic environment simulating 2650 m elevation. During stage 2 sleep, repetitive central apneas alternate with arousal, and oxygen saturation $SaO_2$ declines after apneas. Twenty five per cent of the trained cyclists experienced periodic breathing, which occupied nearly one-third of their nights. Modified with permission from reference 13

even without symptoms, is a consensus definition of OSAS[19].

The prevalence of OSAS limited to those with AHI ≥ 5/h and with sleep symptoms has been estimated to be between 3 and 28%, and is probably about 5% in Western countries[20]. Independent risk factors for OSAS include age, increasing body mass index (BMI), African-American ethnicity, male gender and pregnancy. Prevalence of OSAS increases with age until about 65 years old, after which it remains constant at about 20% (Figure 8.13). Excess adipose tissue, reflected in increased BMI, alters respiratory function by changes in upper airway geometry and worsened ventilation–perfusion matching, caused by obesity-associated decreases in pulmonary functional residual capacity. Neck circumference is correlated with increased AHI, especially if exceeding 16.5 inches (40 cm) in men. Although the prevalence in women is never quite as high as in males, it increases after the menopause. Studies have estimated that the African-American risk for OSAS is about 2.0–2.5 times that of Caucasians and Asians.

Various conditions have been associated with increased prevalence of OSAS, either because of associated craniofacial abnormalities, or through complex interactions of neuromuscular tone and anatomy (Table 8.4). Other diseases associated with a high

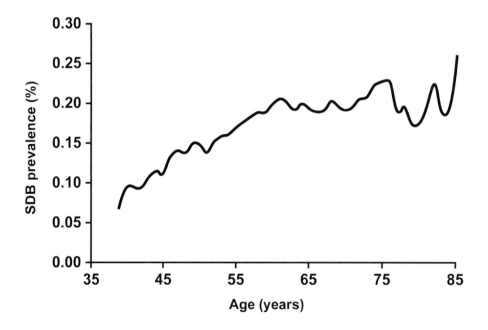

**Figure 8.13** Age and prevalence of sleep-disordered breathing. The prevalence of sleep-disordered breathing (SDB), especially obstructive sleep apnea syndrome, increases with age until the age of about 70 years. Reproduced with permission from reference 20

**Table 8.4** Conditions associated with increased risk of obstructive sleep apnea syndrome

Obesity

Alcohol use

Hypertension

Congestive heart failure

Coronary artery disease

Stroke

Cardiac transplantation

Myxedema

Acromegaly

Cushing's syndrome (exogenous or endogenous)

Trisomy 21

Pierre–Robin syndrome

Crouzon syndrome

Klippel–Feil syndrome

Prader–Willi syndrome

Arnold–Chiari malformation

Post-polio syndrome

prevalence of OSAS include hypertension, congestive heart failure, coronary artery disease and stroke, but these disorders are probably complications of OSAS rather than causative factors.

## Definition and epidemiology of CSAS and Cheyne–Stokes respiration

There is even less consensus in the definitions of CSAS and Cheyne–Stokes respiration (CSR), but CSAS is commonly considered to be present when the frequency of central apneas or hypopneas exceeds 5/h and there are symptoms of either excessive sleepiness or disrupted sleep. Central apneas frequently coexist with obstructive or mixed apneas and hypopneas. If more than half the events are purely central, the patient is usually considered to have CSAS. The diagnosis of CSR requires a crescendo–decrescendo ventilatory pattern, most often punctuated by central apneic pauses, with the patient often having congestive heart failure (CHF) or cerebral disease. Because CSAS and CSR often coexist, definitional boundaries become blurry, and authors often use the terms almost synonymously. Some patients who chronically hypoventilate during sleep (central alveolar hypoventilation syndromes, see Table 9.9) experience central apneas. They tend to manifest with daytime hypercapnia ($PaCO_2 \geq 45\%$) and differ from the more eucapnic or hypocapnic CSAS/CSR patients (Chapter 9).

The prevalence of CSAS/CSR in the general population is low, but is substantial in patients with cardiac and neurological disease. In patients with left ventricular dysfunction, the prevalence of disease is estimated at between 40 and 80%[21]. Eighty-two per cent of 45 consecutive acutely ill patients admitted to a heart failure unit with left ventricular ejection fractions < 45% had sleep-disordered breathing, including 62% with CSR[22]. In another prospective evaluation of sleep-disordered breathing in men with stable heart failure, 51% had an AHI $\geq$ 15/h, with 40% having CSAS/CSR and 11% having OSAS[23]. Risk factors for CSAs in patients with CHF include male gender (odds ratio 3.5), atrial fibrillation (odds ratio 4.13), age > 60 years (odds ratio 2.37) and hypocapnia (odds ratio 4.33)[24]. Among patients with CHF, those with CSAS/CSR have increased mortality and transplant rates compared with those without, even after adjusting for confounding factors (relative risk 2.53, 95% confidence index (CI) 1.08–5.94)[25]. Several short trials show physiological improvements after treating cardiac patients who have CSAS/CSR with CPAP. Multicenter prospective trials are underway to determine whether treatment of CSAS/CSR will improve outcomes.

Forty to ninety per cent of patients admitted to hospital with acute stroke have sleep-disordered breathing, with average AHI ranging from 30 to 60/h[26,27]. Up to half of the apneas are central at the time of admission, but it appears that over 1 month the frequency of central apneas declines, and obstructive apneas and hypopneas become more dominant[28]. Patients admitted with acute coronary syndromes also have a high frequency of CSAS/CSR[29].

## CLINICAL PRESENTATION OF SLEEP APNEA SYNDROMES

### Symptoms

*Obstructive sleep apnea syndrome*

Patients with OSAS may present with daytime or nocturnal complaints, but, not uncommonly, close companions are more aware of symptoms than the patient (Table 8.5). Disruptive snoring and excessive daytime sleepiness are most common, each being present in nearly 70% of patients[30]. While snoring is exceedingly common in patients with OSAS and upper airway resistance syndrome, its absence does not exclude these diagnoses. Most daytime symptoms are not specific for OSAS and can be found in patients with sleep deprivation from a variety of causes. Morning headaches, although found in only 48% of patients with OSAS, are somewhat more specific[31]. Apneas are witnessed in about 75% of patients with OSAS if there is a reliable observer, but are not specific for OSAS[30].

**Table 8.5**  Symptoms of obstructive sleep apnea syndrome

| Daytime symptoms | Nocturnal symptoms |
| --- | --- |
| Sleepiness | snoring |
| Morning headaches | witnessed apneas |
| Poor concentration | choking spells |
| Cognitive dysfunction | restless sleep |
| Personality changes | insomnia |
| Erectile dysfunction | nocturia |
| Lower extremity edema | diaphoresis |
|  | reflux |
|  | drooling |
|  | moaning |

Apneas may also be observed in CSAS, as well as in asymptomatic patients with a low frequency of obstructive events[24].

The medical history may show the presence of predisposing disorders (Table 8.4). A medication history may also be helpful. Many patients have either concurrent depression or have been treated with antidepressants for symptoms ultimately related to OSAS rather than affective disorders. Because patients may have complained of insomnia, hypnotics or sedating, antidepressants such as trazodone may have been prescribed prior to a diagnosis of OSAS having been considered. Alcohol use may predispose to sleep-disordered breathing. As there is a familial association of OSAS, a family history should be obtained[20].

Nocturia is common in patients with OSAS, but the mechanism is uncertain. In one study, pathological nocturia (defined as two or more episodes per night) had an overall prevalence of nearly 50% in patients with OSAS, and was slightly more common in females than in males (60% vs. 40.9%)[32]. It has been suggested that the nocturia episodes may be a response to arousals from other causes such as apneas, rather than caused by a primary need to urinate[33]. This seems plausible given the findings that 76% of nocturia episodes were preceded by apneas or snoring episodes, and 3% by periodic limb movements. Other hypotheses include hypoxia or atrial stretch leading to increased atrial natriuretic peptide secretion and subsequent alterations in intravascular volume, with increased nocturia[32]. Similarly, the pathophysiology of erectile dysfunction, reported to be present in between 30 and 50% of patients with OSAS, is not entirely clear[34,35]. Potential mechanisms include hypoxia-mediated neuropathy, decreased testosterone levels (also associated with obesity alone) and the vascular effects of comorbid hypertension or diabetes. In any event, impotence often improves when OSAS is treated[35].

Many clinicians are aware of the associations between OSAS and cardiovascular diseases, atrial fibrillation and especially hypertension. Patients often minimize sleep complaints, and may not have reliable observers to comment on sleep behaviors. Some clinicians order screening ambulatory oximetries, or ask patients to make audio or video recordings of themselves during sleep, and if abnormalities are found, refer them for sleep evaluations even in the absence of significant sleep complaints. Occasionally the results of an ambulatory cardiac rhythm analysis demonstrating nocturnal arrhythmias prompt referral. Other less common reasons to consider sleep-related breathing disorders include unexplained polycythemia or pulmonary hypertension, motor vehicle accidents, acute delirium during hospitalization or other unusual nocturnal behaviors.

*Central sleep apnea and Cheyne–Stokes respiration*

Daytime symptoms of central sleep apnea (CSA)/CSR are similar to those of OSAS, but patients may complain more of sleep-onset and sleep-maintenance insomnia. In one study, snoring and sleep disturbance could not distinguish between CSA/CSR and OSAS, while other studies have found that patients with OSAS are heavier and more likely to be habitual snorers than those with CSA[23,24].

Because so many patients with CSA/CSR have underlying cardiac or neurological disease, the medical history may be dominated by these associated conditions. Many patients will already have established diagnoses of congestive heart failure, or may be undergoing evaluation for exertional dyspnea or atrial fibrillation. Periodic breathing may have been noted during hospitalization for stroke or heart failure. Because insomnia is prevalent, hypnotics may have already been tried.

### Upper airway resistance syndrome

When RERAs, rather than apneas or hypopneas, are responsible for arousals, then the term 'upper airway resistance syndrome' (UARS) is sometimes used. Some authorities consider this syndrome to be part of the spectrum of OSAS and feel the term should be abandoned. The main complaint of patients with UARS is hypersomnolence[36]. Snoring is very common but not invariably present, and in some slender patients, the bed partner may describe only noisy or irregular breathing patterns. Although there have been no large epidemiological studies of UARS, some find that patients with UARS are less obese, more often female and generally younger when compared with OSAS populations. Because snoring and other symptoms frequently noted in OSAS (Table 8.5) may occasionally be absent, the possibility of UARS must at least be considered in all patients complaining of hypersomnolence.

### Case 8.2

A 74-year-old patient followed for congestive heart failure and hypertension was questioned about sleep on a routine visit. He reported snoring for many years and disrupted sleep for at least 5 years. His wife had noted repetitive apneas and occasional snort arousals for at least 2 years. He went to bed around 11:00 p.m. and usually had no difficulty initiating sleep. However, on four out of seven nights he awakened 1 h later and would not sleep soundly for the rest of the night, taking several naps during the day to compensate. On the other nights of the week, he was able to sleep through until around 7:00 a.m., but regardless he always awakened feeling poorly refreshed. He was aware occasionally that his 'breathing seems to slow down' at night. He was obese, had fine rales at the bases of his lungs and had mild pitting edema of both lower extremities. During the first half of 'split-night' polysomnography, he slept for 120 min with a sleep latency of 16 min. Obstructive apneas and hypopneas occurred 33 times per hour, and central apneas occurred once per hour, resulting in severely disrupted sleep. Oxygen saturation ranged from 73 to 97%, nearly two-thirds of the time falling below 90%. The electrocardiogram (ECG) showed sinus rhythm with frequent unifocal ventricular ectopics. During the second half of the night, a therapeutic trial of CPAP was begun at 5 cmH$_2$O. When the pressure was titrated up to 8–9 cmH$_2$O, most obstructive events were eliminated, but some central events supervened. Higher pressures seemed to cause more central apneas and impaired sleep quality. A pressure of 8–9 cmH$_2$O appeared to be optimal and maintained oxygen saturation generally greater than 90%. Sleep architecture improved on this setting. He was provided with CPAP at

$9 \text{ cmH}_2\text{O}$. At follow-up, his wife still reported fairly frequent apneic pauses without snoring and his sleep was still not restorative. Compliance data downloaded from the machine indicated that he was using it regularly. A bilevel positive airway pressure titration was performed during a second polysomnogram, and at an inspiratory positive airway pressure (IPAP) of $12 \text{ cmH}_2\text{O}$ and expiratory positive airway pressure (EPAP) of $7 \text{ cmH}_2\text{O}$ and back-up rate of 10/min, nearly all sleep-disordered breathing was eliminated. At subsequent follow-up, his alertness returned to normal, observed apneas had ceased and his sleep was now continuous and refreshing.

Split studies are often successful for usual OSAS, but in patients with more complicated problems, a second night's study may be necessary to obtain an adequate treatment formulation. In this case, the patient's OSAS was easily improved with CPAP, but he manifested CSA/CSR on CPAP. He had underlying risk factors for CSA/CSR, including male gender, CHF and age over 60 years[24]. Sometimes CPAP therapy produces CSA, through mechanisms that are not well understood. Bilevel positive airway pressure, usually with a mandatory back-up rate, is often effective.

## Signs and associated findings in sleep apnea syndromes

Examination of the patient with suspected sleep apnea syndrome begins with the observation of breathing pattern while the patient is relaxed but awake. While taking the history, the absence or presence of CSR, respiratory effort or tachypnea, and facial or jaw abnormalities should be observed. If a Cheyne–Stokes pattern is present while awake, one can anticipate that this is aggravated during sleep. Underlying respiratory or neuromuscular disease may be suggested by a rapid shallow breathing pattern, by alterations in gait or muscle strength, or by use of accessory respiratory muscles. Often, while the patient is relaxed and not focused on the examination process, one may note a moderate retrognathia that is not as apparent when asking the patient to demonstrate their bite. Some have suggested the term 'dynamic retrognathia' be used to describe this characteristic.

Physical examination should include the patient's build, height, weight, blood pressure and pulse. Hypercapnia may be suggested by conjunctival injection. The jaw should be inspected for overjet or overbite (Figure 3.1). The oropharynx should be examined for macroglossia, tonsillar tissue, size and appearance of the uvula and soft palate, and narrowing of the anteroposterior and lateral diameters of the oropharyngeal space. One study found the most predictive oropharyngeal finding for OSAS to be tonsillar pillar narrowing and tonsillar enlargement[37]. The tongue should be carefully inspected for enlargement (demonstrated by dental nicking) or fasciculations (found in patients with amyotrophic lateral sclerosis). The degree of patency of the nasal passages and any septal deviation should be judged. Neck size should be noted. The presence of systemic hypertension and any signs of pulmonary disease or pulmonary arterial hypertension should be sought. Lower extremity edema and other signs of right heart failure should be noted. Slow relaxation of deep tendon reflexes may be an indicator of occult hypothyroidism. Following clinical assessment, a decision is made whether to proceed with laboratory testing.

Besides the selection of appropriate sleep testing, it may be helpful to obtain additional laboratory tests in some circumstances. If hypercapnia is suspected on clinical grounds, arterial blood gas testing is sensible prior to any planned sleep study. If history and examination suggest previously undiagnosed cardiac or pulmonary disease, evaluation of these disorders first is prudent, and may include electrocardiogram, echo-cardiogram, B-type natiuretic peptide level, pulmonary function testing, chest radiography or specialty evaluation.

Because diagnostic testing for OSAS is not always readily available, clinical prediction rules have been developed to assist the clinician in estimating the probability of the presence of disease using only clinical data[38]. For example, one clinical model uses the patient's neck circumference, presence of habitual snoring or frequent nocturnal choking or apneas, and history of hypertension to arrive at the probability of having OSAS (Figure 8.14)[39]. Most clinical predic-

| | Sleep Apnea Clinical Score | | | | | |
|---|---|---|---|---|---|---|
| | Not hypertensive | | | Hypertensive | | |
| | Historical features* | | | Historical features* | | |
| Neck circumference (cm) | None | One | Both | None | One | Both |
| <30 | 0 | 0 | 1 | 0 | 1 | 2 |
| 30/31 | 0 | 0 | 1 | 1 | 2 | 4 |
| 32/33 | 0 | 1 | 2 | 1 | 3 | 5 |
| 34/35 | 1 | 2 | 3 | 2 | 4 | 8 |
| 36/37 | 1 | 3 | 5 | 4 | 6 | 11 |
| 38/39 | 2 | 4 | 7 | 5 | 9 | 16 |
| 40/41 | 3 | 6 | 10 | 8 | 13 | 22 |
| 42/43 | 5 | 8 | 14 | 11 | 18 | 30 |
| 44/45 | 7 | 12 | 20 | 15 | 25 | 42 |
| 46/47 | 10 | 16 | 28 | 21 | 35 | 58 |
| 48/49 | 14 | 23 | 38 | 29 | 48 | 80 |
| >49 | 19 | 32 | 53 | 40 | 66 | 110 |

*Historical Features: 1 habitual snoring, 2 partner reports of gasping, choking or snorting

**Probability of sleep apnea**

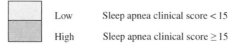

Low    Sleep apnea clinical score < 15

High    Sleep apnea clinical score ≥ 15

**Figure 8.14**  Algorithm for the diagnosis of obstructive sleep apnea syndrome. Reproduced with permission from reference 39

tion rules are not sensitive and specific enough to 'rule out' or 'rule in' OSAS, but may be helpful in raising or lowering clinical suspicion or in prioritizing the urgency of study required. Clearly, in patients whose symptoms dictate rapid evaluation, such as unsafe driving due to hypersomnolence, nocturnal angina or heart failure, the urgency of evaluation is dictated by the complaints, not by probability analysis.

## Diagnostic testing for sleep apnea syndromes

### Use of polysomnography

Diagnostic polysomnogram (PSG) is the standard test for suspected sleep-disordered breathing, and is most frequently performed at an attended sleep laboratory. Estimates of the sensitivity of one night of polysomnography to detect an AHI $\geq 5$ in patients with OSAS range between 75 and 88%[40]. Night-to-night variability, sleep position, sleep environment, medications and underlying respiratory or neurological diseases are some of the variables that might affect the frequency and severity of disordered breathing. In patients with a strong suspicion of sleep apnea and exclusion of other causes for the symptoms, a second PSG may be necessary to diagnose the disorder correctly[41].

During the early days of sleep medicine, a full night of diagnostic polysomnography followed by a full night of therapeutic positive airway pressure titration was routine. More recently, it has become accepted that if a diagnosis is certain after only part of a night (usually more than 120 min of sleep), a CPAP titration can often be completed during the remainder of the study (Table 8.9)[42]. This 'split-night' testing strategy is successful in over 80% of patients with OSAS, and implementing this strategy saves the patient time and conserves the resources of the sleep laboratory. However, one must not hesitate to utilize a second night for therapeutic trials if a satisfactory diagnostic answer has not been obtained half-way through the first study. One of the advantages of attended PSG is that the qualified attendant can apply various interventions during the study. The clinician should consider the patient's likely diagnoses in advance, so that appropriate interventions can be ordered. For example, if OSAS is considered likely, a trial of CPAP therapy should be anticipated. If neuromuscular weakness or hypoventilation from other causes seems likely, a bilevel device with a back-up rate should be available during testing.

### Polysomnographic findings in OSAS

The findings in patients with OSAS are summarized in Table 8.6 and a typical epoch demonstrating features found in OSAS is shown in Figure 8.15. Sleep architecture is affected by arousals caused by obstructive apneas and hypopneas. In addition to the characteristic pattern of obstructive apneas and hypopneas demonstrated on respiratory channels, one usually finds an increase in arousals, increase in stage 1 sleep and decreases in slow-wave and REM sleep. Surprisingly, the termination of some apneas and hypopneas do not appear to result in electroencephalogram (EEG) detectable arousals. Oxyhemoglobin saturation usually fluctuates in response to apneas and

**Table 8.6** Polysomnographic findings in obstructive sleep apnea syndrome

| | |
|---|---|
| Respiratory channels | indirect measures of airflow show apneas or hypopneas |
| | nasal pressure transducer or thermocouple shows decline in magnitude or flattening/concavity of inspiratory curve |
| | snore microphone may show snoring with mild obstruction, and silence with apneas or non-obstructed breathing |
| | respiratory effort recordings demonstrate thoracoabdominal paradox with apneas or hypopneas |
| | esophageal manometer (if used) shows progressively negative pressures with obstruction, and abrupt return to normal levels ($-5$ to $-10$ cmH$_2$O) following arousal or relief of upper airway obstruction |
| ECG channels | respiratory-related sinus arrhythmia accentuated |
| | with significant obstructive apneas or hypopneas, may demonstrate increasing bradycardia or increasing heart block |
| | relative or absolute tachycardia following arousal and resumption of unobstructed breathing (Figure 8.15) |
| | may show arrhythmias, such as supraventricular tachycardia, ventricular ectopy or tachycardia, atrial fibrillation, especially if oxyhemoglobin levels fall below 65% or if patient has underlying heart disease |
| EMG channels | chin EMG may show accentuated phasic increases in amplitude corresponding to activation of pharyngeal and neck muscles to maintain patency |
| | tibial EMG may show leg muscle activity with arousals |
| Oxyhemoglobin saturation channel | shows episodic decline in saturation with hypopneas (by definition) and usually with apneas. Saturation usually returns towards baseline, but if events are frequent or severe, complete recovery may not occur until period of wakefulness |
| EEG channels | most (but not all) apneas and hypopneas terminate with EEG arousal |
| Sleep architecture | increase in arousals and stage 1 sleep and decline in slow-wave and REM sleep; often with CPAP initiation there is a compensatory increase in REM sleep, and to a lesser extent, slow-wave sleep; REM sleep latency may be shortened |

ECG, electrocardiogram; EMG, electromyogram; EEG, electroencephalogram; REM, rapid eye movement; CPAP, continuous positive airway pressure hypopneas, and subsequent hyperpneas. The electrocardiogram usually shows rate variation, with relative slowing during obstructive episodes mediated by increased vagal tone from negative intrathoracic pressure, followed by increases in rate linked to catecholamine excess and declines in venous return after resumption of ventilation ('bradycardia–tachycardia') (Figure 8.15). Sinus arrhythmia is most common, but occasionally heart block, ventricular ectopy or frank ventricular tachycardia can ensue, usually in association with more severe hypoxemia[43]. Although not routinely measured during clinical polysomnography in OSAS, measures of end-tidal $CO_2$ may rise during repetitive obstructive apneas and hypopneas, and systemic blood pressure may show transient increases in response to hypoxemia and arousals.

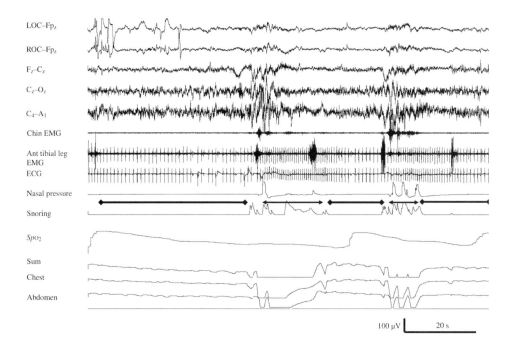

**Figure 8.15** Obstructive sleep apnea. This 120-s polysomogram (PSG) tracing in rapid eye movement (REM) sleep demonstrates the typical findings of obstructive sleep apnea. Apneas are accompanied by paradoxical chest and abdominal movement and oxyhemoglobin desaturation. Electroencephalogram (EEG) arousals are associated with restoration of airflow and snoring. There is a gradual decline in heart rate during the apneas (segments between diamonds), seen by the increase in the R to R interval in the electrocardiogram (ECG) lead. Following arousal, relative tachycardia results (segments between arrows). Channel labels as in Figure 4.1

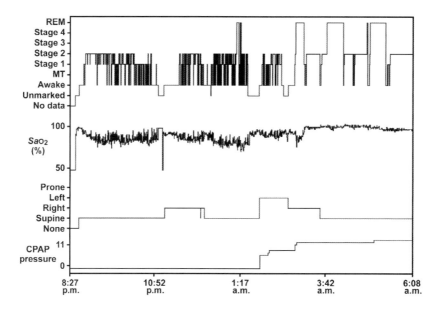

**Figure 8.16** Sleep architecture in obstructive sleep apnea syndrome (OSAS). In this patient, OSAS caused arousals, increase in stage 1 non-rapid eye movement (NREM) sleep, absent slow-wave sleep and decrease in rapid eye movement (REM) sleep compared with expected values in the first portion of testing. After the application of continuous positive airway pressure (CPAP), there is a substantial increase in REM sleep ('REM-rebound'), and reduction in arousals. Concurrent improvements in oxygen saturation $SaO_2$ are also apparent. MT, movement time

Polysomnography performed during initial therapeutic trials of CPAP therapy often records dramatic changes in sleep architecture with elimination of disordered breathing. A marked increase in the proportion of REM sleep ('REM-rebound') is common (Figure 8.16), and slow-wave sleep, although uncommon in the latter half of normal sleep, may be abundant.

*Polysomnographic findings in UARS*

Patients with UARS share some polysomnographic findings with patients having OSAS, including multiple arousals, and a decrease in slow-wave sleep. REM sleep is less affected than in OSAS[36,44]. Snoring is not uniformly present. By definition, a high frequency of overt apneas and hypopneas is absent from PSG recordings in patients with UARS. Thus, a PSG finding of repetitive arousals without apparent cause in a sleepy patient, especially if there is snoring, should prompt consideration of UARS. Heart rate variability may be a clue to increases in airway resistance. If UARS is suspected clinically, one may wish to place an esophageal pressure monitor, which is required for a definitive diagnosis[44]. Because of the invasive nature of esophageal monitoring, many surrogate markers for airway obstruction have been proposed. Some feel that a diagnosis of UARS can be tentatively made by the association of repetitive crescendo snore patterns terminating in arousal with otherwise unexplained hypersomnolence. Nasal pressure transducers are suggested to be quite sensitive in detecting subtle flow limitation, and a pattern of repetitive flow limitation terminating in arousals may also suggest the diagnosis. When a surrogate marker is used tentatively to diagnose UARS, it is wise to ensure that a positive treatment effect occurs following the relief of airway resistance.

### Polysomnographic findings in CSA/CSR

Patients with CSA/CSR demonstrate increased arousals and stage 1 sleep, but slow-wave and REM sleep may be less affected than in patients with OSAS. Apneas with arousals occur repetitively in stage 1 sleep, less frequently in stage 2 and only very rarely in slow-wave sleep. Breathing often normalizes during REM sleep. An esophageal pressure monitor is required for definitive diagnosis, but, in clinical practice, cessation of airflow measured by a thermocouple or nasal pressure transducer associated with the absence of respiratory effort measured indirectly by inductive plethysmography, strain-gauge recordings or intercostal electromyogram (EMG) is considered sufficient to establish the diagnosis. In contrast to central apneas, it may be extremely difficult to differentiate obstructive from central hypopneas without an esophageal pressure monitor. It is not uncommon for both CSA/CSR and components of airway obstruction to coexist. When central apneas are responsible for more than 75% of respiratory events, the patient may be thought of as having CSA/CSR (Figure 8.17). In contradistinction to OSAS where arousals are usually required to terminate the apnea, in CSA/CSR spontaneous breathing begins in response to rising $PaCO_2$, and the arousal occurs during the ensuing hyperpneic phase.

### Home-based polysomnography

Because laboratory-based polysomnography may be poorly accessible or expensive, several other testing strategies have been developed. Home unattended polysomnography with portable units is available, and is used in some health-care systems. One study found that the use of such a device produced an uninterpretable result in 33% of patients for varied reasons[45]. Another study found similar results if the patient applied the sensing equipment, but improved data quality (93%) if a technician applied equipment in their home prior to bedtime[46]. The quality of sleep itself has not been shown to be better during home PSG compared with laboratory studies[45].

### Portable cardiorespiratory monitoring for OSAS

Portable devices that monitor only breathing and cardiac signals, called cardiorespiratory monitors, are also available in a variety of forms. The technologies for cardiorespiratory monitors are not as standardized as for polysomnography, and there is not an extensive literature evaluating their performance as home portable devices. Nonetheless, some appear to provide adequate information to diagnose OSAS, especially if there are few other differential diagnostic

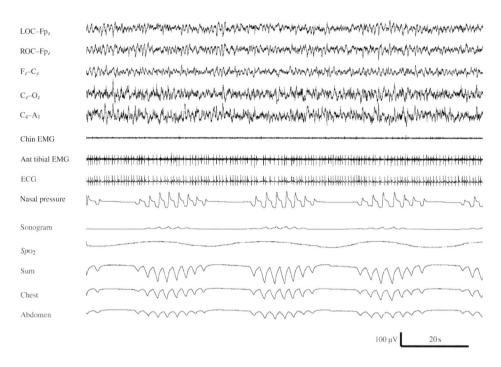

LOC–Fp$_z$

ROC–Fp$_z$

F$_z$–C$_z$

C$_z$–O$_z$

C$_4$–A$_1$

Chin EMG

Ant tibial EMG

ECG

Nasal pressure

Sonogram

SpO$_2$

Sum

Chest

Abdomen

100 μV      20 s

**Figure 8.17** Central sleep apnea (CSA) and Cheyne–Stokes respiration (CSR). The 120-s polysomno-graph tracing demonstrates a breathing pattern with decreasing tidal volume that progresses to central apneas. Note that during apneas there is no movement of the chest or abdomen, indicating no effort to breathe. Following apnea, breathing resumes in a crescendo manner, consistent with the Cheyne–Stokes pattern. The patient is in atrial fibrillation, a risk factor for CSA/CSR. The sonogram demonstrates snoring, which can be present and does not help differentiate CSA/CSR from obstructive sleep apnea syndrome. Channel labels as in Figure 4.1

considerations. Until the performance characteristics are better understood, they are probably best used only when PSG is not available in an appropriate time frame, when there is a very high clinical probability of OSAS without other conflicting considerations and when further testing can be arranged in the event of test results that conflict with clinical impressions, or the patient fails to improve on therapy[47]. The reliability of portable cardiorespiratory monitors in evaluating CSA has not been studied.

*Ambulatory oximetry*

Ambulatory oximetry has been suggested as a tool to screen for OSAS. Recording oximetry devices are inexpensive, can usually be managed by the patient alone at home without much data loss and provide a recorded tracing of oxyhemoglobin saturation trends during the recording period. For the detection of OSAS, sensitivities ranging from 25 to 99% and specificities from 41 to 100% have been published[48–54]. Even with this apparently wide range of diagnostic

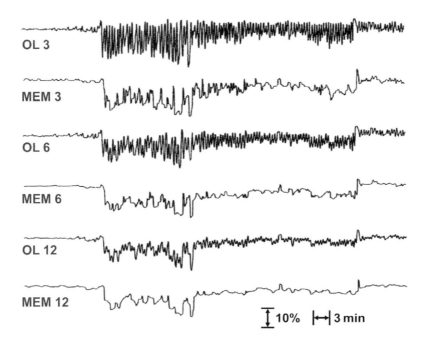

**Figure 8.18** Effect of operational characteristics on oximetry display and sensitivity. The figure shows simultaneous output from an oximeter with different settings in a single patient. OL 3, OL 6 and OL 12 correspond to 'online' recordings with the oximeter averaging time (also called the response time) set at 3, 6 and 12 s, respectively. This means that although the saturation is sampled rapidly, only a representative value is displayed on the chart recorder over a 3-, 6- or 12-s interval. MEM 3, MEM 6 and MEM 12 show the output of the value stored in the memory. Major variations in the tracings can be appreciated. Reproduced with permission reference 55

accuracy, ambulatory oximetry can be very useful, but one must be aware of what factors influence the sensitivity and specificity of the test, and decide ahead of time how one will use the results. Keeping in mind that typical apneas and hypopneas average about 15 s in duration, declines in oxyhemoglobin saturation are most likely to occur when there are reduced alveolar oxygen stores, or the oxyhemoglobin saturation starts on the steep portion of the oxyhemoglobin saturation curve. Obesity or restrictive diseases are

likely to find the patient with a reduced functional residual capacity, and hence reduced alveolar oxygen stores. Those with underlying pulmonary or cardiac disease, or those at high altitude, are more likely to begin testing with oxyhemoglobin saturation on the steep portion of the saturation curve. One should anticipate that oximetry will be more sensitive in these patients (and less specific), and less sensitive in slender persons with healthy cardiopulmonary status. Technical factors, such as sampling and data storage rates, can

**Table 8.7** Factors influencing sensitivity and specificity of ambulatory oximetry for the detection of obstructive sleep apnea syndrome

| | | |
|---|---|---|
| Patient factors | body habitus | obese individuals have decreased functional residual capacity, and thus decreased oxygen stores, and altered V/Q matching leading to hypoxemia |
| | underlying pulmonary disease | patients with pulmonary disease may have $PaO_2$ reduced and close to the steep part of the oxyhemoglobin dissociation curve |
| | patient asleep or awake | oximetry records only oxygen saturation and pulse; if the patient does not sleep, there will be no observation of oximetry effects of sleep-related breathing disorders |
| Technical factors | oximetry sampling rate | See Figure 8.18 |
| | oximetry recording rate | See Figure 8.18 |
| | oximetry probe positioning | oximetry may be missing, or record artifact |
| Varied definitions of abnormalities | definition of apneas and hypopneas and selection of abnormal AHI threshold vary between studies | if desaturations are a necessary part of the definition of disease, sensitivity of oximetry will increase |
| | definition of oximetry abnormalities differs between studies | oximetry abnormalities may be overt (e.g. > 4% desaturation from baseline) or subtle (e.g. fine oscillations in saturation); definition will affect calculation of sensitivity and specificity |

V/Q, ventilation–perfusion; $PaO_2$, oxygen arterial tension; AHI, apnea–hypopnea index

also create substantial differences in conclusions drawn from ambulatory oximetry (Figure 8.18)[55]. Furthermore, there are differing reports of what abnormalities to measure with oximetry. Fine oscillations in oxyhemoglobin saturation tracing (less than 2%) are thought to be due to variations in intrathoracic pressure, and may be a very sensitive indicator of increased work of breathing owing to increased upper airway resistance. Others note the 2–3% accuracy of oximetry, and count only desaturations that exceed 2–3%. All of these factors contribute to the varied reports of sensitivity and specificity (Table 8.7).

Oximetry does not record sleep or position. Occasionally patients may wear the device while unable to sleep or not in bed. Patient-provided information about quality and quantity of sleep, alcohol ingestion and any oxygen or breathing apparatus used is very helpful in interpreting the data.

Given all the variables involved in oximetry, it remains useful under several conditions. First, if clinical suspicion is low, a normal oximetry virtually excludes significant sleep-disordered breathing from consideration. However, in patients with excessive sleepiness, further evaluation is merited. Second, if clinical suspicion is intermediate, a positive oximetry result could persuade a reluctant patient or physician to proceed with formal sleep testing. Third, substantially abnormal oximetry results may help to triage patients with more severe disease towards more expeditious testing when there are constraints on test availability. In other patients with high pretest likelihood of OSAS, oximetry is unlikely to contribute to care. In patients with heart failure where CSA/CSR is suspected, oximetry is fairly sensitive. Finally, in patients with known abnormalities in oximetry (for example, before or during diagnostic polysomnography), oximetry may be useful in follow-up if effectiveness of treatment is uncertain.

## THERAPY OF SLEEP APNEA SYNDROMES

## Treatment of obstructive sleep apnea syndrome: medical therapies

### Life-style modifications

Therapy for OSAS begins with educating the patient about their disease. It is important for them to understand how their disease impacts upon their health and quality of life, emphasizing that, left untreated, they are at increased risk for motor vehicle accidents, may have cognitive and mood disturbances and are increasing their probability of experiencing cardiovascular events. Patients should avoid driving when drowsy and, in the case of professional drivers or pilots, should be aware that their licensing and employment may require proof that therapy is adequate.

Many of the risk factors for developing OSAS have behavioral components. Patients should be advised to drink alcohol moderately at most, and preferably well before bedtime. Weight reduction in obese patients often reduces the frequency of apneas and hypopneas, as well as risk of hypertension and cardiovascular events. In a group of obese patients, weight reduction of about 10% resulted in a 26% reduction in the AHI[56]. Weight loss with the aid of bariatric surgery reduces AHI, but since OSAS is usually manageable with CPAP, this is rarely the sole indication for bariatric procedures.

### Positional therapy

Some patients exhibit sleep-disordered breathing that is largely positional, having apneas, hypopneas and RERAs while supine, but having preserved sleep quality when non-supine. If the patient is able to tolerate sleeping only on the side, then using devices to help ensure a side-sleeping position can be well tolerated and effective. A simple solution is to place wiffle or tennis balls in a pocket sewn onto the back of a nightshirt to prevent sleep in the supine position, but more elaborate devices have been marketed to achieve the same result. For some patients, positional therapy is not possible owing to neck, shoulder, hip or back pain[57].

*Pharmacological therapy*

Ventilatory drive stimulants, central nervous system stimulants, tricyclic antidepressants, serotonin reuptake inhibitors and opioid antagonists have all been suggested for management of OSAS[58]. Although some studies of medroxyprogesterone, a respiratory stimulant, show benefit in OSAS, it appears mostly effective in patients who are hypercapnic and have concurrent alveolar hypoventilation syndrome. Acetazolamide and theophylline are not helpful in OSAS, but are discussed under therapy for CSA/CSR. Opioid antagonists such as doxapram, naloxone and nicotine appear to influence the duration and at times the frequency of obstructive events, but not to a clinically significant degree. Protriptyline, the most studied of the tricyclic antidepressants, is most effective in decreasing REM-related obstructive events. It may be helpful in the treatment of patients with predominantly REM-associated OSAS, but there are only scant data to support this practice, and many patients have difficulty tolerating the side-effects. Serotonergic agents such as fluoxetine, paroxetine, buspirone and imipramine have all been reported to reduce the AHI by about 30% in patients with OSAS, but whether this is clinically significant is uncertain. Specific therapies such as treatment of hypothyroidism may be beneficial.

*Positive airway pressure therapy*

Positive airway pressure (PAP) therapy for OSAS was first described in 1981, and was quickly recognized as an effective and preferred therapy for most patients[59]. Prior to the widespread availability of positive airway pressure, most often delivered as nasal CPAP, only the most severely affected patients were diagnosed, and tracheostomy was often the only therapy offered.

*How does PAP work?* PAP works as a pneumatic splint to maintain an open airway. One of the primary physiological abnormalities in patients with OSAS is the tendency for the airway to collapse, with the relaxation of oropharyngeal muscles, after sleep begins. Patients with OSAS have a positive $P_{crit}$, that is, when muscle tone is relaxed, the airway collapses unless a positive intraluminal pressure is applied (see *'The upper airway during respiration in wakefulness and sleep'* above). Application of PAP $\geq P_{crit}$ has been shown to open the airway using endoscopy, computed tomography and magnetic resonance imaging techniques. When the oropharyngeal airway is splinted open in this manner, airway patency is maintained, and obstructive apneas and hypopneas are eliminated.

Devices for delivering PAP consist of at least three, and sometimes four components (Table 8.8):

**Table 8.8** Components of positive airway therapy

| Component | Implementation |
|---|---|
| The PAP pump: provides and maintains inspiratory and expiratory air at a controlled pressure | continuous positive airway pressure (CPAP): provides a constant airway pressure |
| | bi-level positive airway pressure: provides independently set inspiratory (IPAP) and expiratory (EPAP) pressures |
| | autotitrating positive airway pressure (APAP): uses sensors and feedback algorithms to adjust PAP depending on the degree of obstruction |
| | variable profile PAP: adjusts not only pressure level, but contour of delivery to achieve varied goals |
| Interface with patient: connects the patient's airway with the positive pressure produced by the pump | nasal mask<br>nasal pillows<br>oral mask<br>oronasal mask |
| Vent for expired air | venting via holes in the mask, augmented by continuous wash-out by pressurized air from the pump |
| | venting via exit port next to mask connection, augmented by continuous wash-out |
| Air quality treatments or supplementation | supplemental oxygen, if needed, can be added via ports on the tubing or mask |
| | passive humidity devices: the pressurized air passes over a water reservoir en route to the patient |
| | heated humidity devices: the pressurized air passes through a reservoir where water is heated to augment relative humidity |
| | filters: nearly all PAP devices have filters at the intake to filter air prior to pressurization |

PAP, positive airway pressure

(1) A pump that provides a controlled air pressure;

(2) An interface that seals with the patient's airway and connects to the pump (usually a mask);

(3) A vent for expired air;

(4) Sometimes a device to add humidification or oxygen to the pressurized air.

Although there are many different types of PAP devices and interfaces, the important issue is providing a PAP therapy that effectively reduces sleep-disordered breathing, improves sleep quality and is comfortable enough that the patient can comply with therapy. By far the most common modality is CPAP, and the most common interface is a nasal mask.

*How does one begin CPAP therapy?* CPAP is applied during a PSG, beginning at a low pressure (usually 2–5 cmH$_2$O) and adjusting upwards to eliminate obstructive apneas, hypopneas and RERAs. Monitoring of flow or pressure profiles directly from transducers in the CPAP device can demonstrate flattening consistent with airway resistance, despite the elimination of apneas and hypopneas, and some practitioners feel that such flow restriction should be eradicated to improve treatment effectiveness. Because obstruction tends to be worst with supine posture and REM sleep, a final CPAP pressure should not be chosen until these conditions are recorded on treatment. Often, both diagnostic portions and CPAP titration can be accomplished in a single night. Recommended criteria for proceeding with a 'split-night study' are listed in Table 8.9. Typical treatment pressures average 9–10 cmH$_2$O (range 5–20 cmH$_2$O). Once a treatment

**Table 8.9** Suggested criteria for performing a 'split-night study'

The testing period allows at least 2 h of recorded sleep, or marked hypoxemia with cardiac arrhythmias is noted prior to this period

Recorded apneas and hypopneas occur, producing an AHI usually required to be at least 20/h over the record

A PAP titration period of at least 3 h is recorded. It is desirable to observe effective treatment supine and in REM to assure adequate treatment pressure

AHI, apnea–hypopnea index; UARS, upper airway resistance syndrome; PAP, positive airway pressure; REM, rapid eye movement

pressure is decided, a completed prescription indicates the device, treatment pressure and interface, and whether to add air quality modification such as heated humidity.

CPAP is foreign to every patient initially, and proper introduction is essential to long-term success in CPAP therapy. Although there are no studies evaluating the impact of pre-polysomnographic patient education, nearly all patients and busy sleep laboratories can testify to the benefits of educating the patient about OSAS and CPAP therapy, and introducing and fitting CPAP prior to the sleep study. At our facility, patients are allowed to sit with a CPAP device on at low pressures before their study. This allows adjustments to fit, and if needed, desensitization to the apparatus.

CPAP does not suit every patient with OSAS. There are many steps to successful CPAP therapy (Table 8.10), starting with the

**Table 8.10** The road to successful continuous positive airway pressure (CPAP) therapy

| Milestone | Definition | Range |
|---|---|---|
| Acceptance* | the proportion of patients deemed appropriate for CPAP therapy who allow CPAP titration | 70–76% |
| Prescription* | the proportion of patients accepting CPAP prescription and who begin home therapy | 50 to > 80% |
| Adherence* | the proportion of patients who report that they are continuing to use CPAP | 65–90% |
| Compliance* | the proportion of patients actually using CPAP at a treatment pressure measured objectively (the device is on, with the pressure delivered to the patient via the interface) | 45–70% |
| Effectiveness | target symptoms and signs are improved or resolved, e.g. sleepiness or oxygen saturation is improved to a specified level | ? |

*Some terms adapted from reference 62

patient first accepting the initial trial of CPAP and then deciding whether to begin using it at home. Finally, evaluation of treatment effectiveness must follow, so that adjustments or trouble-shooting can occur.

*What are the benefits of CPAP therapy?* There is ample evidence showing that CPAP use improves AHI, subjective sleepiness, cognitive performance and quality of life for patients with OSAS[60]. Most studies also indicate improvement in objective sleepiness as measured by the multiple sleep latency test (MSLT) or maintenance of wakefulness test (MWT), and some, but not all, studies suggest that CPAP improves control of systemic hypertension. CPAP therapy appears to reduce hospital admissions and health-care costs[61]. Many anticipate that CPAP therapy will lower the morbidity and mortality of patients with OSAS, but results of prospective trials are not yet available. Because CPAP is so effective, it is considered the 'gold standard' against which other therapies are compared.

*How does one improve CPAP compliance and manage CPAP failure?* Initial patient education and preparation help to improve CPAP acceptance and prescription, but careful follow-up and management of challenges increase the likelihood of success. Several studies suggest that factors that favorably influence CPAP compliance include increasing severity of pretreatment sleepiness, more severe hypoxemia during PSG, higher educational level, intensity of health-care support and follow-up with problem-solving and reinforcement 1 month or sooner after CPAP initiation[63–67]. Several other factors

Table 8.11   Modifiable factors influencing PAP tolerance and compliance

| Factor | Management strategies |
| --- | --- |
| Mask discomfort | assure proper fit by careful mask design and size selection<br>avoid over-tightening of straps<br>use hypoallergenic mask and strap materials |
| Nasal mucosal irritation | ensure good mask seal; consider need for chin strap or, rarely, full-face mask<br>use humidifier, especially if risk factors for nasal dryness present (see text for details)<br>consider use of topical nasal steroid spray<br>consider topical decongestants<br>optimally manage allergic rhinitis |
| Pressure-related problems | consider use of 'ramp' feature<br>consider use of alternative PAP device, such as bilevel PAP, autotitrating or variable profile PAP |
| Problems related to bed partner and body image | educate both patient and bed partner<br>careful selection of apparatus to meet particular needs |
| Inconvenience | careful selection of apparatus to meet particular needs |
| Claustrophobia | consider use of nasal pillows or smallest possible mask with least intrusive headgear<br>consider desensitization techniques, relaxation training and biofeedback |

PAP, positive airway pressure

may also influence tolerance and compliance (Table 8.11).

Proper fit allows a good air seal without excessive tightening of the harness. Poor fit not only is uncomfortable, but also can lead to pressure sores or focal nasal bridge necrosis. Up to 65% of patients using CPAP report upper airway side-effects, especially dryness or rhinorrhea, and occasionally epistaxis. Many of these patients benefit from the addition of humidity. Two types of humidifiers are available, cold passover humidity and heated humidity. In one study, a humidifier was added for patients unable to tolerate CPAP use owing to mucosal dryness. Cool humidity was sufficient in about 25% of CPAP users, while heated humidity was needed in another 25%. Age > 60 years, use of drying medications, the presence of underlying chronic nasal mucosal diseases and previous uvulopalatolaryngoplasty predicted the need for heated humidity[68]. Heated humidity results in an improvement in compliance[69], and many recommend its use from the start, especially if any identified risk factors are present. Other empirical interventions to minimize nasal irritation include decongestants, topical nasal steroids and room vaporizers, but these measures have not been rigorously evaluated. Oronasal symptoms are occasionally caused by mouth leaks that produce high unidirectional airflow over nasal and oral mucosa; improving mask fit, adding a chin strap or occasionally using a full-face mask can be helpful. Patients with persistent nasal obstruction may require consultation with an otorhinolaryngologist for consideration of corrective surgery.

Paradoxically tolerance and compliance do not usually fall as target CPAP pressures rise[66,70]. On the contrary, inadequate treatment pressure will adversely affect compliance and benefit[71]. Nevertheless, some patients experience difficulty breathing with CPAP, especially during exhalation. The mechanism and frequency of CPAP-induced dyspnea is not well understood. A 'ramp' feature, available on most CPAP units, begins the pressure level low and increases it to the target pressure over 10–20 min, allowing gradual acclimatization and acceptance. If this is not successful, trials of bilevel, autotitrating or variable profile PAP devices may prove helpful. Aerophagia, sinus discomfort and mask leak owing to high pressures are all related primarily to mean airway pressure, which can often be reduced by the use of such devices, all of which appear to be equivalent to CPAP in reducing AHI. Bilevel devices have not been shown to improve actual compliance, but clearly some patients prefer this modality. Autotitrating PAP has been shown to afford better initial acceptance and may result in better initial compliance[72], but long-term studies are not yet available.

Some bed partners complain of the noise from CPAP machines. Noise can be reduced by repositioning the CPAP machine to below the mattress level or even in an adjacent closet, but if non-standard tubing is used one must check calibration, since there will be a loss of pressure along the length of the CPAP tubing. If the CPAP vent blows air towards a bed partner, disrupting their sleep, the vent can be repositioned or a different mask selected. For patients who complain that the straps muss their hair, alternatives in mask and harness types are available, and some devices require no straps at all. The ongoing innovative efforts of manufacturers continue to provide new alternatives to respond to these practical and important challenges, and knowledge of the full range of devices may make all the difference to a given patient.

The prescribing physician must be sensitive to the travel needs of the patient. Some units are smaller and more portable than others, and are thus easier to carry through airports. International travelers require units with an ability to utilize the available power supplies. Overland truck drivers or camping enthusiasts require voltage converters that enable the use of direct-current power from vehicle batteries. Most modern units have automatic altitude adjustment, but some devices may require calibration if the patient travels between sites of widely different isobars of pressure.

PAP is successful in managing the majority of patients with OSAS. Compliance with CPAP has been studied, but the results are somewhat variable between studies owing to different definitions of compliance. In one study using a covert compliance monitor, patients used CPAP for at least 4 h per night on 70% of nights[73]. Other studies confirm that patients can be grouped into generally compliant or non-compliant patients after about 1 month, and that early success is somewhat predictive of long-term success[74]. Most modern PAP units now have built-in compliance monitoring, and download into software that allows a detailed analysis of usage patterns. The long-term effect of having this information available is not known, but it can potentially be valuable in addressing the problem of the patient whose symptoms do not improve after CPAP prescription.

## Case 8.3

A 50-year-old man complaining of excessive sleepiness, loud snoring and morning headaches underwent polysomnography that showed findings of OSAS, with an AHI of 43 (Figure 8.17). His apneas, hypopneas and RERAs were eliminated with a nasal CPAP of 9 cmH$_2$O, and he accepted a prescription for CPAP. At 1-month follow-up, he explained that he was no better, and that he was having mild difficulties with nasal dryness that made him unable to wear CPAP for more than about 3 h at a time. His wife claimed he had no snoring while using the device. A heated humidifier was added, he was asked to return in 1 month and he was asked to bring his machine and mask with him to the next visit. One month later he again complained that he was no better. A download of compliance data from his CPAP machine found that he had applied the device only on the first night that it was in his possession over 2 months ago, and that it had not been turned on since.

After a frank discussion about his real feelings about CPAP, it was evident he did not intend to use it. A surgical referral was made.

When appropriately diagnosed patients with OSAS fail to improve on therapy, the reason is often poor compliance, but may also be insufficient sleep, inadequate control of sleep-disordered breathing with current settings, faulty equipment or a coexisting but unsuspected additional sleep disorder. Compliance meters can be helpful in beginning to understand the problem. If the patient is compliant but still symptomatic, further evaluation is merited. Abnormal overnight oximetry while on treatment may reveal evidence of inadequate treatment. Occasionally, repeat polysomnography on treatment followed by multiple sleep latency testing is required to diagnose concurrent narcolepsy or idiopathic hypersomnia. Empirical treatment of somnolent but compliant patients with modafinil has recently been approved by the US Food and Drug Administration but remains somewhat controversial[75–78].

*What can be done for PAP failure?* Despite the interventions outlined above, some patients cannot be managed with PAP. In these cases, surgical or oral appliance therapy must be considered. At times, the addition of surgical or oral appliance therapy can supplement PAP and result in success. In the most severe cases, consideration of tracheostomy, at least until other surgical correction can be implemented, may be appropriate. In milder cases, the patient may decide that the risks of remaining untreated are preferable to alternative treatments. For such decisions to be truly informed, thorough education relating to the whole range of alternatives and potential consequences is essential.

*Oral appliances*

Oral appliances work by reshaping the oronasopharynx to promote patency despite muscle relaxation. This is accomplished by two general methods: first, holding the tongue forward, and second, repositioning the mandible forward along with the attached tongue, thus increasing the dimension of the airway during sleep. They can be used for primary snoring without a prior sleep study, but if the oral appliance is intended to treat OSAS, a full evaluation as outlined above is necessary prior to referral to a dental or orthodontic practitioner with experience in fashioning these prostheses.

There are currently over 56 devices marketed for snoring, and not all have received Food and Drug Administration approval for treating OSAS. Devices that allow sequential adjustment of the degree of mandibular protrusion appear favorable, since they allow for gradual 'titration' without the need to refashion a device with

each progressive advancement of the mandible. Some of the more commonly used mandibular repositioning devices for OSAS include the Herbst (Orthodontics, State University of New York at Buffalo), the Klearway (Great Lakes Orthodontics, Ltd), the Adjustable PM Positioner (Jonathan A. Parker, DDS) and the Elastic Mandibular Advancement (EMA) device (Frantz Design, Inc). Tongue-retention devices, such as the Tongue-Retaining Device (TRD) (Advanced Medical Equipment) are less commonly used, but have also been shown to be effective in some cases. Other features considered in recent designs include an allowance for lateral mobility to decrease temporomandibular joint discomfort, and vertical mobility to allow for speaking while wearing the device. There is no clear consensus on what features or configurations are most important to treatment success, and in practice, fitting and adjustment are a dynamic process. This highlights the desirability for devices that are inherently adjustable and for skillful dentists and orthodontists with experience in managing OSAS. Table 8.12

**Table 8.12** Advantages and disadvantages of oral appliances compared with positive airway pressure therapy

| *Advantages of oral appliances* | *Disadvantages of oral appliances* |
| --- | --- |
| Very portable | requires follow-up sleep evaluation to ensure efficacy |
| No need for electrical power | requires suitable dentition |
| No nasal discomfort issues | may cause temporomandibular pain or headaches |
| No straps/headgear required | dental migration may preclude ongoing use |
| Less body-image adjustment required | may cost more than PAP therapy |
| Can be used for concurrent treatment of bruxism | |

**Table 8.13** Indications for oral appliance (OA) therapy

| |
|---|
| Snoring |
| Mild to moderate OSAS |
| Alternative therapy for patients who periodically are unable to use CPAP (travel to remote areas without electricity, etc.) |

OSAS, obstructive sleep apnea syndrome; CPAP, continuous positive airway pressure

summarizes advantages and disadvantages of oral appliances compared with PAP therapy.

It is generally accepted that oral appliances can be effective as primary therapy for patients with mild OSAS, and can be considered as an alternative primary therapy for those with moderate OSAS who will not succeed with CPAP (Table 8.13)[79]. More recent studies show some success when used as primary treatment of moderate or even in some cases of severe OSAS[80]. A subjectively successful treatment result can be expected in about 60% of appropriate patients with mild OSAS, and some studies show patient preference for an oral appliance over PAP therapy[81,82]. Several devices produce effective reduction in AHI, while cephalometric and endoscopic studies document increases in airway dimension. However, there are few prospective trials evaluating overall effectiveness, and one must be careful in generalizing the results obtained with one device to the use of another. Studies analyzing compliance with oral appliances so far rely on patient report, since covert objective compliance measures are not yet developed. Until more is known about patient and device

selection, patients who choose oral appliance therapy require careful follow-up, most often including clinical assessment and either polysomnography or portable studies to evaluate efficacy.

Oral appliance use can initially lead to excessive salivation, xerostomia, pain in muscles of mastication and early-morning malocclusion in as many as one-third of patients[83]. Concern exists over long-term effects of oral appliances on dental caries, periodontal disease, the temporomandibular joint and dental migration, but the frequency and significance of these potential complications is unclear. Considering the cumulative costs of fashioning the device, follow-up for adjustment by a dental practitioner and usually a subsequent sleep study, oral appliance is not always less expensive than PAP therapy. However, it deserves full consideration along with the other modalities in therapy for OSAS.

## Treatment of obstructive sleep apnea syndrome: surgical procedures

Surgical management for OSAS falls into three categories:

(1) Bypass the site of obstruction (e.g. tracheostomy);

(2) Modify the site of obstruction;

(3) Treat OSAS indirectly (e.g. bariatric surgery).

Tracheostomy was the initial therapy for severe OSAS and remains completely successful in eliminating obstruction[84–86]. However, acceptance of tracheostomy is difficult for many, and in most cases, less invasive treatments achieve therapeutic goals. Tracheostomy is reserved for a limited

**Table 8.14** Surgical management for obstructive sleep apnea syndrome

| Goal of procedure | Procedures | | |
|---|---|---|---|
| Bypass all obstructions | tracheostomy | | |
| Modify site of obstruction | *phase I procedures* | | |
| | Fujita type* | Obstruction location | Surgical procedure |
| | 1 | palatal abnormality (tongue normal) | UPPP adenotonsillectomy (more often useful in children) |
| | 2 | palate and base of tongue abnormal | UPPP + GAHM, or UPPP + TCRF |
| | 3 | base of tongue abnormal (palate normal) | GAHM TCRF |
| | *phase II procedure* maxillomandibular advancement (MMA) | | |
| Indirect surgical treatment | bariatric surgery | | |

*Fujita types of anatomical abnormality (see text)[87]; UPPP, uvulopalatopharyngoplasty; GAHM, genioglossus advancement and hyoid myotomy; TCRF, temperature-controlled radiofrequency tongue-base reduction

number of applications, usually when other treatments have failed or are not applicable.

Most surgical management for OSAS seeks first to identify the site or sites of anatomical obstruction, and then use staged procedures to attempt correction of the abnormalities, with phase I procedures addressing soft tissues, and if needed, phase II procedures modifying the maxillo-mandibular skeletal structures that support the soft tissues (Table 8.14, Figure 8.19).

Preoperative evaluation of the upper airway anatomy involves careful inspection, fiberoptic nasopharyngolaryngoscopy and at times various imaging modalities. Lateral cephalometric radiographs are most commonly used, and provide views of soft tissue and bony configuration. Other methods to image the upper airway include magnetic resonance imaging (MRI), volumetric computed tomography (CT) scans and cine studies. Acoustic techniques have also been promoted to map out the airway dimensions. Imaging techniques have provided insight into airway physiology, but there is not unanimity in their clinical utility. Limitations to their interpretation include that the techniques are performed mostly in awake and sometimes upright patients, and that there is poor correlation between imaging results and surgical outcomes[89–92].

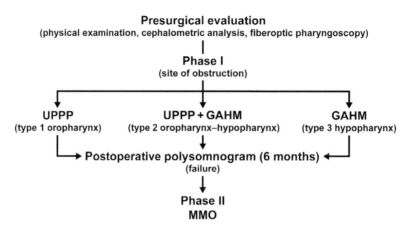

## Surgical protocol

**Presurgical evaluation**
(physical examination, cephalometric analysis, fiberoptic pharyngoscopy)

**Phase I**
(site of obstruction)

**UPPP**
(type 1 oropharynx)

**UPPP + GAHM**
(type 2 oropharynx–hypopharynx)

**GAHM**
(type 3 hypopharynx)

→ Postoperative polysomnogram (6 months) ←
(failure)

**Phase II**
**MMO**

**Figure 8.19**  Staged approach for surgical management of obstructive sleep apnea syndrome. The staged approach is based upon the site of obstruction (types according to Fujita, see text), as determined after careful clinical evaluation. UPPP, uvulopalatopharyngoplasty; GAHM, genioglossus advancement with hyoid myotomy; MMO, maxillomandibular advancement osteotomy. Reproduced from reference 88

Nasal reconstruction is performed when nasal patency influences the ability to comply with PAP therapy, or when obstruction contributes to overall airway obstruction. Septoplasty, polypectomy and turbinate reduction can contribute to improved nasal patency. More recently, temperature-controlled radiofrequency reduction has been used to reduce turbinate size in a less invasive manner. While nasal surgery alone improves the subjective quality of sleep in patients complaining of nasal obstruction, it does not materially affect AHI or desaturation indexes in patients with OSAS, and is rarely effective sole therapy.

Fujita has proposed a classification system to describe the site of anatomical narrowing or abnormality below the nose, with type 1 being exclusively retropalatal, type 2 being a combination of retropalatal and retrolingual and type 3 being exclusively retrolingual (Table 8.14, Figure 8.19)[93]. For example, in Fujita type 1 abnormalities, most surgeons would anticipate that a uvulopalatopharyngoplasty (UPPP) or a UPPP combined with tonsillectomy might be effective. For Fujita type 3 narrowing or collapse, mandibular osteotomy with genioglossus advancement with hyoid myotomy (GAHM) is usually performed. In a Fujita type 2 abnormality, combined UPPP and

GAHM are typically employed. Other procedures may be added to enhance anatomical modification as the surgeon feels is indicated.

Several less invasive approaches to site-specific surgeries have been proposed. Laser-assisted uvuloplasty (LAUP) is aimed at type 1 abnormalities, and was introduced as an office-based procedure for snoring. Studies evaluating the application of LAUP to patients with OSAS have been methodologically flawed, and at present, LAUP does not appear to be effective for OSAS[94,95]. Temperature-controlled radiofrequency tongue-base reduction (TCRF) is another out-patient procedure that strives to achieve reduction of soft tissue size and improve airway patency. This is achieved by creating controlled tissue injury with a special radiofrequency probe inserted into the base of the tongue. Thermal energy is limited to a small area, resulting in tissue injury, interstitial edema and focal hemorrhage within 24 h of treatment. Subsequent fibrotic healing and scar retraction results in reduced tissue mass and volume. Similar applications are being attempted with the soft palate ('somnoplasty'). Efficacy in patients with OSAS is not yet clarified, but initial results suggest that the procedure can be as effective as some more invasive procedures.

Phase I procedures inevitably result in tissue loss, local edema and subsequent healing with scar formation. The immediate

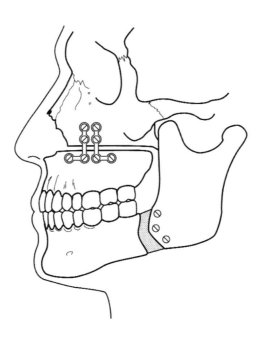

**Figure 8.20** Maxillomandibular advancement for treatment of obstructive sleep apnea syndrome. This diagram shows a Lefort I maxillary osteotomy and sagittal split mandibular osteotomy. The mandible is advanced at least 10 mm, and because of the maxillary advancement, occlusion is preserved. Modified from reference 96 with permission

postoperative period finds the patient at increased risk for respiratory compromise. Patients are best served if they can be acclimatized and treated with PAP treatments prior to surgery, and then use PAP postoperatively until repeat PSG demonstrates resolution of OSAS. Most of the healing will be accomplished by 2–4 months, but many surgeons prefer the patient to wait for 6 months before evaluating success with PSG.

If phase I surgeries are not successful in curing the patient of OSAS, phase II involves maxillomandibular advancement (MMA) (Figure 8.20). Forward movement of the mandible mimics the effect of the 'jaw thrust' maneuver of basic airway protection, opening the retrolingual space and relieving hypopharyngeal obstruction. The maxilla is advanced to preserve bite, improve facial appearance and reduce stress on the temporomandibular joint. Advancement is often greater than 10 mm from the originating position. Often, optimal results require the co-operation of an otorhinolaryngologist, maxillofacial surgeon and orthodontist.

Complications related to the phased protocol may include pain, bleeding, infection, palatal stenosis, paresthesia, nasal speech, mild loss of taste and nasal reflux.

The success of surgical interventions is difficult to predict. Older surgical literature defined 'success' as a reduction of the postoperative AHI to less than 20/h or a 50% reduction compared with the preoperative level, or combinations of such criteria. Unfortunately, by current standards, many treated patients would be considered to be still suffering from OSAS. One group reported results using 50% reduction in AHI *and* AHI less than 20 as criteria for success (Table 8.15). More recent literature is using a goal AHI such as 10 or 15, and often includes an additional parameter such as improvement in sleepiness, snoring and quality of life. Given these limitations, the reported success rate of phase I surgeries averages around 50–60% initially, and may decrease with time or weight gain[86,98]. The addition of phase II usually results in over

**Table 8.15** Success* of phased surgical approach in treatment of obstructive sleep apnea syndrome (OSAS). Adapted from reference 97

| Surgical therapy | | Total success*/total patients | Success* rate (%) |
|---|---|---|---|
| Phase I | GAHM + UPPP | 133/223 | 60 |
| | GAHM | 4/6 | 66 |
| | UPPP | 8/10 | 80 |
| | Total | 145/239 | 61 |
| Phase II (after phase I) | MMO | 24/24 | 100 |

*Success defined as postoperative apnea–hypopnea index (AHI) reduced to less than 20 *and* a 50% reduction compared with preoperative AHI measured 6 months after surgery; GAHM, genioglossus advancement and hyoid myotomy; UPPP, uvulopalatopharyngoplasty; MMO, maxillomandibular advancement osteotomy

90% treatment success. However, not all patients agree to MMA.

Some surgical therapy indirectly improves OSAS. Bariatric surgery for medically complicated obesity can result in dramatic weight loss. There is often a concurrent reduction in AHI, and many patients are at least transiently 'cured' of their OSAS. Unfortunately, OSAS appears to return in many of these patients, at times in the absence of significant weight gain. Rarely, an enlarged thyroid gland or even a neoplastic growth will impinge on the upper airway, and surgical therapy can improve or cure the resultant OSAS.

A surgical cure to OSAS ensures compliance, and is desirable because of the freedom from apparatus it affords the patient. At present, however, surgical treatment success is difficult to predict unless the patient is willing to follow through with potentially extensive surgery and follow-up. Because of the complexities involved, all alternatives, medical, PAP and surgical must be explained and considered prior to selecting a given patient's treatment.

## Treatment of central sleep apnea syndrome

Therapy for CSA/CSR begins with attempts to improve any underlying condition. For example, aggressive management of CHF improves sleep-disordered breathing[99]. With recovery from stroke, CSA/CSR is reduced. However, when CSA/CSR persists or contributes to the underlying disorder, additional therapeutic options include pharmacological, supplemental gases and PAP modalities.

*Pharmacological treatment*

Pharmacological agents studied for treatment of CSA/CSR include acetazolamide, theophylline and benzodiazepines. Acetazolamide is a carbonic anhydrase inhibitor that causes a mild metabolic acidosis. This results in an increase in respiratory drive, even while asleep. Usually, providing a single dose of 250 mg prior to bedtime minimizes the side-effects of paresthesias, anorexia and metallic taste. In one study, this dose led to a progressive significant decline over 1 month from an initial central AHI of $25.5 \pm 6.8$ to $6.8 \pm 2.8$ along with a concurrent improvement in sleep[100]. Higher doses, up to 250 mg four times daily, have been used, especially in cases of high altitude-related central sleep apnea, but many patients suffer side-effects.

Theophylline appears to act as a non-specific ventilatory stimulant in some patients, and in one small randomized, placebo-controlled study improved CSA/CSR[101]. In this trial, stable patients thought to be on optimal CHF therapy were treated with theophylline and oxygen, or placebo. In the treatment group, repeat PSG showed improvement in sleep quality and a significant reduction in the central AHI from $26 \pm 20$ to $6 \pm 14$. It was difficult to determine how much oxygen contributed to this result. Other trials have found theophylline of modest help in patients with idiopathic CSA or CSR. Many remain concerned over the adverse effects of theophylline on sleep and gastroesophageal reflux, and its relatively narrow therapeutic window.

Benzodiazepines may improve the AHI in CSA/CSR and improve sleep quality[102,103]. In one prospective trial, triazolam in doses of 0.125 mg and 0.25 mg at bedtime improved sleep quality, reduced central apnea frequency and improved daytime function[102]. Possible mechanisms include raising the arousal threshold or increasing $PaCO_2$ by mild respiratory drive depression. One cautionary concern is that concurrent obst-ructive breathing events may worsen with benzodiazepine use. There are no data yet regarding the effect of pyrolone-derivative hypnotic drugs such as zolpidem on CSA/ CSR. In non-snoring patients with mild idiopathic CSA/CSR, a trial of a short- or moderately long-acting benzodiazepine such as triazolam or temazepam may be appropriate. As with all pharmacological management, close follow-up is needed to assess efficacy.

### Supplemental gases in treatment of CSA/CSR

Supplemental $CO_2$ is effective in eliminat-ing CSA/CSR in some patients, but it is not readily available for therapeutic use. Oxygen on the other hand is often helpful in reducing AHI and oxyhemoglobin satura-tion nadir in patients with idiopathic CSA, and with CSA/CSR associated with heart failure. In one study, 20 patients with CSA/CSR were studied first without and then with oxygen[104] sufficient to eliminate desat-uration events on oximetry. On retesting, CSA/CSR was reduced in all patients, but total sleep time, sleep efficiency, awakening frequency and sleep architecture did not improve. After 3 months on oxygen, subjec-tive ratings of sleep quality and daytime alertness improved. In another prospective study of patients with stable heart failure treated with oxygen at flows of 2–4 l/min, the AHI was reduced by 41%, but the frequency of obstructive events and arrhythmias did not change[105].

Response to oxygen therapy is not consis-tent in all reports. Even when oxygen reduces the central apnea rate and periodic breathing time, some patients continue to have impaired sleep[106]. Oxygen therapy appears most likely to be of benefit in eucap-nic patients, is less likely to be of much help in hypocapnic patients and should be avoided in unsupervised situations in hyper-capnic patients. When oxygen is helpful, it not only improves sleep, but may also improve exercise tolerance and cognitive function[107]. Oxygen is easily tolerated and often provides a practical treatment option. A common error in trying oxygen therapy is that use of too low flow rates, less than 2 l/min, via nasal cannula is not always effec-tive, and higher flows are often necessary. Whether treatment of CSA/CSR with oxygen results in improvement of mortality remains unknown.

### Positive airway pressure therapy for CSA/CSR

PAP therapies evaluated in patients with CSA/CSR include CPAP, bilevel PAP, non-invasive positive pressure ventilation (NIPPV) and novel forms of regulated venti-lators. CPAP has been noted to be beneficial in patients with acute and chronic decom-pensated congestive heart failure[108]. Mech-anisms probably include afterload reduction, improvement in respiratory function by reducing airway resistance and augmenting inspiratory muscle function, increase in functional residual volume and reducing physiological shunt. Several studies now show that use of CPAP in patients with CSA/CSR and CHF over time results in improvement in AHI, improvement in nocturnal oxygen and symptoms and im-provement in left ventricular ejection fraction[25,108]. The $PaCO_2$ tends to increase, and there is a reduction in sympathetic activity and mitral regurgitant fraction. These effects are often not apparent during one night of CPAP titration, and may not be measurable for many weeks. Thus, other than ensuring elimination of obstructive events, there is no widely accepted protocol for CPAP titration in patients with CSA/CSR. Beyond eliminating obstruction, we titrate to tolerance, striving for levels of 8–12 $cmH_2O$, and assess progress in 2–3 months. Often oximetry and clinical enquiry is sufficient to evaluate treatment tolerance and efficacy. A large prospective trial to determine whether CPAP im-proves mortality in patients with CHF and CSA/CSR is currently under way.

NIPPV, usually delivered as bilevel PAP via nasal mask with spontaneous-timed (ST) mode, is very effective in improving AHI. In one prospective, randomized study, oxygen, CPAP, NIPPV and adaptive servoventilation (ASV) were compared. ASV, not currently available commercially, is a novel form of PAP where inspiratory assistance is varied from breath to breath to dampen variations in minute ventilation from the mean minute ventilation. This smooths the hypopnea/hyperpnea cycling of CSA/CSR. All four treatments lowered AHI[109], but NIPPV and ASV were more effective than oxygen or CPAP, both in lowering AHI and in improving sleep parameters. However, NIPPV can be used if oxygen or CPAP is not sufficient, and may be a preferable choice since it is often more effective and less expensive than domiciliary oxygen. Like CPAP, titration of NIPPV is somewhat empirical. The EPAP level is set to eliminate any obstructive events if present, and the IPAP is often gradually increased as tolerated to 6–8 $cmH_2O$

above EPAP. Most often this will result in EPAP at around 5–7 $cmH_2O$ and the IPAP at 11–15 $cmH_2O$. Ventilation rate is usually set to be 1–2 breaths per minute less than the patient's spontaneous awake respiratory rate. If NIPPV is more effective than $O_2$ during a PSG, it is often well tolerated by patients, who appreciate improvements in subjective quality of sleep more quickly than when using CPAP.

*Approach to the patient with CSA/CSR*

Patients with underlying disorders that perpetuate CSA/CSR should be aggressively treated. If additional therapy is thought to be desirable, owing to sleep complaints, desaturation or concerns about the contribution of CSA/CSR to morbidity and mortality, then one should proceed with polysomnography. Often the PSG is designed with a diagnostic phase, and then with intervals for therapeutic trials of $O_2$, CPAP or NIPPV. Usually there is only time for one or two diagnostic trials in a given night, so repeat polysomnography may be necessary if the question regarding best therapy is unresolved. Pharmacological therapy, if used, may be added synchronously with or sequentially prior to PAP or gas modalities. Whichever treatments are used, follow-up with clinical inquiry and either oximetry or PSG is important to determine treatment success.

## SLEEP APNEA IN HOSPITALIZED PATIENTS

Postoperative episodic hypoxemia during sleep is common, and has been considered a risk factor for myocardial ischemia and cardiac arrhythmias[110]. Supplemental oxygen of up to 37% improves the mean oxyhemoglobin saturation but not the frequency or depth of desaturation events in patients following total hip arthroplasty[111]. Perhaps this is because most of the significant episodic desaturation events are associated with obstructive apneas and hypopneas, and are worsened by use of narcotic analgesia, which further reduces upper airway tone and increases the arousal threshold to hypoxemia[112]. Sleep-disordered breathing may be common even in young and otherwise healthy postoperative patients. A study evaluating breathing patterns in 30 otherwise healthy postoperative general surgery patients on room air with an average BMI of 24.4 found an average AHI of 12 with an average minimum oxygen saturation of 80%[113]. Neither history of snoring nor the type of anesthesia used correlated with breathing events. Sleep-disordered breathing is more common in obese patients postoperatively.

The largest study examining the effects of OSAS on postoperative outcome retrospectively compared 101 patients with OSAS with 101 matched control patients undergoing total joint surgery. Complications were significantly different in the OSAS patients (39%), compared with the control group, (18%)[114]. Serious complications occurred in 24% of cases versus 9% of the control group, and hospital stay was longer in patients with OSAS than in controls. Those who habitually used CPAP preoperatively experienced similar outcomes to the control group. Smaller retrospective studies have not found a consistent relationship between OSAS and hospital complications or mortality, but this remains an area of grave concern in intra- and postoperative management.

Critically ill patients have severely fragmented sleep, and even when ventilated, sleep-disordered breathing can contribute to arousals and abnormal sleep architecture. Patients ventilated with pressure-support modalities may develop central sleep apnea with sleep fragmentation. This is thought to occur because augmentation of tidal volume amplifies ventilatory overshoot following an apneic episode, decreasing the $PaCO_2$, and thus causing the subsequent apnea. In one study of ventilated patients, changing to an assist-control ventilator mode improved CSA/CSR and sleep[115]. Since arousals from apneic events are known to cause sympathetic activation and hemodynamic changes, some hypothesize that targeting measures that improve sleep in acutely ill patients will result not only in more rested patients, but also in improved outcomes.

Many patients hospitalized with stroke, acute myocardial and cerebral ischemic events and congestive heart failure develop, or are newly noted to have sleep apnea syndromes. The effect of sleep apneas on recovery from acute illness is not known, but it is reasonable to assume that their presence is adverse, and it seems prudent to treat significant and identified apnea syndromes. For non-ventilated patients, evaluation and treatment may prove extremely challenging. Sleep studies in acutely ill patients routinely reveal highly fragmented and restricted sleep, with an average of 4–5 h sleep per 24-h period, and only about 50% of sleep occurring at night. Such studies are rarely of high diagnostic quality, and the patient, who is usually focusing on other issues and may have difficulty accepting a PAP mask and pressure, often resists initiating PAP therapy. One strategy is to provide empirical PAP during recovery, and then to arrange a PSG when the patient is less ill or recovered. Autotitrating PAP may be a reasonable choice for patients with suspected OSAS, but should not be attempted if CSA/CSR is thought probable[116]. Empirical choice of CPAP or bilevel PAP or use of APAP is appealing, but there are no data to show that this is effective in the long run. Patients who have a bad initial CPAP experience while ill may be reluctant to accept long-term PAP therapy after recovery.

Patients who are known, or who are suspected, to have OSAS ideally will be allowed 2 or more weeks of appropriate PAP therapy prior to any planned surgical procedures, and PAP will be a planned part of postoperative care. In patients with severe OSAS or observed deep desaturations, close observation in a monitoring unit and anesthetic and pain management approaches that minimize narcotic or respiratory depressant use are appropriate.

## REFERENCES

1. Sleep-related breathing disorders in adults: recommendations for syndrome definition and measurement techniques in clinical research. The report of an American Academy of Sleep Medicine Task Force. *Sleep* 1999;22:667–89

2. Douglas NJ, White DP, Pickett CK, Weil JV, Zwillich CW. Respiration during sleep in normal man. *Thorax* 1982;37:840–4

3. Berger AJ, Mitchell RA, Severinghaus JW. Regulation of respiration [First of three parts]. *N Engl J Med* 1977;297:92–7

4. Douglas NJ. Control of ventilation during sleep. *Clin Chest Med* 1985;6:563–75

5. Berthon-Jones M, Sullivan CE. Ventilation and arousal responses to hypercapnia in normal sleeping humans. *J Appl Physiol* 1984;57:59–67

6. Bowes G, Townsend ER, Bromley SM, Kozar LF, Phillipson EA. Role of the carotid body and of afferent vagal stimuli in the arousal response to airway occlusion in sleeping dogs. *Am Rev Respir Dis* 1981;123:644–7

7. Gold AR, Schwartz AR. The pharyngeal critical pressure. The whys and hows of using nasal continuous positive airway pressure diagnostically. *Chest* 1996;110:1077–88

8. Schwartz AR, Smith PL, Wise RA, Gold AR, Permutt S. Induction of upper airway occlusion in sleeping individuals with subatmospheric nasal pressure. *J Appl Physiol* 1988; 64:535–42

9. Gold AR, Marcus CL, Dipalo F, Gold MS. Upper airway collapsibility during sleep in upper airway resistance syndrome. *Chest* 2002;121:1531–40

10. Beninati W, Harris CD, Herold DL, Shepard JW Jr. The effect of snoring and obstructive sleep apnea on the sleep quality of bed partners. *Mayo Clin Proc* 1999; 74:955–8

11. Wilson K, Stoohs RA, Mulrooney TF, Johnson LJ, Guilleminault C, Huang Z. The snoring spectrum: acoustic assessment of snoring sound intensity in 1139 individuals undergoing polysomnography. *Chest* 1999; 115:762–70

12. Young T, Finn L, Kim H. Nasal obstruction as a risk factor for sleep-disordered breathing. The University of Wisconsin Sleep and Respiratory Research Group. *J Allergy Clin Immunol* 1997;99:S757–62

13. Kinsman TA, Hahn AG, Gore CJ, Wilsmore BR, Martin DT, Chow C-M. Respiratory events and periodic breathing in cyclists

sleeping at 2650-m simulated altitude. *J Appl Physiol* 2002;92:2114–18

14. Guilleminault C, Tilkian A, Dement WC. The sleep apnea syndromes. *Annu Rev Med* 1976;27:465–84

15. Roehrs T, Zorick F, Wittig R, Conway W, Roth T. Predictors of objective level of daytime sleepiness in patients with sleep-related breathing disorders. *Chest* 1989; 95:1202–6

16. Mathur R, Douglas NJ. Frequency of EEG arousals from nocturnal sleep in normal subjects. *Sleep* 1995;18:330–3

17. Young T, Palta M, Dempsey J, Skatrud J, Weber S, Badr S. The occurrence of sleep-disordered breathing among middle-aged adults. *N Engl J Med* 1993;328:1230–5

18. Shahar E, Whitney CW, Redline S, *et al.* Sleep-disordered breathing and cardiovascular disease: cross-sectional results of the Sleep Heart Health Study. *Am J Respir Crit Care Med* 2001;163:19–25

19. Tunis S, Shuren J, Spencer FC, Sheridan J. *Continuous Positive Airway Pressure (CPAP) Therapy Used in the Treatment of Obstructive Sleep Apnea (OSA)* (CAG-00093R), Vol 2001. Baltimore, MD: Centers for Medicare and Medicaid Services (CMS), 2001

20. Young T, Peppard PE, Gottlieb DJ. Epidemiology of obstructive sleep apnea: a population health perspective. *Am J Respir Crit Care Med* 2002;165:1217–39

21. Leung RS, Bradley TD. Sleep apnea and cardiovascular disease. *Am J Respir Crit Care Med* 2001;164:2147–65

22. Tremel F, Pepin JL, Veale D, *et al.* High prevalence and persistence of sleep apnoea in patients referred for acute left ventricular failure and medically treated over 2 months. *Eur Heart J* 1999;20:1201–9

23. Javaheri S, Parker TJ, Liming JD, *et al.* Sleep apnea in 81 ambulatory male patients with stable heart failure. Types and their prevalences, consequences, and presentations. *Circulation* 1998;97:2154–9

24. Sin DD, Fitzgerald F, Parker JD, Newton G, Floras JS, Bradley TD. Risk factors for central and obstructive sleep apnea in 450 men and women with congestive heart failure. *Am J Respir Crit Care Med* 1999; 160:1101–6

25. Sin DD, Logan AG, Fitzgerald FS, Liu PP, Bradley TD. Effects of continuous positive airway pressure on cardiovascular outcomes in heart failure patients with and without Cheyne–Stokes respiration. *Circulation* 2000; 102:61–6

26. Turkington PM, Bamford J, Wanklyn P, Elliott MW. Prevalence and predictors of upper airway obstruction in the first 24 hours after acute stroke. *Stroke* 2002; 33:2037–42

27. Harbison J, Ford GA, James OF, Gibson GJ. Sleep-disordered breathing following acute stroke. *Q J Med* 2002;95:741–7

28. Hui DS, Choy DK, Wong LK, *et al.* Prevalence of sleep-disordered breathing and continuous positive airway pressure compliance: results in Chinese patients with first-ever ischemic stroke. *Chest* 2002; 122:852–60

29. Moruzzi P, Sarzi-Braga S, Rossi M, Contini M. Sleep apnoea in ischaemic heart disease: differences between acute and chronic coronary syndromes. *Heart* 1999;82:343–7

30. Strohl KP, Redline S. Recognition of obstructive sleep apnea. *Am J Respir Crit Care Med* 1996;154:279–89

31. Loh NK, Dinner DS, Foldvary N, Skobieranda F, Yew WW. Do patients with obstructive sleep

apnea wake up with headaches? *Arch Intern Med* 1999;159:1765–8

32. Hajduk IA, Strollo PJ Jr, Jasani RR, Atwood CW Jr, Houck PR, Sanders MH. Prevalence and predictors of nocturia in obstructive sleep apnea–hypopnea syndrome – a retrospective study. *Sleep* 2003;26:61–4

33. Pressman MR, Figueroa WG, Kendrick-Mohamed J, Greenspon LW, Peterson DD. Nocturia. A rarely recognized symptom of sleep apnea and other occult sleep disorders. *Arch Intern Med* 1996;156:545–50

34. Hirshkowitz M, Karacan I, Gurakar A, Williams RL. Hypertension, erectile dysfunction, and occult sleep apnea. *Sleep* 1989;12:223–32

35. Fanfulla F, Malaguti S, Montagna T, *et al.* Erectile dysfunction in men with obstructive sleep apnea: an early sign of nerve involvement. *Sleep* 2000;23:775–81

36. Exar EN, Collop NA. The upper airway resistance syndrome. *Chest* 1999;115:1127–39

37. Schellenberg JB, Maislin G, Schwab RJ. Physical findings and the risk for obstructive sleep apnea. The importance of oropharyngeal structures. *Am J Respir Crit Care Med* 2000;162:740–8

38. Rowley JA, Aboussouan LS, Badr MS. The use of clinical prediction formulas in the evaluation of obstructive sleep apnea. *Sleep* 2000;23:929–38

39. Flemons WW, Whitelaw WA, Brant R, Remmers JE. Likelihood ratios for a sleep apnea clinical prediction rule. *Am J Respir Crit Care Med* 1994;150:1279–85

40. Littner M. Polysomnography in the diagnosis of the obstructive sleep apnea–hypopnea syndrome: where do we draw the line? *Chest* 2000;118:286–8

41. Le Bon O, Hoffmann G, Tecco J, *et al.* Mild to moderate sleep respiratory events: one negative night may not be enough. *Chest* 2000;118:353–9

42. Chesson AL Jr, Ferber RA, Fry JM, *et al.* The indications for polysomnography and related procedures. *Sleep* 1997;20:423–87

43. Shepard JW Jr. Hypertension, cardiac arrhythmias, myocardial infarction, and stroke in relation to obstructive sleep apnea. *Clin Chest Med* 1992;13:437–58

44. Guilleminault C, Stoohs R, Clerk A, Cetel M, Maistros P. A cause of excessive daytime sleepiness. The upper airway resistance syndrome. *Chest* 1993;104:781–7

45. Portier F, Portmann A, Czernichow P, *et al.* Evaluation of home versus laboratory polysomnography in the diagnosis of sleep apnea syndrome. *Am J Respir Crit Care Med* 2000;162:814–18

46. Golpe R, Jimenez A, Carpizo R. Home sleep studies in the assessment of sleep apnea/hypopnea syndrome. *Chest* 2002;122:1156–61

47. Practice parameters for the use of portable recording in the assessment of obstructive sleep apnea. Standards of Practice Committee of the American Sleep Disorders Association. *Sleep* 1994;17:372–7

48. Williams AJ, Yu G, Santiago S, Stein M. Screening for sleep apnea using pulse oximetry and a clinical score. *Chest* 1991;100:631–5

49. Ryan PJ, Hilton MF, Boldy DA, *et al.* Validation of British Thoracic Society guidelines for the diagnosis of the sleep apnoea/hypopnoea syndrome: can polysomnography be avoided? *Thorax* 1995;50:972–5

50. Levy P, Pepin JL, Deschaux-Blanc C, Paramelle B, Brambilla C. Accuracy of

oximetry for detection of respiratory disturbances in sleep apnea syndrome. *Chest* 1996;109:395–9

51. Schafer H, Ewig S, Hasper E, Luderitz B. Predictive diagnostic value of clinical assessment and nonlaboratory monitoring system recordings in patients with symptoms suggestive of obstructive sleep apnea syndrome. *Respiration* 1997;64:194–9

52. Olson LG, Ambrogetti A, Gyulay SG. Prediction of sleep-disordered breathing by unattended overnight oximetry. *J Sleep Res* 1999;8:51–5

53. Golpe R, Jimenez A, Carpizo R, Cifrian JM. Utility of home oximetry as a screening test for patients with moderate to severe symptoms of obstructive sleep apnea. *Sleep* 1999;22:932–7

54. Vazquez JC, Tsai WH, Flemons WW, *et al.* Automated analysis of digital oximetry in the diagnosis of obstructive sleep apnoea. *Thorax* 2000;55:302–7

55. Davila DG, Richards KC, Marshall BL, *et al.* Oximeter performance: the influence of acquisition parameters. *Chest* 2002;122:1654–60

56. Peppard PE, Young T, Palta M, Dempsey J, Skatrud J. Longitudinal study of moderate weight change and sleep-disordered breathing. *J Am Med Assoc* 2000;284:3015–21

57. Jokic R, Klimaszewski A, Crossley M, Sridhar G, Fitzpatrick MF. Positional treatment vs continuous positive airway pressure in patients with positional obstructive sleep apnea syndrome. *Chest* 1999;115:771–81

58. Hudgel DW, Thanakitcharu S. Pharmacologic treatment of sleep-disordered breathing. *Am J Respir Crit Care Med* 1998;158:691–9

59. Sullivan CE, Issa FG, Berthon-Jones M, Eves L. Reversal of obstructive sleep apnoea by continuous positive airway pressure applied through the nares. *Lancet* 1981;1:862–5

60. Tousignant P, Cosio MG, Levy RD, Groome PA. Quality adjusted life years added by treatment of obstructive sleep apnea. *Sleep* 1994;17:52–60

61. Peker Y, Hedner J, Johansson A, Bende M. Reduced hospitalization with cardiovascular and pulmonary disease in obstructive sleep apnea patients on nasal CPAP treatment. *Sleep* 1997;20:645–53

62. Grunstein RR. Sleep-related breathing disorders. 5. Nasal continuous positive airway pressure treatment for obstructive sleep apnoea. *Thorax* 1995;50:1106–13

63. Chervin RD, Theut S, Bassetti C, Aldrich MS. Compliance with nasal CPAP can be improved by simple interventions. *Sleep* 1997;20:284–9

64. Hoy CJ, Vennelle M, Kingshott RN, Engleman HM, Douglas NJ. Can intensive support improve continuous positive airway pressure use in patients with the sleep apnea/hypopnea syndrome? *Am J Respir Crit Care Med* 1999;159:1096–100

65. McArdle N, Devereux G, Heidarnejad H, Engleman HM, Mackay TW, Douglas NJ. Long-term use of CPAP therapy for sleep apnea/hypopnea syndrome. *Am J Respir Crit Care Med* 1999;159:1108–14

66. Meurice JC, Dore P, Paquereau J, *et al.* Predictive factors of long-term compliance with nasal continuous positive airway pressure treatment in sleep apnea syndrome. *Chest* 1994;105:429–33

67. Sin DD, Mayers I, Man GC, Pawluk L. Long-term compliance rates to continuous positive airway pressure in obstructive sleep apnea: a population-based study. *Chest* 2002;121:430–5

68. Rakotonanahary D, Pelletier-Fleury N, Gagnadoux F, Fleury B. Predictive factors for the need for additional humidification during nasal continuous positive airway pressure therapy. *Chest* 2001;119:460–5

69. Massie CA, Hart RW, Peralez K, Richards GN. Effects of humidification on nasal symptoms and compliance in sleep apnea patients using continuous positive airway pressure. *Chest* 1999;116:403–8

70. Hoffstein V, Viner S, Mateika S, Conway J. Treatment of obstructive sleep apnea with nasal continuous positive airway pressure. Patient compliance, perception of benefits, and side effects. *Am Rev Respir Dis* 1992;145:841–5

71. Meurice JC, Paquereau J, Denjean A, Patte F, Series F. Influence of correction of flow limitation on continuous positive airway pressure efficiency in sleep apnoea/hypopnoea syndrome. *Eur Respir J* 1998;11:1121–7

72. Konermann M, Sanner BM, Vyleta M, *et al.* Use of conventional and self-adjusting nasal continuous positive airway pressure for treatment of severe obstructive sleep apnea syndrome: a comparative study. *Chest* 1998;113:714–18

73. Kribbs NB, Pack AI, Kline LR, *et al.* Objective measurement of patterns of nasal CPAP use by patients with obstructive sleep apnea. *Am Rev Respir Dis* 1993;147:887–95

74. Pepin JL, Krieger J, Rodenstein D, *et al.* Effective compliance during the first 3 months of continuous positive airway pressure. A European prospective study of 121 patients. *Am J Respir Crit Care Med* 1999;160:1124–9

75. Pollak CP. Con: modafinil has no role in management of sleep apnea. *Am J Respir Crit Care Med* 2003;167:106–7

76. Black J. Pro: modafinil has a role in management of sleep apnea. *Am J Respir Crit Care Med* 2003;167:105–6

77. Pack AI, Black JE, Schwartz JR, Matheson JK. Modafinil as adjunct therapy for daytime sleepiness in obstructive sleep apnea. *Am J Respir Crit Care Med* 2001;164:1675–81

78. Arnulf I, Homeyer P, Garma L, Whitelaw WA, Derenne JP. Modafinil in obstructive sleep apnea–hypopnea syndrome: a pilot study in 6 patients. *Respiration* 1997;64:159–61

79. Practice parameters for the treatment of snoring and obstructive sleep apnea with oral appliances. American Sleep Disorders Association. *Sleep* 1995;18:511–13

80. Mehta A, Qian J, Petocz P, Darendeliler MA, Cistulli PA. A randomized, controlled study of a mandibular advancement splint for obstructive sleep apnea. *Am J Respir Crit Care Med* 2001;163:1457–61

81. Ferguson KA, Ono T, Lowe AA, al-Majed S, Love LL, Fleetham JA. A short-term controlled trial of an adjustable oral appliance for the treatment of mild to moderate obstructive sleep apnoea. *Thorax* 1997;52:362–8

82. Ferguson K. Oral appliance therapy for obstructive sleep apnea: finally evidence you can sink your teeth into. *Am J Respir Crit Care Med* 2001;163:1294–5

83. Clark GT, Sohn JW, Hong CN. Treating obstructive sleep apnea and snoring: assessment of an anterior mandibular positioning device. *J Am Dent Assoc* 2000;131:765–71

84. Myatt HM, Croft CB, Kotecha BT, Ruddock J, Mackay IS, Simonds AK. A three-centre prospective pilot study to elucidate the effect of uvulopalatopharyngoplasty on patients with mild obstructive sleep apnoea

due to velopharyngeal obstruction. *Clin Otolaryngol* 1999;24:95–103

85. Hamazoe R, Furumoto T, Kaibara N, Inoue Y. Vertical banded gastroplasty for sleep apnea syndrome associated with morbid obesity. *Obes Surg* 1992;2:271–4

86. Sher AE, Schechtman KB, Piccirillo JF. The efficacy of surgical modifications of the upper airway in adults with obstructive sleep apnea syndrome. *Sleep* 1996;19:156–77

87. Fujita S. Pharyngeal surgery for obstructive sleep apnea and snoring. In Fairbanks D, Fujita S, Ikematsu T, eds. *Snoring and Obstructive Sleep Apnea*. New York: Raven Press, 1987:101–28

88. Riley RW, Powell NB, Guilleminault C, *et al.* Obstructive sleep apnea. Trends in therapy. *WJM* 1995;162:143–8

89. Li KK, Guilleminault C, Riley RW, Powell NB. Obstructive sleep apnea and maxillomandibular advancement: an assessment of airway changes using radiographic and nasopharyngoscopic examinations. *J Oral Maxillofac Surg* 2002;60:526–30, discussion 531

90. Millman RP, Carlisle CC, Rosenberg C, Kahn D, McRae R, Kramer NR. Simple predictors of uvulopalatopharyngoplasty outcome in the treatment of obstructive sleep apnea. *Chest* 2000;118:1025–30

91. Woodson BT. Predicting which patients will benefit from surgery for obstructive sleep apnea: the ENT exam. *Ear Nose Throat J* 1999;78:792–5, 798–800

92. Schwab RJ, Goldberg AN. Upper airway assessment: radiographic and other imaging techniques. *Otolaryngol Clin North Am* 1998;31:931–68

93. Fujita S. Obstructive sleep apnea syndrome: pathophysiology, upper airway evaluation and surgical treatment. *Ear Nose Throat J* 1993;72:67–72, 75–6

94. Ferguson KA, Heighway K, Ruby RR. A randomized trial of laser-assisted uvulopalatoplasty in the treatment of mild obstructive sleep apnea. *Am J Respir Crit Care Med* 2003;167:15–19

95. Littner M, Kushida CA, Hartse K, *et al.* Practice parameters for the use of laser-assisted uvulopalatoplasty: an update for 2000. *Sleep* 2001;24:603–19

96. Fairbanks D, Fujita S. *Snoring and Obstuctive Sleep Apnea Syndrome*. New York: Raven Press, 1994:205

97. Riley RW, Powell NB, Guilleminault C. Obstructive sleep apnea syndrome: a review of 306 consecutively treated surgical patients. *Otolaryngol Head Neck Surg* 1993;108:117–25

98. Practice parameters for the treatment of obstructive sleep apnea in adults: the efficacy of surgical modifications of the upper airway. Report of the American Sleep Disorders Association. *Sleep* 1996;19:152–5

99. Solin P, Bergin P, Richardson M, Kaye DM, Walters EH, Naughton MT. Influence of pulmonary capillary wedge pressure on central apnea in heart failure. *Circulation* 1999;99:1574–9

100. DeBacker W, Verbraecken J, Willemen M, Wittesaele W, DeCock W, Van deHeyning P. Central apnea index decreases after prolonged treatment with acetazolamide. *Am J Respir Crit Care Med* 1995;151:87–91

101. Javaheri S, Parker TJ, Wexler L, Liming JD, Lindower P, Roselle GA. Effect of theophylline on sleep-disordered breathing in heart failure. *N Engl J Med* 1996;335:562–7

102. Bonnet MH, Dexter JR, Arand DL. The effect of triazolam on arousal and respira-

tion in central sleep apnea patients. *Sleep* 1990;13:31–41

103. Hanly P, Powles P. Hypnotics should never be used in patients with sleep apnea. *J Psychosom Res* 1993;37:59–65

104. Franklin KA, Eriksson P, Sahlin C, Lundgren R. Reversal of central sleep apnea with oxygen. *Chest* 1997;111:163–9

105. Javaheri S, Ahmed M, Parker TJ, Brown CR. Effects of nasal $O_2$ on sleep-related disordered breathing in ambulatory patients with stable heart failure. *Sleep* 1999;22:1101–6

106. Staniforth AD, Kinnear WJ, Starling R, Hetmanski DJ, Cowley AJ. Effect of oxygen on sleep quality, cognitive function and sympathetic activity in patients with chronic heart failure and Cheyne–Stokes respiration. *Eur Heart J* 1998;19:922–8

107. Andreas S, Clemens C, Sandholzer H, Figulla HR, Kreuzer H. Improvement of exercise capacity with treatment of Cheyne–Stokes respiration in patients with congestive heart failure. *J Am Coll Cardiol* 1996;27:1486–90

108. Naughton M, Liu P, Bernard D, Goldstein R, Bradley T. Treatment of congestive heart failure and Cheyne–Stokes respiration during sleep by continuous positive airway pressure. *Am J Respir Crit Care Med* 1995;151:92–7

109. Teschler H, Dohring J, Wang YM, Berthon-Jones M. Adaptive pressure support servo-ventilation: a novel treatment for Cheyne–Stokes respiration in heart failure. *Am J Respir Crit Care Med* 2001;164:614–19

110. Rosenberg J, Kehlet H. Postoperative episodic oxygen desaturation in the sleep apnoea syndrome. *Acta Anaesthesiol Scand* 1991;35:368–9

111. Rosenberg J, Pedersen MH, Gebuhr P, Kehlet H. Effect of oxygen therapy on late postoperative episodic and constant hypoxaemia. *Br J Anaesth* 1992;68:18–22

112. Catley DM, Thornton C, Jordan C, Lehane JR, Royston D, Jones JG. Pronounced, episodic oxygen desaturation in the postoperative period: its association with ventilatory pattern and analgesic regimen. *Anesthesiology* 1985;63:20–8

113. Rosenberg J, Rasmussen GI, Wojdemann KR, Kirkeby LT, Jorgensen LN, Kehlet H. Ventilatory pattern and associated episodic hypoxaemia in the late postoperative period in the general surgical ward. *Anaesthesia* 1999;54:323–8

114. Gupta RM, Parvizi J, Hanssen AD, Gay PC. Postoperative complications in patients with obstructive sleep apnea syndrome undergoing hip or knee replacement: a case–control study. *Mayo Clin Proc* 2001;76:897–905

115. Parthasarathy S, Tobin MJ. Effect of ventilator mode on sleep quality in critically ill patients. *Am J Respir Crit Care Med* 2002;166:1423–9

116. Littner M, Hirshkowitz M, Davila D, *et al.* Practice parameters for the use of auto-titrating continuous positive airway pressure devices for titrating pressures and treating adult patients with obstructive sleep apnea syndrome. An American Academy of Sleep Medicine report. *Sleep* 2002;25:143–7

# Chapter 9

# Sleep in patients with respiratory diseases and respiratory failure

*And now I see with eye serene*
*The very pulse of the machine;*
*A being breathing thoughtful breath,*
*A traveller between life and death.*

**William Wordsworth,** *Lost in the Gloom*
*of Uninspired Research*

## RESPIRATORY DISEASE AND SLEEP

During sleep, minute ventilation is reduced and hypercapnic and hypoxic respiratory drive is decreased, especially during rapid eye movement (REM) sleep (Chapter 8). Patients with respiratory disease who are well compensated during waking hours may develop marked hypoxemia or hypercapnia during sleep that may contribute to morbidity and mortality. Thus, sleep can be a challenging time for patients with respiratory disease. Conversely, respiratory diseases adversely affect sleep, causing disruptive symptoms (cough, dyspnea, chest pain, anxiety) and disturbed gas exchange (hypoxemia, hypercapnia). Being aware of how individual respiratory diseases and sleep affect one another can help the physician anticipate the needs of the patient and appropriate therapeutic alternatives.

## RESPIRATORY FAILURE AND NON-INVASIVE POSITIVE PRESSURE VENTILATION

### Respiratory failure

When the respiratory system is unable to maintain adequate oxygenation of the circulating blood or elimination of metabolically produced carbon dioxide, the patient is said to be in respiratory failure. Arterial oxygen tension ($PaO_2$) less than 50 mmHg and arterial carbon dioxide tension ($PaCO_2$) greater than 45 mmHg are generally accepted criteria for the presence of respiratory failure. Acute respiratory failure is usually the result of severe pneumonia, acute respiratory distress syndrome or acute cardiopulmonary disease. In contrast, chronic respiratory failure develops more insidiously, and the patient may not provide symptoms or signs to suggest its presence until it has reached an advanced state. Chronic respiratory failure

**Table 9.1**  Differential diagnosis of respiratory failure

|  | Hypoxemic respiratory failure | Ventilatory respiratory failure |
|---|---|---|
| Acute | acute respiratory distress syndrome<br>acute pulmonary embolism<br>acute pulmonary edema<br>severe pneumonia<br>traumatic chest wall contusion | drugs that depress CNS or respiratory center (e.g. narcotics, alcohol, benzodiazepines, γ-hydroxybutyrate)<br>cervical spinal cord or brain stem injury<br>exacerbation of COPD or asthma<br>acute neuromuscular disease (e.g. Guillain–Barré syndrome)<br>pharmacological or toxic neuromuscular blockade (e.g. organophosphate toxicity, botulism) |
| Chronic | interstitial lung disease (e.g. interstitial pneumonitis, hypersensitivity pneumonitis)<br>arteriovenous or intracardiac shunt bronchiectasis (e.g. cystic fibrosis, post-infectious bronchiectasis)<br>emphysema | chronic obstructive pulmonary disease<br>neuromuscular disease (e.g. amyotrophic lateral sclerosis, myotonic dystrophy, phrenic neuropathies, etc.)<br>kyphoscoliosis<br>obesity hypoventilation syndrome<br>severe obstructive sleep apnea syndrome<br>severe pulmonary fibrosis<br>primary alveolar hypoventilation syndrome |

CNS, central nervous system; COPD, chronic obstructive pulmonary disease

can be anticipated under certain clinical circumstances (e.g. severe chronic obstructive pulmonary disease, pulmonary fibrosis or neuromuscular disease), but at times is apparent only after an arterial blood gas determination is performed.

Respiratory failure may be physiologically divided not only into acute and chronic categories, but also into hypoxemic and ventilatory failure categories (Table 9.1). In hypoxemic respiratory failure, physiological or anatomical shunt leads to inadequate oxygenation of circulating blood with little effect on exchange of carbon dioxide. The result is decreased $PaO_2$ and often compensatory increased ventilatory drive, which results in a relative preservation or even decline of $PaCO_2$. During sleep, increased ventilatory drive may be evident as persistent tachypnea. However, the underlying pulmonary physiology is often such that, during periods of decreased ventilation, for example REM sleep, oxygen desaturation may be more pronounced than at baseline.

In ventilatory failure, reduced central nervous system drive to breathe, neuromuscular dysfunction, altered chest wall mechanics or increased dead space reduces alveolar ventilation. There is a consequent rise in alveolar $CO_2$ and $PaCO_2$, and mild alveolar hypoxia develops, reflecting the inverse relationship between alveolar $PaO_2$ and $PaCO_2$ defined by the alveolar gas equation. Thus, decreased $PaO_2$ and oxygen saturation ($SaO_2$) accompany the increase in $PaCO_2$. Compensation for sustained hypercapnia is relatively slow, taking place over

hours and days, and involves retention of bicarbonate by the kidneys to buffer the elevation in carbonic acid resulting from retained $CO_2$. In chronic ventilatory failure, not only is the serum bicarbonate increased, but a decreased sensitivity to hypercapnia often develops (see below). Gas exchange abnormalities are usually magnified during sleep because of changes in ventilatory drive and mechanical factors (Figure 9.1). The physiological changes of chronic hypo-

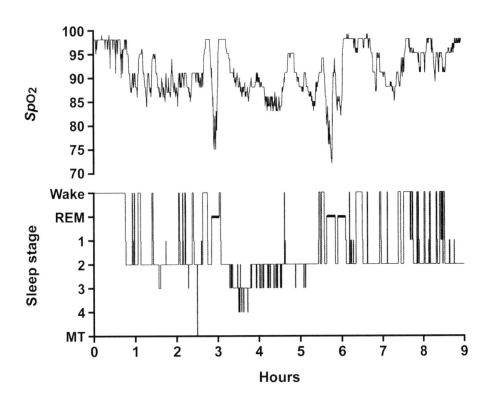

**Figure 9.1** Nocturnal oxygen saturation in a patient with severe chronic obstructive pulmonary disease (COPD). Desaturation begins with drowsiness and is established with non-rapid eye movement (NREM) sleep. More severe desaturation is noted with rapid eye movement (REM) sleep. Also demonstrated is the abnormal sleep architecture, with reduced REM and slow-wave sleep, reduced sleep efficiency, increased awakenings typically noted in patients with COPD and oxygen desaturation. $SaO_2$, oxygen saturation; MT, movement. Reproduced from reference 1

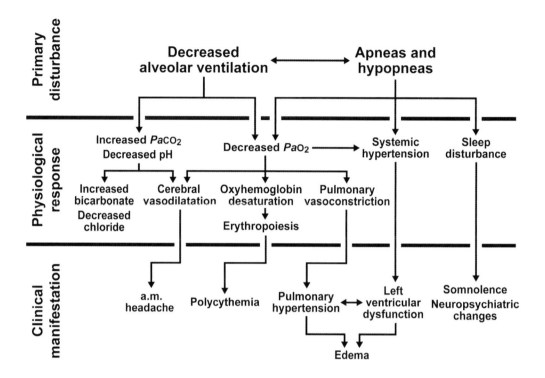

**Figure 9.2** The syndrome of alveolar hypoventilation. Primary disturbances from all etiologies of alveolar hypoventilation lead to the physiological responses noted in the diagram. The clinical manifestations of chronic hypoventilation proceed from these physiological effects and adaptations. $PaCO_2$, arterial $CO_2$ tension; $PaO_2$, arterial $O_2$ tension

ventilation lead to clinical manifestations that are similar, regardless of underlying cause (Figure 9.2).

## Evaluation of chronic ventilatory failure

The laboratory evaluation of patients with chronic alveolar hypoventilation includes various tests to evaluate the components of the respiratory system, including pulmonary function tests, tests of respiratory muscle strength and tests of ventilatory control (Table 9.2).

*Pulmonary function tests*

The ratio of the forced expiratory volume in 1 s ($FEV_1$) to the forced vital capacity (FVC) is greater than 0.7 in the absence of lower airway obstruction. In restrictive disease from whatever cause, there is often a reduction in FVC and a reduction in the total lung

**Table 9.2** Results of tests in chronic alveolar hypoventilation

| Tests | Failure of central respiratory control | Failure of neuromuscular respiratory function* | Abnormalities of thoracic cage or pulmonary disease |
|---|---|---|---|
| $PaCO_2$ | $\uparrow$, or may $\downarrow$ by voluntary hyperventilation | $\uparrow$ | $\uparrow$ |
| Chest X-ray | N or findings of pulmonary hypertension | N or poor expansion or hemidiaphragm elevation | N or abnormal depending on underlying disease |
| Diaphragm fluoroscopy | N | may be abnormal if diaphragm paralysis | N |
| Pulmonary function | N | restriction | abnormal (depends on disease[†]) |
| MIP/MEP, or $P_{di}$[‡] | N | decreased | N |
| EMG | N | abnormal | N |
| $CO_2$ and $O_2$ response | abnormal | N or slightly decreased | N or slightly decreased |
| Polysomnography | disturbed sleep, hypoventilation, central apneas, may be less severe in REM | disturbed sleep, hypoventilation, central or obstructive apneas, much worse in REM | disturbed sleep, hypoventilation worse in REM |

*Respiratory motorneurons, spinal cord, phrenic nerves, muscles; [†]pulmonary function test may show obstruction, restriction, increased or decreased compliance depending on disease; [‡]maximal inspiratory pressure (MIP), maximal expiratory pressure (MEP), transdiaphragmatic pressure ($P_{di}$); $PaCO_2$, arterial $CO_2$ tension; EMG, electromyogram; $\uparrow$, increase; $\downarrow$, decrease; N, normal; REM, rapid eye movement

capacity (TLC), a measurement that requires techniques beyond usual spirometry. Restrictive abnormalities may be seen with neuromuscular weakness, chest wall abnormalities or pulmonary diseases that decrease lung compliance. A disproportionate decline in the peak expiratory flow (PEF) or in the maximum voluntary ventilation (MVV) may provide a clue to neuromuscular weakness, but may alternatively indicate poor co-operation or co-ordination during testing.

*Respiratory muscle testing*

Aggregate respiratory muscle strength may be assessed by measuring the maximum inspiratory pressure (MIP) and maximum expiratory pressure (MEP). It is sensitive, but not always specific, in detecting neuromuscular weakness. Healthy adults most often produce an MIP greater than 100 cmH$_2$O and an MEP greater than 150 cmH$_2$O. Production of less than 50% of normal values usually indicates disease, while MIP less than 15 cmH$_2$O is usually incompatible with adequate ventilation, and MEP less than 40 cmH$_2$O makes coughing and clearance of secretions difficult. With diaphragm weakness or paralysis, MIP is more severely reduced than in generalized neuromuscular weakness. The test relies on patient effort and the ability to provide a seal on the manometer, so either poor effort or mouth co-ordination may result in submaximal measurements.

Measurement of transdiaphragmatic pressure is less effort-dependent, but requires placement of esophageal and gastric pressure manometers. With sniff maneuvers, either under voluntary control or generated by phrenic nerve stimulation, the difference in gastric ($P_{ga}$) and esophageal pressure ($P_{es}$) is measured. The transdiaphragmatic pressure, calculated as the difference between $P_{ga}$ and $P_{es}$, is usually greater than 30 cmH$_2$O, while with diaphragmatic paralysis it is typically $0 \pm 3$ cmH$_2$O[2]. Diaphragm fluoroscopy may also be helpful in detecting diaphragm paralysis. Paradoxical movement of one or both diaphragms with a sniff maneuver usually indicates diaphragm paralysis or severe weakness, but results may occasionally be misleading[3,4].

Phrenic nerve conduction studies and electromyographic needle examination of the diaphragm may provide helpful diagnostic information. Such evaluation can indicate the presence of phrenic neuropathies, as well as systemic neuromuscular diseases, such as amyotrophic lateral sclerosis, myopathies or myasthenia gravis.

### Tests of ventilatory control

A patient's response to hypoxia or hypercapnia may be measured and compared with the normal response curves as an assessment of function of the ventilatory control system (Figure 8.5). When challenged by hypoxia, a normal subject will increase ventilation by 1 l/min for each 1% decrease in oxygen saturation. Superimposed hypercapnia increases the response, while decreased responsiveness is noted with age, in circumstances of chronic hypoxia, such as living for many years at high altitude, and in sleep. The normal ventilatory response to a hypercapnic challenge is 2–5 l/min for each mmHg increase in $Pa$CO$_2$. Hypoxia increases the response, as does anxiety or pain. The response is decreased in sleep, as well as whenever the central respiratory control center is impaired. Chronic exposure to hypercapnia or excessive ventilatory loads may also lead to decreased sensitivity of ventilatory responsiveness to CO$_2$.

The pattern of test results will usually reveal the location of the underlying defect in chronic ventilatory failure (Table 9.2).

The remainder of this chapter discusses the effects of specific causes of respiratory disease and failure and their known effect on sleep, and, where possible, treatment strategies which may be helpful. The principles employed for management of any of the given disorders are often applicable to the care of patients with disorders manifesting similar physiologies.

## Non-invasive positive pressure ventilation

Many forms of chronic respiratory failure are first manifest or worsen during sleep, and thus support of oxygenation and ventilation during sleep has received much attention. The means of providing support may be in the form of nocturnal supplemental oxygen, continuous positive airway presure (CPAP), bilevel positive airway pressure (PAP) or mechanical ventilatory support. With the advent of non-invasive positive pressure ventilation (NIPPV), only rarely are tracheostomy and mechanical ventilation required. NIPPV is also sometimes referred to as bilevel PAP in the spontaneous-timed (ST) mode (see below).

CPAP and bilevel PAP (spontaneous mode) are discussed elsewhere (Chapter 8) and not reviewed here. NIPPV often uses similar patient interfaces, such as nasal or oronasal masks secured with elastic bands. A machine programmed to deliver a set volume of gas (volume control) or a set inflation pressure (pressure control) can provide positive pressure ventilatory assistance. However, volume control devices are usually not well tolerated via a mask interface, so most NIPPV is delivered with pressure control. The actual ventilator devices are similar to a bilevel PAP, cycling between an expiratory and an inspiratory airway pressure, except that the device can deliver a mandatory inspiratory pressure at a set rate. When bilevel PAP is used without the timed back-up rate, it is often said to be in the 'S' or spontaneous mode. To be considered NIPPV, a back-up minimum respiratory rate must be set ('T' or 'ST' mode). When the device delivers an inspiratory pressure at a predetermined rate and duration independent of patient effort, it is set in a timed only, or 'T' mode. Most often, patients are supported with the spontaneous-timed or 'ST' mode, with which each initiated breath is recognized and augmented by the ventilator, but a back-up respiratory rate is also set.

To prescribe NIPPV, one needs to specify the expiratory positive airway pressure (EPAP), the inspiratory positive airway pressure (IPAP), the back-up or mandatory respiratory rate and the inspiratory fraction or supplemental flow of oxygen desired. Typically, the EPAP is set at a minimum of $3–4 \, cmH_2O$ to ensure an adequate wash-out of the nasal or oronasal mask, reducing the tendency for the patient to rebreathe $CO_2$-rich air. If there is evidence for upper airway obstruction on polysomnogram (PSG), EPAP can be adjusted to obtain and maintain upper airway patency. The difference between IPAP and EPAP can be thought of as a 'pressure support' to augment patient-initiated breaths during the S mode, or as a 'pressure control' breath when the device does not detect an inspiratory effort and applies the IPAP to inflate the patient's lungs. The obtained tidal volumes will depend on the patient's effort, the compliance of the respiratory system and the airway resistance, and will vary from breath to breath.

The optimal settings must be individualized to the patient's clinical situation, tolerance and pathophysiology. Most patients can tolerate pressure support of $5 \, cmH_2O$ easily, but acceptance of higher pressures is variable. Titration of NIPPV is done during polysomnography or other direct

**Table 9.3**   Non-invasive positive pressure ventilation (NIPPV) for chronic respiratory failure

| Underlying disease | Effectiveness | Level of evidence* |
|---|---|---|
| COPD | may be effective for selected patients | I, although some variability in RCT |
| Interstitial lung disease | may be effective for selected patients | V |
| Neuromuscular and chest wall disease | effective | III |
| Sleep disordered breathing | CPAP effective, NIPPV may be effective if CPAP fails | II |

*Level I, randomized controlled trials (RCT) with low false-positive and false-negative errors; level II, RCT with high false-positive and false-negative errors; level III, non-randomized, concurrent-cohort comparison; level IV, non-randomized, historical-cohort comparison; level V, case series without control subjects; CPAP, continuous positive airway pressure

monitoring (such as an in-patient ventilatory unit), to determine whether therapeutic goals, such as improved oxygenation, ventilation and sleep quality are achieved. However, some patients adapt to NIPPV slowly, and weeks of follow-up and adjustment are needed to assess success. The effectiveness of NIPPV in chronic respiratory diseases is a subject of ongoing study, and varies with different causes of respiratory failure (Table 9.3)[5].

## OBSTRUCTIVE RESPIRATORY DISEASES

The hallmark of obstructive respiratory diseases is airflow limitation demonstrated by spirometric measurements. Obstructive diseases have reduced expiratory flow rates, often represented by the forced expiratory volume in 1 s ($FEV_1$), that are proportionately greater than any observed decrease in forced expiratory volume (forced vital capacity, FVC). The $FEV_1/FVC$ ratio is less than 0.7. As the degree of airflow obstruction worsens, the $FEV_1$ decreases, and ultimately there may be an inability to expire all inhaled gases completely. The trapped air leads not only to hyperinflation, with increases in total lung capacity (TLC), but also to intrinsic alveolar positive end expiratory pressure (PEEP). The changes brought about by hyperinflation, intrinsic PEEP and increased airway resistance increase the work of breathing by as much as three-fold at rest[6]. The unique changes in posture and respiratory control during sleep commonly interact with obstructive diseases to worsen gas exchange and sleep quality. Asthma, chronic obstructive pulmonary disease (COPD) and cystic fibrosis are the more common examples of obstructive respiratory diseases.

## Asthma

Asthma is characterized by airway inflammation, and is most often accompanied by variable airflow obstruction. This airway inflammation causes recurrent episodes of wheezing, breathlessness, chest tightness and cough. There is a tendency towards bronchoconstriction, resulting from an increased bronchial responsiveness to non-specific respiratory irritants such as histamine, methacholine and adenosine, and at times to specific allergens such as dust mite or cat antigens. Most patients afflicted with asthma preserve or have only mild abnormalities in their pulmonary function when not involved in exacerbations. During severe exacerbations, acute ventilatory failure can develop. Only a very few progress to persistent severe pulmonary function abnormalities; chronic ventilatory failure is not common in asthma.

### Asthma and sleep

Asthma manifestations do not distribute uniformly across the circadian cycle. Many patients with asthma suffer worsening of their symptoms during sleep, particularly during the early hours of the morning. The presence and frequency of nocturnal symptoms are so ubiquitous that they are used to categorize the severity of asthma and degree of control in contemporary asthma treatment guidelines[7]. In one large study, 74% of 7729 patients with asthma symptoms noted nocturnal awakenings at least once per week[8], and patients with asthma report more difficulty initiating and maintaining sleep than those without asthma[9]. Polysomnographic studies have generally demonstrated more arousals and awakenings, decreased total sleep time and decreased sleep efficiency compared with controls[10]. Patients with nocturnal asthma have increased mortality, often have poorer asthma control, and exhibit decreased quality of life compared with those without nocturnal asthma.

Airway resistance, often inferred from peak flow measures, is influenced by circadian factors in both normal subjects and asthmatic patients[11]. Peak flow is highest in the mid- to late afternoon, while the nadir occurs most often close to 4:00 a.m. The circadian variability appears to be more pronounced with age. In normal patients, peak to nadir differences rarely exceed 10%, and those with swings in p.m. to a.m. peak flow of more than 20% are said to have nocturnal asthma (see case 9.1 below).

Many potential mechanisms for the 'nocturnal' or sleep-related worsening of asthma have been suggested (Table 9.4). Some

**Table 9.4** Mechanisms for sleep-related worsening of asthma

| |
|---|
| Airway cooling |
| Allergen exposure (dust, dust mite, pet dander, etc.) |
| Gastroesophageal reflux |
| Decreased plasma epinephrine |
| Decreased plasma cortisol |
| Increased plasma histamine |
| Increased circulating and airway eosinophils |
| Increased cholinergic tone |
| Increased airway resistance caused by mechanical changes of obesity |
| Obstructive sleep apnea syndrome |

studies have suggested that sleep itself is the potent trigger for airway narrowing, noting that shift workers exhibit rapid inversion of resistance cycle phase when they reverse sleep times[12]. However, sleep-related variability in airway resistance does not appear to be reliably related to sleep stage[13,14]. Several studies show that inflammation worsens in subjects with nocturnal asthma in a circadian fashion. Compared with normals or even non-nocturnal asthma patients, there are increases in a variety of inflammatory markers, including interleukin-1β, circulating and lung eosinophils and alveolar lymphocytes[15]. The mechanisms for the circadian regulation of inflammation are not well understood.

Several disorders that may disrupt sleep have been associated with worsening asthma control including gastroesophageal reflux disease (GERD) and obstructive sleep apnea. GERD is associated with both nocturnal and daytime asthma symptoms and reflex bronchospasm[16,17]. In one cross-sectional study, over 2600 subjects were evaluated for GERD symptoms, which were identified in 4.6% of the sample population. Those with GERD were more likely to report nocturnal respiratory symptoms than those without, and asthma was twice as prevalent in those with GERD (9%)[16]. Obstructive sleep apnea syndrome (OSAS) has been associated with increased bronchial hyper-responsiveness, with therapeutic PAP ameliorating this hyper-reactivity[18]. The triad of GERD, asthma and OSAS are commonly encountered in clinical practice, and at times, optimal asthma control can be achieved only after OSAS and GERD are managed.

## Asthma treatment and sleep

Most patients with asthma, as well as their physicians, underestimate the severity of their disease, and much of the morbidity of asthma could be reduced with more aggressive treatment[19]. Goals of asthma therapy include reduction of symptoms, preservation of lung functon and avoidance of troublesome exacerbations. Nocturnal asthma is generally an indication for long-acting bronchodilators and inhaled corticosteroids in addition to short-acting 'rescue' inhaled bronchodilators[7].

There are several alternative inhaled corticosteroids (budesonide, beclomethasone, fluticasone, triamcinolone), with differing potencies, delivery mechanisms, pharmacokinetics and bioavailabilities. However, there is no compelling evidence that they influence sleep directly. Long-acting bronchodilators currently available and tested for their effect on lung function, asthma symptoms and sleep include theophylline, and the inhaled agents, salmeterol and formoterol. Several studies with oral theophylline in asthmatics have shown an increase in the number of arousals, decrease in stage 2 sleep and decreased total sleep time, while others show no effects on sleep[10, 20–24]. In one important study, effects of oral theophylline were studied in non-asthmatic subjects, thus eliminating the contributions of asthma to sleep disruption[23]. As might be predicted from the fact that theophylline is a methylxanthine in the same class as caffeine, total sleep time decreased and the number of arousals increased.

In contrast, salmeterol appears to be at least as effective in controlling asthma symptoms and slightly more effective in preventing nocturnal declines in airflow, and may be associated with fewer awakenings and arousals than theophylline[10,24,25]. Subjectively, sleep quality as judged by the Pittsburgh Sleep Quality Index is better in patients with nocturnal asthma using salmeterol, compared with theophylline or placebo[10]. Formoterol appears comparable to salmeterol in terms of effects on sleep, pulmonary function and asthma symptoms[20,25]. Long-acting anticholinergic inhalants are available, but their effects on sleep in asthmatics have not been studied.

## Case 9.1

A 35-year-old woman with a longstanding stable history of intermittent cough and allergic rhinitis developed increased nasal congestion, cough, wheeze and intermittent dyspnea over a 1-month period. Particularly bothersome were coughing paroxysms at night and dyspnea waking her from sleep. She had a history of childhood asthma and a family history of atopy, and described an average of two episodes of 'bronchitis' per year. On examination, her nasal mucosa was boggy, erythematous and glistening. She did not use accessory muscles, but on auscultation, expiratory wheezing was present bilaterally. Spirometry showed an $FEV_1/FVC$ ratio of 0.65, with an $FEV_1$ of 75% of the predicted normal which improved acutely to 90% of predicted with albuterol. Peak expiratory flow (PEF) was 450 l/s. Inhaled budesonide 200 $\mu$g twice daily and an albuterol metered-dose inhaler, two puffs every 4 h as needed, resulted in an improvement of daytime symptoms. However, she was still experiencing frequent awakenings with scantily productive cough, almost nightly attacks of dyspnea and wheezing at about 3:30 a.m., requiring albuterol. A peak flow diary showed more than 20% variability between p.m. and a.m. peak flows. Her symptoms of nocturnal asthma and the peak flow record indicated that her asthma was poorly controlled. Adding inhaled salmeterol did not improve her nocturnal symptoms or peak flow record significantly. It was then discovered that her son's hamster had been brought into the house shortly before her asthma had worsened. Removal of the hamster to a friend's house resulted in peak flow improvement and prompt relief of her nocturnal symptoms. In the coming months, it became apparent that she required 400 $\mu$g of budesonide once per day to maintain normal spirometry and to be symptom-free.

The case illustrates several aspects of asthma care. Nocturnal symptoms, often very bothersome to the patient, must be sought and may be present in the absence of significant daytime symptoms. Peak flow diaries can be useful in determining asthma control. In addition to intrinsic factors, specific environmental allergen exposure may contribute to nocturnal asthma, and a careful history is often more successful than potent medicines. Asthma is frequently more severe than either the patient or the physician expects; this asthmatic woman had remained untreated for many years.

## Chronic obstructive pulmonary disease (COPD)

Chronic obstructive pulmonary disease (COPD), as defined by the Global Initiative

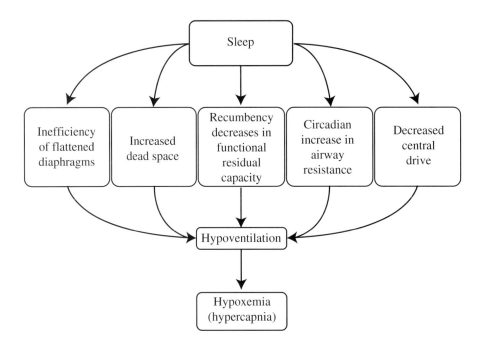

**Figure 9.3** Mechanisms of nocturnal hypoxemia in patients with chronic obstructive pulmonary disease (COPD)

for Chronic Obstructive Lung Disease (GOLD), is 'a disease state characterized by airflow limitation that is not fully reversible. The limitation is usually both progressive and associated with an abnormal inflammatory response of the lungs to noxious particles or gases'[26]. It is the fourth leading cause of death in the USA, and is ranked twelfth worldwide for burden of disease. The primary cause is smoking cigarettes, and both the physiological impairment of smoking-related diseases such as COPD, heart disease and stroke, as well as the nicotine in tobacco, can disrupt sleep.

Like patients with asthma, COPD patients have both subjective and objective reductions in sleep quality compared with healthy subjects[27–29]. Patients with severe COPD have decreased sleep time, reduced REM sleep and sleep fragmentation. This poor sleep quality probably contributes to chronic fatigue and reduced quality of life[30]. Sleep disruption is probably multifactorial, associated with oxygen desaturation, cough, dyspnea, medicine effects and anxiety[31].

### Sleep and hypoxemia in COPD

Patients with severe COPD have worsening gas exchange during sleep, with increasing $PaCO_2$ and decreasing $SaO_2$ (Figure 9.1)[32]. The degree of desaturation can be profound, often twice that experienced by COPD patients at peak exercise[33]. Factors contributing to sleep-related hypoxemia in patients with COPD include hypoventilation, ventilation–perfusion mismatching and decreased functional residual capacity.

Hypoventilation is the most important of these mechanisms (Figure 9.3). Ventilation decreases during both REM and non-rapid eye movement (NREM) sleep in normal subjects, but patients with COPD are likely to exhibit more profound hypoventilation for a number of reasons. First, during wake and NREM sleep, accessory muscles of respiration provide a substantial contribution to

ventilation in patients with advanced COPD who have hyperinflation. During REM sleep, these muscles relax, and the patient with COPD becomes more dependent on the diaphragm for ventilation. If the diaphragm is already flattened and lengthened due to hyperinflation, it will not be very effective, and marked hypoventilation results[34]. Second, patients with COPD have an increased 'dead space', or portion of each breath that does not participate in active gas exchange. With the rapid shallow breathing

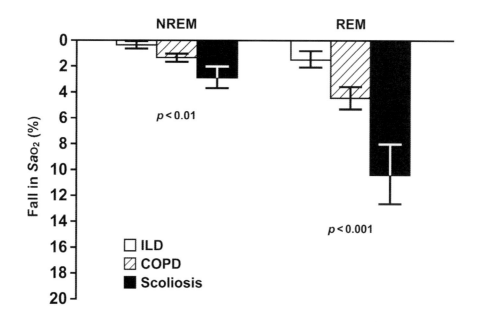

**Figure 9.4** Nocturnal hypoxemia in patients with different pulmonary diseases. Patients with interstitial lung disease (ILD), chronic obstructive pulmonary disease (COPD) and scoliosis were selected for similar wake oxygen saturation ($SaO_2$), and then studied during sleep. Oxygen saturation falls more in patients with scoliosis than in COPD, and more in COPD than in ILD. ILD patients tend to have increased respiratory drive during both wake and sleep, while those with COPD and severe scoliosis have decreased respiratory drive. Additionally, patients with COPD and scoliosis are greatly affected by rapid eye movement (REM) sleep, when because of the deformity of their lungs (hyperinflation in the case of COPD, compression in the case of scoliosis) their ventilation becomes very dependent on the diaphragm. NREM, non-rapid eye movement. Modified with permission from reference 36

**Table 9.5** Mechanisms and consequences of sleep-related hypoxia in chronic obstructive pulmonary disease

---

A. Mechanisms of sleep-related hypoxia

    a  Hypoventilation

    b  Effects of the oxyhemoglobin dissociation curve

    c  Ventilation–perfusion mismatching

    d  Increased airway resistance

    e  Superimposed obstructive sleep apnea syndrome

B. Consequences of sleep-related hypoxia

    a  Pulmonary hypertension

    b  Impaired sleep quality

    c  Increased nocturnal arrhythmias

    d  Polycythemia

    e  Peripheral edema

    f  Increased all-cause mortality

---

pattern of phasic REM sleep, a greater fraction of total ventilation will be dead space, and alveolar ventilation will fall proportionally[34]. Third, patients with COPD may have exaggerated increases in airway resistance during sleep, but to a lesser degree than those with asthma. Finally, hypoxic and hypercapnic ventilatory responses, usually blunted in NREM and especially in REM sleep, may be more blunted than usual in patients with COPD[35]. These factors probably explain why patients with COPD become more hypoxemic with sleep than patients with pulmonary fibrosis with similar baseline wake oxygenation (Figure 9.4)[36].

The oxygen saturation at rest while awake is the best predictor of sleep desaturation in subjects with COPD[37,38]. If resting $SaO_2$ is greater than 95%, nocturnal desaturation is rare[37]. Lung function is also somewhat predictive. In a population-based study of over 6000 subjects, desaturation was more common in those whose ratio of $FVC/FEV_1$ was less than 65%[39], and the more severely abnormal lung function predicted more severe desaturation. Other factors associated with the degree of nocturnal desaturation in patients with COPD include obesity and hypercapnia.

What is the significance of reduced sleep-related oxygen saturation in patients with COPD (Table 9.5)? In one study of patients with COPD, sleep-related hypoxemia caused acute increases in pulmonary artery pressure from a mean of 37 mmHg during wakefulness to 55 mmHg during sleep[32]. Patients with COPD and sustained oxygen desaturation have increased pulmonary vascular resistance, and a more impaired hemodynamic response to exercise[40,41]. These observations have led to the hypothesis that isolated nocturnal hypoxemia in COPD leads to diurnal pulmonary hypertension and subsequent risk for cor pulmonale. However, trials to date have not demonstrated this progression, and sustained pulmonary hypertension may be reflective of the underlying disease rather than consequences of episodic hypoxemia[42].

Nocturnal hypoxemia may be associated with impaired survival in patients with COPD[43], but the mechanism is unclear. The Nocturnal Oxygen Therapy Trial and the British Research Council domiciliary oxygen treatment trial established that patients with daytime hypoxemia have reduced mortality and improvement in quality of life and neurocognitive function when oxygen therapy is

**Table 9.6** Accepted criteria for long-term oxygen therapy in chronic obstructive pulmonary disease

| | |
|---|---|
| Absolute | $PaO_2 \leq 55$ mmHg (or $SaO_2 \leq 88\%$) on room air, awake, or |
| In the presence of cor pulmonale | $PaO_2 \leq 59$ mmHg ($SaO_2 \leq 90\%$) with any of the following:<br>polycythemia (Hct > 55%)<br>ECG evidence of pulmonary hypertension<br>congestive heart failure<br>mental status changes due to hypoxemia |
| Specific circumstances | $PaO_2 > 55$ mmHg (or $SaO_2 > 88\%$) at rest, but $PaO_2 \leq 55$ mmHg (or $SaO_2 \leq 88\%$) with exercise on room air, with improved oxygen saturation during exercise using supplemental oxygen (prescribe oxygen with exercise)<br>$PaO_2 > 55$ mmHg (or $SaO_2 > 88\%$) at rest, but $PaO_2 \leq 55$ mmHg (or $SaO_2 \leq 88\%$) during sleep (prescribe oxygen during sleep) |

$PaO_2$, arterial oxygen tension; $SaO_2$, oxygen saturation; Hct, hematocrit; ECG, electrocardiogram

applied to correct hypoxemia[44,45]. Table 9.6 lists accepted indications for long-term oxygen therapy, which is the only treatment that improves mortality in patients with COPD. These recommendations for oxygen therapy were not initially based on nocturnal measures of oxygenation, and to date there is no convincing evidence that oxygen supplementation for COPD patients with isolated nocturnal hypoxemia improves survival or even quality of sleep, despite improvement in oxygen saturation and pulmonary pressures[46–48]. The practice of 'screening' otherwise asymptomatic patients with COPD for isolated nocturnal hypoxemia is not fully supported by available evidence, but oxygen therapy is still often recommended at this time. Patients with daytime $PaO_2 \geq 60$ mmHg but evidence of cor pulmonale or complaints of headache or dyspnea on awakening merit oximetry. If deep desaturations are present, oxygen therapy or polysomnography seems reasonable (see Case 9.2).

**Case 9.2**

A 66-year-old previously smoking farmer was hospitalized for severe dyspnea following a viral upper respiratory infection with purulent bronchitis. He had experienced many years of exertional dyspnea, and over the previous year had noted anorexia, weight loss, difficulties sleeping, poor concentration, anhedonia and ankle edema. Not uncommonly, he noted headache on awakening. He did not snore or have witnessed apneas. On examination, he was cachectic and used accessory respiratory muscles and pursed lip breathing while he leaned on the bedside table. His chest was hyperexpanded and there was increased resonance to percussion bilaterally. Breath sounds were diminished, and the expiratory phase was increased. Cardiac auscultation revealed distant heart sounds and he had mild bilateral ankle edema. Chest X-ray showed changes consistent with severe apical bullous emphysema and flattened diaphragm but no infiltrate. Hematocrit was 57%, electrocardiogram (ECG) showed a p-pulmonale pattern, and awake on room air his arterial blood gases showed a pH of 7.48, $PaCO_2$ of 46 mmHg, and $PaO_2$ of 48 mmHg. Oxygen delivered via nasal cannula at 2 l/min brought his waking $SaO_2$ to 91%, but during sleep, nursing staff noted that he required 3 l/min to keep $SaO_2$ over 86%. He was discharged home with oxygen at 2 l/min during wakeful rest, and 3 l/min with exertion or sleep. On return 6 weeks later, his edema had resolved, and he noted improvement in daytime mood and concentration. His resting oxygen requirement was the same. Appetite was marginally better. His sleep was still poor, but he no longer noted morning headache.

Chronic COPD with hypoxemia is associated with poor sleep, impaired neuropsychiatric function, pulmonary hypertension and ultimately cor pulmonale (Table 9.5, Figure 9.2). Oxygen improves pulmonary hypertension and hemodynamics, neuropsychiatric function, quality of life and mortality in subjects with resting hypoxemia (Table 9.6).

### COPD treatment and sleep

Other than oxygen therapy (discussed above), the main aspects of COPD management include smoking cessation, bronchodilator therapy, immunization, improving or maintaining physical conditioning and prompt treatment of infections or exacerbations. Smoking cessation is so far the only measure that slows disease progression. Both sustained-release bupropion and nicotine replacement therapy improve the likelihood of successful smoking cessation, but these agents can cause insomnia. A side-effect of nicotine transdermal therapy is disturbing dreams, and patients should remove the transdermal patch at bedtime[49].

Recommended bronchodilator therapy includes short- and long-acting inhaled bronchodilators, and theophylline. The effect of short- or long-acting inhaled β-agonists on sleep quality of patients with COPD is not well studied. One randomized, controlled, double-blind study involving 36 patients with moderate-to-severe COPD showed that 4 weeks of treatment with nebulized ipratropium bromide, an anticholinergic bronchodilator, provided modest improvements in minimum oxygen saturation, improvement in perceived sleep quality, increased REM sleep time and improvement in pre-sleep spirometry, compared with placebo. The effects of longer-acting inhaled anticholinergics on sleep quality are not yet available. Theophyllines have many theoretical benefits in patients with COPD, including enhancing central respiratory drive, improving diaphragm contractility, bronchodilatation, improvements in right ventricular contractility and improved gas exchange during sleep[50]. However, theophyllines cause sleep disruption and have other side-effects that often limit their usefulness[51].

Use of NIPPV for acute exacerbations of COPD is well established for carefully selected patients[52,53]. The application of nocturnal NIPPV to patients with severe 'stable' COPD has been more controversial owing to mixed results in clinical trials. A recent consensus conference concluded that hypercapnic COPD patients who desaturate nocturnally may derive the most benefit from NIPPV, but patients should have symptoms attributable to impaired sleep or gas exchange, such as fatigue, dyspnea and morning headache. COPD patients with little or no $CO_2$ retention do not appear to benefit much from NIPPV[5].

*The overlap syndrome: concurrence of obstructive sleep apnea syndrome and COPD*

OSAS is a common disorder, and its prevalence is similar among those with COPD to that in the general population[39,54]. When OSAS and COPD coexist, patients usually have typical symptoms, noted in Chapter 8[38]. However, gas exchange abnormalities may be more profound, and have resulted in recognition of the 'overlap syndrome', where obstructive lung disease combined with OSAS leads to chronic respiratory failure and, when severe, to cor pulmonale. Perhaps because of the increased severity in gas exchange abnormalities, the overlap syndrome is over-represented in pulmonary consultative practices. In one European chest clinic, 11% of patients with an apnea–hypopnea index (AHI) > 20 also had moderate-to-severe COPD[55].

Therapy for patients with concurrent COPD and OSAS involves PAP and, if needed, supplemental oxygen. Some have found that bilevel PAP is needed to achieve therapeutic goals of improving sleep and oxygenation[56]. After a diagnostic PSG establishes the presence of OSAS, CPAP titration should be attempted first, and either oxygen added if needed to correct oxygen saturation to 89–92%, or bilevel PAP tried in a sponta-

neous mode. Arterial blood gas measurements during or after PAP titration are advisable if the patient is severely hypoxic or known to retain $CO_2$, to ensure that hypercapnia is not dangerously worsened. If the goals of improved sleep and gas exchange are achieved at titration and the patient is compliant with PAP use, blood gas values often improve over time. If PAP therapy fails, NIPPV, or even tracheostomy with nocturnal positive pressure ventilation, is sometimes necessary.

**Case 9.3**

A 70-year-old woman followed for peripheral vascular disease became very somnolent (Epworth sleepiness scale score of 18), dyspneic and edematous over a 2-year period. She had a prior history of moderate but largely asymptomatic COPD with an $FEV_1$ measuring 62% of the predicted value. Arterial blood gases 2 years before, performed during a vascular procedure, showed a $PaO_2$ of 62 mmHg with normal $PaCO_2$ and pH. She had gained 35 lb during convalescence from the surgery. No one observed her sleep, so snoring or apnea history was unreliable. On examination, she was plethoric, obese and somnolent, and had marked dependent edema. Breath sounds were diminished, and heart sounds were distant. An overnight oximetry is shown in Figure 9.5.

She was placed on oxygen 3 l/min via nasal cannula, and arterial blood gases measured pH 7.31, $PaCO_2$ 66 mmHg and $PaO_2$ 68 mmHg. Inhaled formoterol and ipratropium were begun. Polysomnography was performed while wearing oxygen

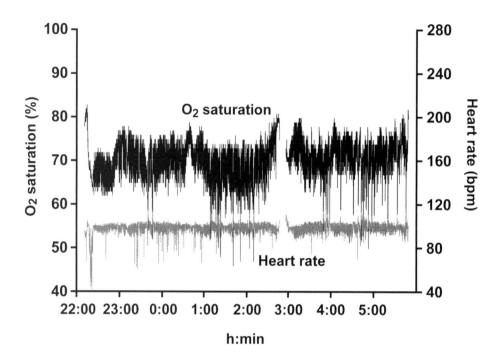

**Figure 9.5** Overnight oximetry for case 9.3 (overlap syndrome). This overnight oximetry was performed on room air. Note both severe nocturnal hypoxemia and repetitive sawtooth type desaturations indicative of superimposed obstructive sleep apnea syndrome. This combination is highly suggestive of the overlap syndrome

at 3 l/min via nasal cannula. The AHI was 36.5, and oxygen saturation fell to a minimum of 48%. On CPAP set at 7 cmH$_2$O combined with oxygen at 2 l/min bled into the CPAP tubing, her oxygen saturation ranged between 88 and 92%, apneas and hypopneas were abated and she slept very well. On CPAP therapy, her sleepiness and daytime concentration improved. Her edema resolved without diuretic, and she was no longer as limited by dyspnea.

Overlap syndrome often produces stigmata of right heart failure, and patients often manifest more severe pulmonary hypertension than do patients with either OSAS or equivalent COPD alone. Not infrequently, CPAP or bilevel PAP therapy without oxygen will prove sufficient. PAP is more economical than long-term oxygen therapy and, when adequate oxygenation is achieved with PAP alone, should be given a trial first. If needed, oxygen may be supplemented to PAP to maintain $Sa$O$_2$ above target levels. This patient required supplemental oxygen along with PAP therapy. Treating COPD is an integral part of the management of overlap syndrome.

## Cystic fibrosis

Cystic fibrosis (CF) is a heritable disorder occurring at a frequency of approximately 1:2000 to 1:2500 live births. Median life span is now nearly 30 years, owing to improvement in patient care. The primary mutations have been located in a single gene locus on the long arm of chromosome 7 that encodes for the CF transmembrane conductance regulator (CFTR), a chloride channel that regulates electrolyte transport and secretion functions in multiple exocrine cells. Although CF is a multisystem disorder, pulmonary disease is the main cause of morbidity and mortality. Defects in mucous secretion and resultant impairment in mucociliary clearance lead to serial infections, recurrent airway inflammation, bronchiectatic changes and inevitably worsening obstructive lung disease. As respiratory function worsens and strength declines, chronic respiratory failure ensues.

Increased sleep-related disability and impairment compared with a normal population was noted in a study of 240 CF patients of all ages[57]. Polysomnographic studies show reduced total sleep time, but no increase in arousals or awakenings[58]. Similar to patients with advanced COPD, some CF patients have significant oxygen desaturation during sleep. Desaturation is most severe during REM sleep, and is thought to be mostly due to hypoventilation[59,60]. Factors predictive of hypoxemia during sleep are resting wake $Pa_{O_2} < 94\%$ and $FEV_1 < 65\%$[61].

Correction of oxygenation and ventilation improve quality of life and sleep[62]. Supplemental oxygen therapy is indicated for hypoxemic patients with CF. Nocturnal NIPPV has been used successfully in patients with CF suffering chronic respiratory failure[63]. In patients with severe CF who had significant gas exchange abnormalities during sleep but were normocapnic in the daytime, NIPPV was able to prevent oxygen-induced hypercapnia. Home NIPPV improves physiological variables and quality of life up to 18 months after initiation of the treatment[62], and has been described as both a treatment and a bridge to transplantation.

## RESTRICTIVE THORACIC CAGE AND LUNG DISEASES

Restrictive respiratory disorders are defined by a reduction in TLC on pulmonary function testing. Typically, the $FEV_1$ and FVC are reduced in proportion to one another. Restriction can result whenever the balance of elastic forces leading to lung collapse increases or when the outward chest wall recoils or muscular forces assisting in lung inflation decrease. Thus, intrathoracic diseases that render the lungs stiffer or less compliant, such as pulmonary fibrosis, lead to restriction, and are usually associated with augmented respiratory center stimulation because of activation of intrapulmonary receptors (see Chapter 8). In early stages, such disorders may be asymptomatic at rest and be noticed as only exertional dyspnea. Gas exchange abnormalities are typically minimal at this stage, and compensatory adaptation usually involves the assumption of a shallow, more rapid breathing pattern. As the disorders progress, rest dyspnea and gas exchange abnormalities become more apparent. Respiratory drive is often high, and $Pa_{CO_2}$ may be low initially, but as dead-space ventilation increases and alveolar ventilation decreases, arterial $O_2$ falls and $Pa_{CO_2}$

193

may normalize or begin to rise. When chest wall stiffness or deformity causes restriction, presentation is more variable. Rest or exertional dyspnea may be present in the absence of blood gas abnormalities, or there may be early evidence of chronic ventilatory failure in patients lacking respiratory symptoms. Some of the earliest symptoms may be the result of sleep-related hypoventilation, such as morning headache, or poorly restorative sleep. Neuromuscular disorders with respiratory muscle weakness also lead to restrictive disorders, but are considered separately.

## Obesity

Obesity is epidemic in developed nations, and is characterized by a body mass index (BMI) exceeding 30.0 $(kg/m^2)$[64,65]. Obese patients have abnormal respiratory function when awake and upright, and more so when supine or asleep[66]. The increased mass of the chest and abdomen decrease the elastic recoil of the chest wall and inhibit diaphragm function. Especially when supine, these changes tend to decrease resting lung volumes (the functional residual capacity, FRC). This 'squeezing' of lungs can cause some airway closure at volumes above FRC, resulting in decreased ventilation of the dependent parts of the lung and subsequent ventilation–perfusion mismatch with hypoxemia. Small airway collapse also leads to increases in airway resistance in obese subjects. Furthermore, the work of breathing may be increased by 60% in uncomplicated obesity when respiratory muscles must work against increased weight and decreases in chest wall recoil, and by up to 250% in some patients with obesity hypoventilation syndrome[67]. Decreases in FVC and TLC are

expected at BMIs that exceed 45, but may occur at a lower level.

### Effects of obesity on sleep

These predictable changes in respiratory mechanics are worse when an obese person lies down because of the upward displacement of the diaphragm caused by the weight overlying the abdomen. The usual hypoventilation of sleep and hypotonia of REM sleep exaggerate breathing problems in obesity, but the individual responses to these challenges vary between persons. A spectrum of sleep problems are seen in obese subjects (Table 9.7).

Obese persons without sleep-disordered breathing have poorer sleep quality, increased sleep latency, decreased sleep efficiency and decreased percentage REM sleep, and are sleepier than non-obese subjects[68]. The mechanism of sleepiness may be related to serum levels of inflammatory cytokines,

**Table 9.7** The spectrum of effects of obesity on sleep

| |
|---|
| Disturbed sleep and daytime sleepiness without sleep-disordered breathing |
| Snoring |
| Obstructive sleep apnea syndrome |
| REM sleep hypoventilation |
| Hypoventilation in REM and NREM sleep without waking hypercapnia |
| Hypoventilation in REM and NREM sleep with waking hypercapnia (obesity hypoventilation syndrome) |
| REM, rapid eye movement; NREM, non-rapid eye movement |

such as interleukin-6 (IL-6) and tumor necrosis factor-α (TNF-α), which are elevated in sleepy subjects in general, and are generally higher in obese than in normal-weight healthy subjects. Both loud snoring and OSAS are more prevalent in obese individuals. In one study, loud snoring was present in 46.7% of obese subjects without apnea, but only in 8.1% of control subjects[68]. In some patients, ventilation is adequate during NREM sleep, but the diaphragm is unable to provide adequate ventilation when challenged by the ponderous abdomen, and hypoventilation and hypoxemia during REM result. In others, mild hypoxia develops even during NREM sleep, with marked worsening during REM sleep. Such patients are at risk for pulmonary hypertension, since they spend significant time with hypoxia-induced pulmonary vasoconstriction. The most severe pattern of obesity-association hypoventilation is the obesity hypoventilation syndrome (OHS), characterized by daytime hypercapnia.

*Obesity hypoventilation syndrome*

Over 40 years ago, Burwell and colleagues described a syndrome characterized by morbid obesity, hypersomnolence, plethora, edema, diurnal hypoventilation, polycythemia and cor pulmonale[69]. The colorful name 'Pickwickian syndrome', chosen because of the seeming characterization of such a patient by Dickens in his novel *The Pickwick Papers*, is still used today, but is an imprecise term. Some have suggested that the syndrome be classified as a specific type of sleep hypoventilation syndrome[70]. The pathophysiology of OHS is complex and not altogether understood. The syndrome results from a combination of increased res-

piratory load and, in some cases, congenital or acquired blunted ventilatory drive. The respiratory load can be resistive (owing to upper airway obstruction), or due to the changes in pulmonary mechanics associated with obesity. Ventilatory response to $CO_2$ and $O_2$ is often reduced[71]. In some but not all studies, first-order relatives have shown decreased response to hypoxia and hypercapnia, suggesting a possible genetic predisposition to the disorder in some patients[72]. The distinction between patients with OHS who do not have upper airway obstruction and those with adult-onset primary alveolar hypoventilation syndrome (PAHS) can be somewhat blurred, except that patients with OHS are by definition always obese (see below).

Patients with OHS manifest symptoms and signs of chronic alveolar hypoventilation, with poorly restorative and disrupted sleep, morning headaches, daytime sleepiness and often snoring. Dyspnea may or may not be present, while hypercapnia and most often mild hypoxia need to be present to make the diagnosis. The physical examination, chest X-ray, electrocardiogram (ECG) and echocardiography may demonstrate findings of pulmonary arterial hypertension and right-sided heart failure. Pulmonary function will most often show restriction, with normal or reduced diffusing capacity.

The contribution of concurrent upper airway obstruction in patients with OHS varies between individuals. In one study of 23 obese patients with diurnal hypercapnia, the average AHI was 62/h, but some had an AHI as low as 9/h. In 11 patients, hypoventilation was corrected immediately by CPAP alone, indicating that the chronic hypoventilation was due predominantly to upper air-

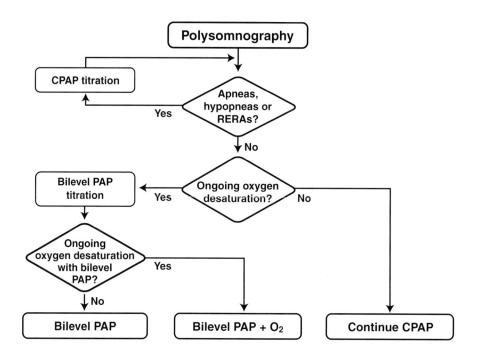

**Figure 9.6** Algorithm for management of obesity hypoventilation syndrome (OHS). Patients with OHS may have components of flow limitation that will respond to continuous positive airway pressure (CPAP) therapy. If hypoventilation persists, a bilevel positive airway pressure (PAP) (spontaneous, S mode) will often result in adequate ventilation to maintain improved oxygen saturation. Occasionally, supplemental oxygen will be required with bilevel PAP to maintain adequate oxygen saturation. An arterial blood gas test at the conclusion of PAP titration is advised if supplemental oxygen is used, since some patients will exhibit severe $CO_2$ retention with oxygen therapy. RERA, respiratory effort-related arousal

way obstruction, while others required bilevel PAP. In this study and others, age, gender, BMI, degree of hypercapnia, ventilatory response to $CO_2$, AHI and lung function did not differ between patients with predominantly severe OSAS and obesity alone, and those with central hypoventilation that remained after upper airway patency was re-established.

From a treatment standpoint, each patient must be approached individually. Usually, following the protocol suggested in Figure 9.6 results in successful management of patients with OHS and gradual improvement of arterial blood gas measurements. NIPPV is sometimes needed if CPAP or bilevel PAP in the S mode with supplemental $O_2$ is insufficient during polysomnography.

**Table 9.8** Causes of kyphoscoliosis

Idiopathic

Poliomyelitis

Pott's disease (tuberculosis of the spine)

Neurofibromatosis

Ehlers–Danlos syndrome

Marfan's syndrome

Muscular dystrophy

## Kyphoscoliosis

Kyphoscoliosis is most often idiopathic and begins in childhood, but can be the result of a variety of diseases (Table 9.8). Kyphosis refers to anteroposterior spinal curvature, and impinges less on pulmonary function, while scoliosis is lateral angulation and rotation of the spine, which can lead to abnormalities in respiratory function and respiratory failure. If kyphoscoliosis is not severe and progressive, it does not limit life. However, when the angle measured between the upper and lower portions of the spine (Cobb's angle) exceeds 100°, chronic respiratory failure is often present. More acute respiratory decompensation can result with infection, respiratory depressant drugs or other concurrent cardiopulmonary disease.

Most patients with significant kyphoscoliosis exhibit a rapid shallow breathing pattern, and show restriction on pulmonary function testing. The abnormal 'squeezing' of the lungs caused by chest wall deformity and decreased chest wall compliance lead to decreased FRC, ventilation–perfusion mismatch, resting hypoxemia and increased work of breathing similar to that in the obese patient. The ventilatory response to hypercapnia or hypoxemia is blunted as an adaptive response to chronic increased mechanical work of breathing. One special circumstance is that of poliomyelitis, which not only can affect motor neurons with paralysis of axial muscles, but also can damage the medullary respiratory center during the initial infection. After seeming partial or complete recovery, some patients manifest central alveolar hypoventilation or develop scoliosis with respiratory failure 20–30 years later as part of the post-polio syndrome. Kyphoscoliotic patients with ventilatory failure can develop pulmonary hypertension and cor pulmonale, which carry a poor prognosis.

All types of sleep-disordered breathing can be observed, with affected patients complaining of sleep disruption and excessive daytime sleepiness[73]. The treatment of scoliosis involves surgical management of altered anatomy, medical management of the adverse health effects, respiratory therapy and social support. Although supplemental oxygen increases $SaO_2$ in kyphoscoliotic patients, it often leads to increased $PaCO_2$. Thus, titration of initial therapy is best done under careful observation utilizing not only oximetry, but also arterial blood gas testing. Nocturnal NIPPV is established therapy for patients with kyphoscoliosis and respiratory failure, improving arterial blood gas values, sleep quality and quality of life measures[5].

## Interstitial lung disease

Interstitial lung disease (ILD) describes a heterogeneous group of disorders associated with fibrosis of alveolar and other connective tissue in the lungs that generally progress over many months or years. The most common ILDs are cryptogenic fibrosing alveolitis (also called idiopathic pulmonary fibrosis), sarcoidosis, ILD associated with connective–tissue disorders, pneumoconioses, hypersensitivity pneumonitis and drug-induced lung diseases[74]. Although of diverse pathophysiologies, they share certain pulmonary function characteristics. As they progress, they all cause restriction by reducing the compliance of the lungs, cause impaired gas exchange by worsening physiological shunt and usually stimulate the respiratory center via vagal afferents, causing mild respiratory alkalosis. As the disease progresses, respiratory mechanics, the work of breathing and physiological shunt worsen to cause hypoxemia mixed with chronic ventilatory failure. Despite new developments in the treatment of ILD, the prognosis of most ILDs is poor, with gradual development of respiratory failure, cor pulmonale and eventually death. Pulmonary infection is a common final cause of death[75,76].

Patients with ILD have characteristically very disturbed sleep, with increased stage 1 sleep, decreased REM sleep and increased arousals[77]. Oxygen desaturation occurs in both NREM and REM sleep, and is most related to awake baseline oxygen saturation. Respiratory rate is typically higher during both wakefulness and sleep in patients with ILD compared with normal subjects. Because of relatively high respiratory drive, supplemental oxygen therapy is usually well tolerated without increased $CO_2$ retention, and in contrast to the situation with kyphoscoliosis, can generally be safely administered without intense monitoring. Supplemental oxygen during sleep improves both oxygen saturation and sleep quality[78]. Nocturnal NIPPV in ILD has not been extensively studied, but is not always well tolerated or associated with sustained improvement in gas exchange. Pharmacological treatment of many ILDs often involves corticosteroids that can disturb sleep and cause insomnia. Furthermore, the long-term use of corticosteroids, and some of the underlying disorders (such as rheumatoid arthritis), are associated with increased risk for OSAS.

**Table 9.9** Neuromuscular disorders with sleep-related breathing disorders

---

Muscular dystrophies
    myotonic dystrophy
    Duchenne muscular dystrophy[79,80]

Congenital myopathies
    nemaline myopathy[81]

Metabolic myopathies
    mitochondrial myopathy[82]
    acid maltase deficiency[83]
    hypothyroidism[84]

Anterior horn cell diseases
    amyotrophic lateral sclerosis
    poliomyelitis

Inflammatory or autoimmune neuropathies
    chronic inflammatory demyelinating
    polyradiculoneuropathy
    Guillain–Barré syndrome

Disorders of the neuromuscular junction
    myasthenia gravis

## NEUROMUSCULAR RESPIRATORY FAILURE

Like restrictive thoracic cage abnormalities, neuromuscular disease affecting respiratory

**Table 9.10** Recommended respiratory monitoring in patients with amyotrophic lateral sclerosis

| Test | Frequency |
| --- | --- |
| Spirometry (FVC, $FEV_1$, MVV) | initially and every 3 months |
| MIP and MEP | initially and every 3 months |
| Overnight oximetry | initially and every 3 months |
| Arterial blood gas testing | initially and with marked change in other measured parameters (overnight oximetry, spirometry or serum chloride levels) |
| Polysomnography | individualized, depending on sleep symptoms, overnight oximetry and facilities for instituting NIPPV |

FVC, forced vital capacity; $FEV_1$, forced expiratory volume in 1 s; MVV, maximum voluntary ventilation; MIP, maximum inspiratory pressure; MEP, maximum expiratory pressure; NIPPV, non-invasive positive pressure ventilation

muscles leads to restrictive ventilatory mechanics and altered respiratory control. The extents to which these changes occur vary with the underlying disease process (Table 9.9). Some neuromuscular diseases may be associated with upper airway obstruction in addition to respiratory mechanical changes. For example, patients with myotonic dystrophy have a higher AHI than do control patients with neuromuscular disease and similar degrees of respiratory muscle weakness[85].

## Amyotrophic lateral sclerosis

Amyotrophic lateral sclerosis (ALS) is a degenerative, progressive, fatal neurological disease associated with bulbar, skeletal and respiratory muscle weakness. Death is usually the result of respiratory failure. Although respiratory involvement typically develops after limb and bulbar muscle involvement, occasionally ALS patients present with respiratory insufficiency as the initial symptom. Chronic respiratory failure usually develops insidiously, and may go unrecognized by patient or physician until the FVC is reduced by more than 50%. Often the respiratory insufficiency first manifests during sleep. Because of insidious onset and insensitivity of the clinical examination, patients diagnosed with ALS should be monitored serially with careful clinical evaluation, pulmonary function tests and overnight oximetry (Table 9.10).

Serial spirometry will show progressive declines in FVC and maximum voluntary ventilation (MVV). Functional declines can be rapid and patients are nearly always symptomatic when FVC falls below 50% of predicted values. Maximal inspiratory pressure (MIP) and maximal expiratory pressure (MEP) also decline sometimes before FVC, perhaps reflective of early diaphragm involvement. MIP values less than 60 $cmH_2O$, usually associated with nocturnal desaturation, can be found in up to 65% of ALS

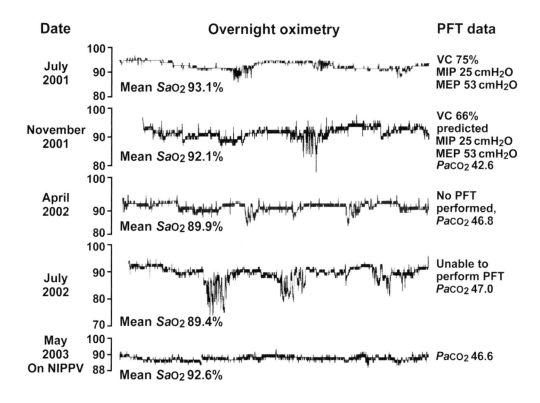

**Figure 9.7** Sequential nocturnal oxygen saturation ($SaO_2$) tracings in a patient with amyotrophic lateral sclerosis. The figure shows overnight oximetry tracings averaging 6 h 43 min in duration in a woman diagnosed with amyotrophic lateral sclerosis in July 2001. All are on room air without breathing assistance except the last, during which the patient used non-invasive positive pressure ventilation (NIPPV) with room air. As neuromuscular function deteriorated (supported by general decline in pulmonary function tests), the episodic desaturations caused by rapid eye movement (REM) sleep became more pronounced and the mean oxygen saturation decreased. See case 9.4 for details. VC, vital capacity; MIP, maximal inspiratory pressure; MEP, maximal expiratory pressure; $PaCO_2$, arterial $CO_2$ tension; PFT, pulmonary function test

patients with FVC > 70% of that predicted. MIP values less than 15 cmH$_2$O are usually associated with respiratory failure. Blood gas analysis will reveal onset of $CO_2$ retention. Serum chloride level < 98 mmol/l has also been suggested as a metabolic indicator of respiratory acidosis and hence a prognostic indicator[86]. The development of diurnal respiratory insufficiency is invariably preceded by sleep-related hypoventilation, first with REM-related hypoxemia, and later with sustained hypoxemia and hypercapnia (Figure 9.7)[87].

Sleep is adversely affected by respiratory decline, with patients noting disturbed sleep and daytime fatigue. In addition to respiratory issues, difficulty in turning to change position, muscle cramps with pain, secretion control and psychological distress all combine to decrease sleep quality. Patients should be questioned regarding sleep on a frequent basis, with emphasis on detecting early symptoms of hypoventilation such as frequent awakenings, nightmares, headaches on awakening and daytime sleepiness, as well as more obvious symptoms such as dyspnea or orthopnea. Many of these symptoms overlap with those of OSAS, which can coexist in patients with ALS[87]. Polysomno-

graphy is essential in establishing the correct diagnosis.

Nocturnal NIPPV improves quality of sleep and quality of life measures in patients with ALS[88]. In some studies, NIPPV improved mortality in ALS patients (Figure 9.8)[89]. However, as many as 50% will not be able to tolerate NIPPV or will be unwilling to use it. A minority of patients opt for tracheostomy with positive pressure ventilation. Others elect to forgo ventilatory support,

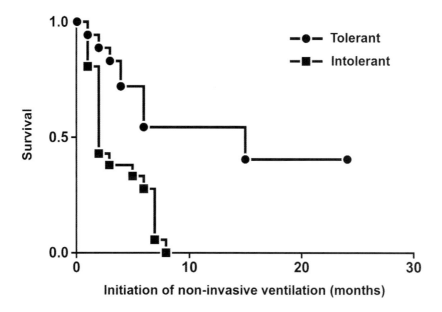

**Figure 9.8** Effect of non-invasive positive pressure ventilation (NIPPV) on mortality in amyotrophic lateral sclerosis. Kaplan–Meier survival plots from initiation of NIPPV in patients with amyotrophic lateral sclerosis. Patients intolerant of NIPPV had a relative risk for death 3.1-fold greater (95% confidence interval, 1.8-fold–9.6-fold) than that in tolerant patients ($p < 0.001$). Median duration of survival in intolerant and tolerant patients was 2 and 15 months, respectively. Reproduced with permission from reference 89

accepting comfort or hospice care at a late stage of their illness.

The timing of initiation of NIPPV is debated. Current US Centers for Medicare and Medicaid Services criteria for initial coverage of respiratory assist devices indicate that the patient must at a minimum have documentation of symptoms of hypoventilation. In addition, the patient must demonstrate at least one of the following: arterial blood gases showing $PaCO_2 > 45$ mmHg while awake, nocturnal oximetry data demonstrating desaturation to $< 88\%$ for at least 5 (continuous) min, an FVC $< 50\%$ of the predicted value or an MIP $< 60$ cmH$_2$O. There are several reasons why it may be prudent to begin at an earlier point in the decline than when FVC is $< 50\%$ of that predicted. First, it allows the patient time to become used to NIPPV and master the mask fit and mechanics of using the device. Second, the inspiratory efforts are often weak later in the disease, leaving the patient dependent on the timed breaths. These may or may not initially match the respiratory rate desired by the patient, so there may be some ventilator–patient dyssynchrony. This is not as noticeable to the patient if they first become accustomed to NIPPV use when spontaneous breaths trigger pressure support, and entrainment and synchronization gradually occur over time.

In our practice, we consider the patient's symptoms, results of oximetry and other tests, and discuss the goals of NIPPV with the patient and their care-givers at the earliest sign of deterioration. Together we make a decision regarding initiation of NIPPV, most often with the guidance of polysomnography. In this way, concurrent OSAS can be excluded, and NIPPV settings can be titrated

to achieve the goals of improving gas exchange, improving sleep quality and maximizing patient comfort. Typical initial settings involve an IPAP of 7–10 mH$_2$O, EPAP of 3–5 cmH$_2$O, and an ST rate of 10–14 breaths/min. Supplemental oxygen is used if needed with NIPPV, but should be used cautiously if at all without NIPPV, since it can lead to hypercapnic failure and death[90]. Pronounced involvement of bulbar muscles can interfere with NIPPV, but is not always a contraindication. A full range of masks can be tried, using whatever is most comfortable. In more advanced disease, an oronasal mask is often tolerated best because of increased mouth leak caused by flaccid oral muscles. If secretions are excessive despite pharmacological management, or if there is evidence of aspiration, NIPPV is contraindicated. Use of NIPPV for patients with ALS often relies on the assistance of domestic care-givers for mask adjustment and other comfort concerns during the sleep period.

NIPPV is only one component of the sleep-related care of patients with ALS. A wedge or hospital bed can help promote a semirecumbent position that facilitates breathing and reduces the likelihood of aspiration. Secretions must also be managed, and home suction devices and cough assistance devices can be useful in maintaining good pulmonary toilet. Patients frequently have concurrent depression and anxiety that require management as well. A multidisciplinary team approach is most helpful in optimizing care of these complex patients.

## Case 9.4

A 67-year-old woman was evaluated for weakness, dysarthria, dysphagia and exertional dyspnea. Neurological examination and electromyogram (EMG) were consistent with a diagnosis of ALS. Her serial oximetry and pulmonary function data are shown in Figure 9.7. When the patient was first diagnosed in June 2001, there were few sleep complaints. By November 2001, the patient had developed mild sleep disruption, but no morning headaches. Upright vital capacity was still above 60%, but there was clear nocturnal desaturation to a minimum of 79%. By April 2002, there was marked sleep disruption and occasional morning headaches, and the patient was wheelchair-dependent. A discussion about NIPPV after the April 2002 results prepared the patient for expected sleep-related difficulties, and informed her of treatment options, but at that time, she was not ready to accept intervention. By July 2002, the patient was more open to consideration of NIPPV, and polysomnography demonstrated not only neuromuscular-related hypoventilation, but some obstructive apneas and hypopneas as well. She tolerated NIPPV (IPAP 14, EPAP 6, respiratory rate 14) very well. She continued using NIPPV successfully, reducing sleep-related interruptions and nocturnal dyspnea complaints, and improved daytime alertness. At a follow-up visit in May 2003, the overnight oximetry showed very good control of nocturnal oxygen saturation. Her $PaCO_2$ indicated ongoing or chronic hypoventilation, as would be expected with a progressive neuromuscular disease. At the return visit, oral and respiratory secretions were noted to be an increasing problem.

ALS is progressive, and by serial testing, one may anticipate respiratory failure and intervene before great discomfort is present. Frequently the pulmonary function and gas exchange abnormalities are more severe than the clinical complaints. NIPPV can improve the quality of life, and may improve mortality.

## Muscular dystrophies and other myopathies

Patients with muscular dystrophies and other myopathies may all experience progressive muscle weakness and consequent respiratory failure similar to patients with ALS. In myotonic dystrophy, patients may have obstructive and central apneas as well as sleep-related hypoventilation, all contributing to sleep fragmentation and sleepiness. The AHI and degree of oxygen desaturation are greater in myotonic dystrophy than in other neuromuscular diseases[85]. Irregular breathing patterns may be evident during wakefulness and in light-sleep, but may improve during slow-wave sleep[91]. PAP therapy is effective for OSAS, and NIPPV has been shown to improve sleep, quality of life and prognosis. However, the sleepiness associated with myotonic dystrophy is often not fully explained by sleep-disordered breathing, and does not always respond to PAP. A central disorder of excessive sleepiness may be present, and modafinil or other stimulant therapy can improve alertness and mood in some cases[92].

Sleep-disordered breathing in Duchenne muscular dystrophy may appear early in the disease as obstructive apneas and hypopneas, but later there may be an increasing proportion of central events[79]. The AHI is generally only modestly elevated, in the 7–10-event/h range. In common with the other neuromuscular diseases, REM-related hypoxemia is first noted, followed by more severe hypoventilation in all stages of sleep, and ultimately respiratory failure. Nocturnal NIPPV improves sleep quality. As in patients with ALS, periodic spirometry should be performed along with careful questioning about sleep quality. Polysomnography should be considered when $PaCO_2$ is $\geq$ 45 mmHg, or if symptoms suggest sleep-disordered breathing[80].

Sleep-disordered breathing may also be seen in other myopathies, such as acid maltase deficiency and nemaline myopathy[93]. In all cases, nocturnal hypoventilation and sleep impairment may be missed if not specifically sought. In one study of eight children with myopathies, symptoms of sleep hypoventilation (often noted retrospectively after ventilation was initiated) included anorexia, weight gain, headaches and poor sleep, and all responded to NIPPV[94].

## Case 9.5

A 57-year-old man noted progressive difficulty staying awake driving and gradually increasing leg edema but no clear dyspnea on exertion, even when climbing stairs. He had developed severe orthopnea and headache on waking, and had been sleeping in a recliner. He denied dysphagia, diplopia or weakness. His past medical history and family history were not contributory. Examination was most notable for orthopnea and the absence of fasciculations. His serum creatinine kinase was elevated. Pulmonary function tests showed an FVC of 72% predicted, an $FEV_1$ of 70% predicted with normal $FEV_1/FVC$ ratio and a normal diffusing capacity, but reduced MVV of 51% pre-

dicted with low MIP. A room air arterial blood gas test at rest had shown $PaO_2$ of 49 mmHg, $PaCO_2$ of 66 mmHg and pH 7.41. The local health system had provided home oxygen before presentation, and on follow-up, arterial blood gases showed that $PaO_2$ had increased to 90 mmHg, but the $PaCO_2$ had risen to 75 mmHg. An EMG demonstrated findings of a very proximal myopathy affecting the respiratory muscles to the greatest extent. Myotonic discharges in the diaphragm and thoracic paraspinal muscles raised the possibility of a storage disease myopathy. A deltoid muscle biopsy confirmed the absence of acid maltase activity. During a brief diagnostic polysomnographic study, the man demonstrated severe fragmentation and desaturation during REM to 50%. He was started on NIPPV during the remainder of his polysomnographic study. His sleep latency on NIPPV measured 8 min while supine, and his overall sleep efficiency was 81%. His architecture showed 50% slow-wave and REM sleep, consistent with prior marked sleep deprivation. At an IPAP of 15 cmH$_2$O and EPAP of 4 cmH$_2$O with back-up rate of 14, his sleep and oxygen saturation improved immensely for all positions and sleep states.

Acid maltase deficiency (AMD) is inherited as an autosomal recessive trait and can present in infancy, childhood or adulthood. Adult-onset AMD usually presents with progressive proximal weakness in a limb–girdle distribution, with associated diaphragmatic involvement leading to respiratory insufficiency early in the course of the disease. Variable presentations may lead to delays in diagnosis. An elevated creatinine kinase is noted in all forms of AMD, and is a clue to diagnosis. Oxygen therapy may lead to marked hypercapnia and death, and should be administered only with careful monitoring. Ventilatory support is more appropriate, more successful and safer.

## Phrenic neuropathies

Unilateral or bilateral phrenic neuropathies are caused by a wide array of traumatic, immune-mediated, infectious, neoplastic or idiopathic etiologies. Unilateral disease is more common than bilateral disease, and in most cases has less severe abnormalities of pulmonary function. The frequency of sleep-related symptoms in patients with unilateral diaphragm dysfunction has not been studied, but in one retrospective study of 12 patients with unilateral disease, there was a decrease in REM and slow-wave sleep, and all had significant oxygen desaturation[95]. Patients with bilateral diaphragm paralysis are nearly always symptomatic awake, and suffer severe orthopnea with marked hypoventilation, especially during REM sleep. Morning headaches and daytime sleepiness are usually present.

Evaluation of patients with suspected diaphragm paralysis should begin with fluoroscopy, pulmonary function tests and measurement of respiratory muscle strength. When bilateral diaphragm paralysis is suspected, EMG is indicated. If sleep-disordered breathing is suspected from symptoms, PSG is indicated. In other cases, overnight oximetry should be performed, since marked abnormalities may be present without symptoms. When oximetry is markedly abnormal, arterial blood gases should be checked. PSG will show thoracoab-dominal paradox, a decrease in REM sleep, increased fragmentation and oxygen desaturation. NIPPV is most often effective in improving sleep and daytime arterial blood gases and may improve daytime dyspnea.

## FAILURE OF RESPIRATORY CONTROL

### Primary alveolar hypoventilation syndrome

Primary alveolar hypoventilation syndrome (PAHS) is characterized by chronic hypercapnia and hypoxia in the absence of an identifiable neurological, neuromuscular,

Table 9.11 Central alveolar hypoventilation syndromes

| |
| --- |
| *Primary alveolar hypoventilation syndromes* |
| Adult-onset primary alveolar hypoventilation syndrome |
| Congenital central hypoventilation syndrome |
| *Secondary alveolar hypoventilation syndromes due to neurological disease* |
| Intracerebral hemorrhage or infarct |
| Multisystem atrophy |
| Bilateral carotid body paraganglioma |
| Sarcoidosis[99] |
| Acoustic neuroma[100] |
| Paraneoplastic encephalitis with anti-Hu antibodies[101] |
| Neurofibromatosis |
| Chronic inflammatory demyelinating polyneuropathy[102] |
| Rett syndrome[103] |
| Leber's disease[104] |

chest wall or pulmonary disease. In common with all causes of central alveolar hypoventilation, the site of failure is in the automatic (central) ventilatory control system, but with PAHS there are no specific identifiable histological or structural defects in the area of the medullary respiratory neurons (Table 9.11)[96–98]. Obstructive apneas and hypopneas do not substantially contribute to the disordered breathing. Patients can maintain rhythmic breathing during wakefulness, but hypoventilation is severe during sleep, and may be accompanied by central apneas.

PAHS may affect children and adults. Congenital central hypoventilation syndrome is a very rare condition presenting in the newborn period, with fewer than 200 patients reported worldwide. There appears to be an increased association with Hirschsprung's disease, as well as abnormalities in the extraocular muscles or eyelids[105]. More common is presentation of PAHS in males aged 20–50 years, although females may also be affected[106].

### Clinical presentation

The disorder is often detected coincident with an unrelated respiratory infection, or after marked respiratory depression complicates usual doses of anesthesia or sedation. Affected patients are often asymptomatic and unaware. Dyspnea is often absent, since depressed ventilatory sensitivity to hypoxia and hypercapnia is blunted. When symptoms are present, they include fatigue, somnolence, disturbed sleep and morning headache. Cyanosis or polycythemia is not uncommon, and other features of cor pulmonale on physical examination may be found as the disorder progresses. Any of these findings should prompt evaluation of arterial blood gases and measures of respiratory function. At times, the pain or anxiety engendered by obtaining arterial blood gases may result in hyperventilation and a normalized $Pa_{CO_2}$. Review of prior serum bicarbonate levels may be a clue to chronic hypoventilation. Overnight oximetry will reveal marked hypoxemia as a result of hypoventilation. Chest X-ray, ECG and echocardiography may reveal evidence of pulmonary hypertension and right heart failure. During polysomnography, most cases of PAHS show hypoventilation to be worst during NREM and especially during slow-wave sleep, owing to nearly exclusive reliance on automatic respiratory control. Identifying the location of the defect as the central respiratory control center depends on the constellation of test results already reviewed (Table 9.2).

The differential diagnosis includes other causes of chronic ventilatory failure (Tables 9.1, 9.11). By meticulous history-taking taking and neurological evaluation, most other causes can be identified or eliminated. Because of the potential for familial forms of PAHS, a careful family history should be obtained[105].

### Management

The primary goal of management is to improve symptoms, improve ventilation and avoid acute and chronic complications of disease. The patient should be advised to exercise caution with alcohol and over-the-counter or prescription sedatives. Physicians must be made aware of the danger of pharmacological blunting of ventilatory drive. Several pharmacological agents have been used to augment respiratory drive, including acetazolamide, progesterone, theophylline and almitrine[107]. While these may work to a variable degree, they may bring unacceptable side-effects, do not have reliable impact and must be individually evaluated in each patient if used at all. Oxygen may improve $SaO_2$, but does not address ventilatory failure, which may worsen with loss of hypoxic drive. If supplemental oxygen is used, it should be initiated when sleep can be monitored carefully, and arterial blood gases should be measured to ensure that hypercapnia does not rise unacceptably. In most patients, mechanical ventilatory assistance is required to ensure adequate ventilation during sleep. This has been accomplished by rocking beds, negative-pressure ventilators, phrenic nerve stimulation and mechanical pressure or volume control ventilation. Ventilatory support can most often be accomplished with NIPPV, which is generally well tolerated and results in improvement in symptoms and arterial blood gases.

## Secondary alveolar hypoventilation due to neurological disease

The central respiratory control center can be affected by a wide number of degenerative, neoplastic and inflammatory neurological conditions (Table 9.11). Among these, multi-system atrophy (MSA) can especially result in a wide variety of sleep-disordered breathing (see Chapter 17). These require evaluation with polysomnography, and when indicated, PAP or NIPPV to correct sleep-related breathing disorders and hypoventilation.

## Sudden infant death syndrome

Sudden infant death syndrome (SIDS) is a disorder of unknown cause, and in the USA is responsible for more infant deaths beyond the neonatal period than any other disorder. The diagnosis is applied to cases where sudden death of an infant under 1 year of age remains unexplained after thorough clinical, autopsy and environmental examination. SIDS is probably caused by a variety of mechanisms, but one of the leading hypotheses is that death occurs because of a failure of respiratory control and arousal mechanisms. Examinations of the brain-stems of SIDS infants have revealed hypoplasia or decreased neurotransmitter binding in certain nuclei involved in ventilatory control and blood pressure responses, and some propose that maldevelopment or delay in maturation of these areas predisposes to SIDS when certain additional risks are present. The risk of SIDS is lowest in the first month, and maximal between the second and fourth months. Identified risks include prone sleeping, soft sleep surfaces or loose bedding, overheating, maternal smoking during pregnancy, bed-sharing, preterm delivery and low birth weight. Recommendations to reduce the risk of SIDS include correction of these factors, especially ensuring infants do not sleep prone. Although electronic cardiac and apnea monitors are available for home use, there is no evidence that the use of such monitors reduces rates of SIDS. Rates of SIDS have declined in the past decade in proportion to reductions in prone infant sleeping.

## ACUTE RESPIRATORY FAILURE AND CRITICAL ILLNESS

Acute respiratory failure, often a component of critical illness, is managed in intensive-care units and often requires the use of mechanical ventilators. Studies of sleep quality show that sleep architecture and quantity are dramatically changed by critical illness, the therapies employed and the care environment. One study of 20 critically ill mechanically ventilated patients found that eight had severely disrupted sleep but interpretable polysomnography, five had atypical sleep with dominant slow-wave activity alternating with more typical sleep epochs and seven showed coma. In the disrupted sleep group, 54.4% of total sleep time occurred during the day, and 40% of all sleep was stage 1, while only 10% was REM sleep[108]. Arousals or awakenings occurred 42 times each hour. Other polysomnographic studies demonstrate a similar pattern, with suppression of slow-wave and REM sleep, increase in stage 1, increased arousals and approximately half of sleep occurring intermittently throughout the daytime.

The adverse changes in architecture can be related to discomfort, care-related interruptions (position change, obtaining vital signs, blood draws and other tests), environmental noise, direct effects of illness or exacerbation of pre-existing sleep-related breathing disorders. Intensive medical therapy may adversely affect sleep. Corticosteroids, adrenergic agonists and invasive or uncomfortable devices may cause discomfort or insomnia. Choice of ventilator modality may influence sleep quality; pressure support ventilation has been shown to cause more central apneas and arousals than assist support ventilation[109].

An early study of sleep in the respiratory-care unit suggested that 54% of sleep disturbances were due to noise from the care unit and personnel intervention[110]. Another study showed that sound levels in the intensive-care unit (ICU) exceeded those recommended by the US Environmental Protection Agency, reaching over 80 dB once each hour[111]. Efforts to reduce ICU noise and light have not uniformly led to improvements in sleep quality, perhaps suggesting that illness-related factors are more important contributors to sleep fragmentation[112].

The ICU environment and intrusiveness of medical care leave much room for improvement. The effects of sleep fragmentation on hard clinical outcomes such as time on the ventilator, days in the ICU or rates of delirium have not yet been determined. However, given the relationship of sleep to cardiovascular, respiratory, neurological, immunological and endocrine function, it is likely that improvements in sleep quality will be reflected in superior clinical outcomes.

## REFERENCES

1. Lewis DA. Sleep in patients with respiratory disease. *Respir Care Clin North Am* 1999;5: 447–60

2. Miller JM, Moxham J, Green M. The maximal sniff in the assessment of diaphragm function in man. *Clin Sci (Lond)* 1985;69: 91–6

3. McCauley RG, Labib KB. Diaphragmatic paralysis evaluated by phrenic nerve stimulation during fluoroscopy or real-time ultrasound. *Radiology* 1984;153:33–6

4. Shochina M, Ferber I, Wolf E. Evaluation of the phrenic nerve in patients with neuromuscular disorders. *Int J Rehab Res* 1983;6:455–9

5. Clinical indications for noninvasive positive pressure ventilation in chronic respiratory failure due to restrictive lung disease, COPD, and nocturnal hypoventilation. A

consensus conference report. *Chest* 1999;116:521–34

6. Laghi F, Tobin MJ. Disorders of the respiratory muscles. *Am J Respir Crit Care Med* 2003;168:10–48

7. National Asthma Education and Prevention Program. Expert panel report: guidelines for the diagnosis and management of asthma update on selected topics – 2002. *J Allergy Clin Immunol* 2002;110:S141–219

8. Turner-Warwick M. Epidemiology of nocturnal asthma. *Am J Med* 1988;85:6–8

9. Janson C, De Backer W, Gislason T, et al. Increased prevalence of sleep disturbances and daytime sleepiness in subjects with bronchial asthma: a population study of young adults in three European countries. *Eur Respir J* 1996;9:2132–8

10. Wiegand L, Mende CN, Zaidel G, et al. Salmeterol vs theophylline: sleep and efficacy outcomes in patients with nocturnal asthma. *Chest* 1999;115:1525–32

11. Hetzel MR, Clark TJ. Comparison of normal and asthmatic circadian rhythms in peak expiratory flow rate. *Thorax* 1980;35:732–8

12. Hetzel MR, Clark TJ. Does sleep cause nocturnal asthma? *Thorax* 1979;34:749–54

13. Kales A, Beall GN, Bajor GF, Jacobson A, Kales JD. Sleep studies in asthmatic adults: relationship of attacks to sleep stage and time of night. *J Allergy* 1968;41:164–73

14. Montplaisir J, Walsh J, Malo JL. Nocturnal asthma: features of attacks, sleep and breathing patterns. *Am Rev Respir Dis* 1982;125:18–22

15. Calhoun WJ. Nocturnal asthma. *Chest* 2003;123:399S–405S

16. Gislason T, Janson C, Vermeire P, et al. Respiratory symptoms and nocturnal gastroesophageal reflux: a population-based study of young adults in three European countries. *Chest* 2002;121:158–63

17. Cibella F, Cuttitta G. Nocturnal asthma and gastroesophageal reflux. *Am J Med* 2001; 111:31S–6S

18. Lin CC, Lin CY. Obstructive sleep apnea syndrome and bronchial hyperreactivity. *Lung* 1995;173:117–26

19. Adams RJ, Fuhlbrigge A, Guilbert T, Lozano P, Martinez F. Inadequate use of asthma medication in the United States: results of the asthma in America national population survey. *J Allergy Clin Immunol* 2002;110:58–64

20. Konermann M, Luck G, Rawert B, Pirsig W. Effect of the long-acting β-2 agonist inhalant formoterol on the quality of sleep of patients with bronchial asthma. *Pneumologie* 2000;54:104–9

21. Man GC, Champman KR, Ali SH, Darke AC. Sleep quality and nocturnal respiratory function with once-daily theophylline (Uniphyl) and inhaled salbutamol in patients with COPD. *Chest* 1996;110:648–53

22. Roehrs T, Merlotti L, Halpin D, Rosenthal L, Roth T. Effects of theophylline on nocturnal sleep and daytime sleepiness/alertness. *Chest* 1995;108:382–7

23. Kaplan J, Fredrickson PA, Renaux SA, O'Brien PC. Theophylline effect on sleep in normal subjects. *Chest* 1993;103:193–5

24. Selby C, Engleman HM, Fitzpatrick MF, Sime PM, Mackay TW, Douglas NJ. Inhaled salmeterol or oral theophylline in nocturnal asthma? *Am J Respir Crit Care Med* 1997; 155:104–8

25. Campbell LM, Anderson TJ, Parashchak MR, Burke CM, Watson SA, Turbitt ML. A comparison of the efficacy of long-acting β2-agonists: eformoterol via Turbohaler and salmeterol via pressurized metered dose inhaler or Accuhaler, in mild to mod-

erate asthmatics. Force Research Group. *Respir Med* 1999;93:236–44

26. Pauwels RA, Buist AS, Calverley PMA, Jenkins CR, Hurd SS. Global strategy for the diagnosis, management, and prevention of chronic obstructive pulmonary disease. NHLBI/WHO Global Initiative for Chronic Obstructive Lung Disease (GOLD) Workshop Summary. *Am J Respir Crit Care Med* 2001;163:1256–76

27. Cormick W, Olson LG, Hensley MJ, Saunders NA. Nocturnal hypoxaemia and quality of sleep in patients with chronic obstructive lung disease. *Thorax* 1986;41: 846–54

28. Douglas NJ. Sleep in patients with chronic obstructive pulmonary disease. *Clin Chest Med* 1998;19:115–25

29. Lewis DA. Sleep in patients with asthma and chronic obstructive pulmonary disease. *Curr Opin Pulm Med* 2001;7:105–12

30. Breslin E, van der Schans C, Breukink S, *et al.* Perception of fatigue and quality of life in patients with COPD. *Chest* 1998;114: 958–64

31. Brezinova V, Catterall JR, Douglas NJ, Calverley PM, Flenley DC. Night sleep of patients with chronic ventilatory failure and age matched controls: number and duration of the EEG episodes of intervening wakefulness and drowsiness. *Sleep* 1982;5: 123–30

32. Coccagna G, Lugaresi E. Arterial blood gases and pulmonary and systemic arterial pressure during sleep in chronic obstructive pulmonary disease. *Sleep* 1978;1:117–24

33. Mulloy E, McNicholas WT. Ventilation and gas exchange during sleep and exercise in severe COPD. *Chest* 1996;109:387–94

34. Millman RP, Knight H, Kline LR, Shore ET, Chung DC, Pack AI. Changes in compartmental ventilation in association with eye

movements during REM sleep. *J Appl Physiol* 1988;65:1196–202

35. Meurice JC, Marc I, Series F. Influence of sleep on ventilatory and upper airway response to $CO_2$ in normal subjects and patients with COPD. *Am J Respir Crit Care Med* 1995;152:1620–6

36. Midgren B. Oxygen desaturation during sleep as a function of the underlying respiratory disease. *Am Rev Respir Dis* 1990;141: 43–6

37. Thomas VD, Vinod Kumar S, Gitanjali B. Predictors of nocturnal oxygen desaturation in chronic obstructive pulmonary disease in a South Indian population. *J Postgrad Med* 2002;48:101–4

38. Connaughton JJ, Catterall JR, Elton RA, Stradling JR, Douglas NJ. Do sleep studies contribute to the management of patients with severe chronic obstructive pulmonary disease? *Am Rev Respir Dis* 1988;138:341–4

39. Sanders MH, Newman AB, Haggerty CL, *et al.* Sleep and sleep-disordered breathing in adults with predominantly mild obstructive airway disease. *Am J Respir Crit Care Med* 2003;167:7–14

40. Fletcher EC, Luckett RA, Miller T, Fletcher JG. Exercise hemodynamics and gas exchange in patients with chronic obstruction pulmonary disease, sleep desaturation, and a daytime $Pa_{O_2}$ above 60 mmHg. *Am Rev Respir Dis* 1989;140:1237–45

41. Fletcher EC, Luckett RA, Miller T, Costarangos C, Kutka N, Fletcher JG. Pulmonary vascular hemodynamics in chronic lung disease patients with and without oxyhemoglobin desaturation during sleep. *Chest* 1989;95:757–64

42. Chaouat A, Weitzenblum E, Kessler R, *et al.* Sleep-related $O_2$ desaturation and daytime pulmonary haemodynamics in COPD

patients with mild hypoxaemia. *Eur Respir J* 1997;10:1730–5

43. Fletcher EC, Donner CF, Midgren B, *et al.* Survival in COPD patients with a daytime *Pa*O$_2$ greater than 60 mmHg with and without nocturnal oxyhemoglobin desaturation. *Chest* 1992;101:649–55

44. Continuous or nocturnal oxygen therapy in hypoxemic chronic obstructive lung disease: a clinical trial. Nocturnal Oxygen Therapy Trial Group. *Ann Intern Med* 1980;93:391–8

45. Long term domiciliary oxygen therapy in chronic hypoxic cor pulmonale complicating chronic bronchitis and emphysema. Report of the Medical Research Council Working Party. *Lancet* 1981;1:681–6

46. Fleetham J, West P, Mezon B, Conway W, Roth T, Kryger M. Sleep, arousals, and oxygen desaturation in chronic obstructive pulmonary disease. The effect of oxygen therapy. *Am Rev Respir Dis* 1982;126:429–33

47. Chaouat A, Weitzenblum E, Kessler R, *et al.* A randomized trial of nocturnal oxygen therapy in chronic obstructive pulmonary disease patients. *Eur Respir J* 1999;14:1002–8

48. Fletcher EC, Luckett RA, Goodnight-White S, Miller CC, Qian W, Costarangos-Galarza C. A double-blind trial of nocturnal supplemental oxygen for sleep desaturation in patients with chronic obstructive pulmonary disease and a daytime *Pa*O$_2$ above 60 mmHg. *Am Rev Respir Dis* 1992;145:1070–6

49. West R. Bupropion SR for smoking cessation. *Expert Opin Pharmacother* 2003;4:533–40

50. Mulloy E, McNicholas WT. Theophylline improves gas exchange during rest, exercise, and sleep in severe chronic obstructive pulmonary disease. *Am Rev Respir Dis* 1993;148:1030–6

51. Mulloy E, McNicholas WT. Theophylline in obstructive sleep apnea. A double-blind evaluation. *Chest* 1992;101:753–7

52. Bott J, Carroll MP, Conway JH, *et al.* Randomised controlled trial of nasal ventilation in acute ventilatory failure due to chronic obstructive airways disease. *Lancet* 1993;341:1555–7

53. Keenan SP, Kernerman PD, Cook DJ, Martin CM, McCormack D, Sibbald WJ. Effect of noninvasive positive pressure ventilation on mortality in patients admitted with acute respiratory failure: a meta-analysis. *Crit Care Med* 1997;25:1685–92

54. Fleetham JA. Is chronic obstructive pulmonary disease related to sleep apnea–hypopnea syndrome? *Am J Respir Crit Care Med* 2003;167:3–4

55. Chaouat A, Weitzenblum E, Krieger J, Ifoundza T, Oswald M, Kessler R. Association of chronic obstructive pulmonary disease and sleep apnea syndrome. *Am J Respir Crit Care Med* 1995;151:82–6

56. Resta O, Guido P, Picca V, *et al.* Prescription of nCPAP and nBIPAP in obstructive sleep apnoea syndrome: Italian experience in 105 subjects. A prospective two centre study. *Respir Med* 1998;92:820–7

57. Congleton J, Hodson ME, Duncan-Skingle F. Quality of life in adults with cystic fibrosis. *Thorax* 1996;51:936–40

58. Bradley S, Solin P, Wilson J, Johns D, Walters EH, Naughton MT. Hypoxemia and hypercapnia during exercise and sleep in patients with cystic fibrosis. *Chest* 1999;116:647–54

59. Tepper R, Skatrud J, Dempsey J. Ventilation and oxygenation changes during sleep in cystic fibrosis. *Chest* 1983;84:388–93

60. Muller NL, Francis PW, Gurwitz D, Levison H, Bryan AC. Mechanism of hemoglobin

desaturation during rapid-eye-movement sleep in normal subjects and in patients with cystic fibrosis. *Am Rev Respir Dis* 1980;121:463–9

61. Braggion C, Pradal U, Mastella G. Hemoglobin desaturation during sleep and daytime in patients with cystic fibrosis and severe airway obstruction. *Acta Paediatr* 1992;81:1002–6

62. Piper A, Parker S, Torzillo P, Sullivan C, Bye P. Nocturnal nasal IPPV stabilizes patients with cystic fibrosis and hypercapnic respiratory failure. *Chest* 1992;102:846–50

63. Serra A, Polese G, Braggion C, Rossi A. Non-invasive proportional assist and pressure support ventilation in patients with cystic fibrosis and chronic respiratory failure. *Thorax* 2002;57:50–4

64. Manson JE, Bassuk SS. Obesity in the United States: a fresh look at its high toll. *J Am Med Assoc* 2003;289:229–30

65. Fontaine KR, Redden DT, Wang C, Westfall AO, Allison DB. Years of life lost due to obesity. *J Am Med Assoc* 2003;289:187–93

66. Zerah-Lancner F, Lofaso F, Coste A, Ricolfi F, Goldenberg F, Harf A. Pulmonary function in obese snorers with or without sleep apnea syndrome. *Am J Respir Crit Care Med* 1997;156:522–7

67. Lazarus R, Sparrow D, Weiss ST. Effects of obesity and fat distribution on ventilatory function: the normative aging study. *Chest* 1997;111:891–8

68. Resta O, Foschino Barbaro MP, Bonfitto P, *et al.* Low sleep quality and daytime sleepiness in obese patients without obstructive sleep apnoea syndrome. *J Intern Med* 2003;253:536–43

69. Burwell CS, Robin ED, Whaley RD, *et al.* Extreme obesity associated with alveolar hypoventilation: a pickwickian syndrome. *Am J Med* 1956;21:811–18

70. Sleep-related breathing disorders in adults: recommendations for syndrome definition and measurement techniques in clinical research. The Report of an American Academy of Sleep Medicine Task Force. *Sleep* 1999;22:667–89

71. Zwillich CW, Sutton FD, Pierson DJ, Greagh EM, Weil JV. Decreased hypoxic ventilatory drive in the obesity-hypoventilation syndrome. *Am J Med* 1975;59:343–8

72. Jokic R, Zintel T, Sridhar G, Gallagher CG, Fitzpatrick MF. Ventilatory responses to hypercapnia and hypoxia in relatives of patients with the obesity hypoventilation syndrome. *Thorax* 2000;55:940–5

73. Guilleminault C, Kurland G, Winkle R, Miles L. Severe kyphoscoliosis, breathing, and sleep: the 'Quasimodo' syndrome during sleep. *Chest* 1981;79:626–30

74. Ryu JH, Olson EJ, Midthun DE, Swensen SJ. Diagnostic approach to the patient with diffuse lung disease. *Mayo Clin Proc* 2002;77:1221–7

75. Douglas WW, Ryu JH, Schroeder DR. Idiopathic pulmonary fibrosis: impact of oxygen and colchicine, prednisone, or no therapy on survival. *Am J Respir Crit Care Med* 2000;161:1172–8

76. Ryu JH, Colby TV, Hartman TE. Idiopathic pulmonary fibrosis: current concepts. *Mayo Clin Proc* 1998;73:1085–101

77. George CF, Kryger MH. Sleep in restrictive lung disease. *Sleep* 1987;10:409–18

78. Vazquez JC, Perez-Padilla R. Effect of oxygen on sleep and breathing in patients with interstitial lung disease at moderate altitude. *Respiration* 2001;68:584–9

79. Khan Y, Heckmatt JZ. Obstructive apnoeas in Duchenne muscular dystrophy. *Thorax* 1994;49:157–61

80. Hukins CA, Hillman DR. Daytime predictors of sleep hypoventilation in Duchenne muscular dystrophy. *Am J Respir Crit Care Med* 2000;161:166–70

81. Falga-Tirado C, Perez-Peman P, Ordi-Ros J, Bofill JM, Balcells E. Adult onset of nemaline myopathy presenting as respiratory insufficiency. *Respiration* 1995;62:353–4

82. Kotagal S, Archer CR, Walsh JK, Gomez C. Hypersomnia, bithalamic lesions, and altered sleep architecture in Kearns–Sayre syndrome. *Neurology* 1985;35:574–7

83. Mellies U, Ragette R, Schwake C, Baethmann M, Voit T, Teschler H. Sleep-disordered breathing and respiratory failure in acid maltase deficiency. *Neurology* 2001;57:1290–5

84. Saarelainen S, Jantti V, Kalimo H, Haapasalo H. Hypotyreoosin aiheuttama alveolaarinen hypoventilaatio ja myopatia. *Duodecim* 1993;109:759–63

85. Gilmartin JJ, Cooper BG, Griffiths CJ, *et al.* Breathing during sleep in patients with myotonic dystrophy and non-myotonic respiratory muscle weakness. *Q J Med* 1991;78:21–31

86. Stambler N, Charatan M, Cedarbaum JM. Prognostic indicators of survival in ALS. ALS CNTF Treatment Study Group. *Neurology* 1998;50:66–72

87. Gay PC, Westbrook PR, Daube JR, Litchy WJ, Windebank AJ, Iverson R. Effects of alterations in pulmonary function and sleep variables on survival in patients with amyotrophic lateral sclerosis. *Mayo Clin Proc* 1991;66:686–94

88. Miller RG, Rosenberg JA, Gelinas DF, *et al.* Practice parameter: the care of the patient with amyotrophic lateral sclerosis (an evidence-based review): report of the Quality Standards Subcommittee of the American Academy of Neurology: ALS Practice Parameters Task Force. *Neurology* 1999; 52:1311–23

89. Aboussouan LS. Effect of noninvasive positive-pressure ventilation on survival in amyotrophic lateral sclerosis. *Ann Intern Med* 1997;127:450–3

90. Gay PC, Edmonds LC. Severe hypercapnia after low-flow oxygen therapy in patients with neuromuscular disease and diaphragmatic dysfunction. *Mayo Clin Proc* 1995; 70:327–30

91. Serisier DE, Mastaglia FL, Gibson GJ. Respiratory muscle function and ventilatory control. I In patients with motor neurone disease. II In patients with myotonic dystrophy. *Q J Med* 1982;51:205–26

92. MacDonald JR, Hill JD, Tarnopolsky MA. Modafinil reduces excessive somnolence and enhances mood in patients with myotonic dystrophy. *Neurology* 2002;59: 1876–80

93. Ragette R, Mellies U, Schwake C, Voit T, Teschler H. Patterns and predictors of sleep disordered breathing in primary myopathies. *Thorax* 2002;57:724–8

94. Khan Y, Heckmatt JZ, Dubowitz V. Sleep studies and supportive ventilatory treatment in patients with congenital muscle disorders. *Arch Dis Child* 1996;74:195–200

95. Patakas D, Tsara V, Zoglopitis F, Daskalopoulou E, Argyropoulou P, Maniki E. Nocturnal hypoxia in unilateral diaphragmatic paralysis. *Respiration* 1991; 58:95–9

96. Plum F, Leigh RJ. Abnormalities of central mechanisms. In Hornbein TF, ed. *Regulation of Breathing, part 2.* New York: Marcel Dekker 1981;17:989–1067

97. Gozal D, Harper RM. Novel insights into congenital hypoventilation syndrome. *Curr Opin Pulm Med* 1999;5:335–8

98. Gozal D. Congenital central hypoventilation syndrome: an update. *Pediatr Pulmonol* 1998;26:273–82

99. Kim H, Bach JR. Central alveolar hypoventilation in neurosarcoidosis. *Arch Phys Med Rehab* 1998;79:1467–8

100. Lee DK, Wahl GW, Swinburne AJ, Fedullo AJ. Recurrent acoustic neuroma presenting as central alveolar hypoventilation. *Chest* 1994;105:949–50

101. Ball JA, Warner T, Reid P, Howard RS, Gregson NA, Rossor MN. Central alveolar hypoventilation associated with paraneoplastic brain-stem encephalitis and anti-Hu antibodies. *J Neurol* 1994;241:561–6

102. Yamamoto T, Ohnishi A, Miyoshi T, Hashimoto T, Murai Y. A case of chronic inflammatory demyelinating polyradiculoneuropathy (CIDP) with bilateral recurrent nerve palsy and primary alveolar hypoventilation – comparative studies of the histological findings of the two sural nerve biopsies with 9 years interval. *Rinsho Shinkeigaku – Clin Neurol* 1994;34:712–16

103. Cirignotta F, Mondini S, Zucconi M, Sforza E, Gerardi R, Petronelli R. Breathing impairment in central alveolar hypoventilation and Rett syndrome. *Funct Neurol* 1987;2:487–92

104. Hunter AR. Idiopathic alveolar hypoventilation in Leber's disease. Unusual sensitivity to mild analgesics and diazepam. *Anaesthesia* 1984;39:781–3

105. Spengler CM, Gozal D, Shea SA. Chemoreceptive mechanisms elucidated by studies of congenital central hypoventilation syndrome. *Respir Physiol* 2001;129:247–55

106. Rhoads GG, Brody JS. Idiopathic alveolar hypoventilation: clinical spectrum. *Ann Intern Med* 1969;71:271–8

107. Antic N, McEvoy RD. Primary alveolar hypoventilation and response to the respiratory stimulant almitrine. *Int Med J* 2002;32:622–4

108. Cooper AB, Thornley KS, Young GB, Slutsky AS, Stewart TE, Hanly PJ. Sleep in critically ill patients requiring mechanical ventilation. *Chest* 2000;117:809–18

109. Parthasarathy S, Tobin MJ. Effect of ventilator mode on sleep quality in critically ill patients. *Am J Respir Crit Care Med* 2002;166:1423–9

110. Hilton BA. Quantity and quality of patients' sleep and sleep-disturbing factors in a respiratory intensive care unit. *J Adv Nurs* 1976;1:453–68

111. Meyer TJ, Eveloff SE, Bauer MS, Schwartz WA, Hill NS, Millman RP. Adverse environmental conditions in the respiratory and medical ICU settings. *Chest* 1994;105:1211–16

112. Walder B, Francioli D, Meyer JJ, Lancon M, Romand JA. Effects of guidelines implementation in a surgical intensive care unit to control nighttime light and noise levels. *Crit Care Med* 2000;28:2242–7

# Section III
# The patient who cannot sleep

# Chapter 10

# Insomnia and its causes

*O sleep, O gentle sleep,*
*Nature's soft nurse, how have I frighted thee,*
*That thou no more wilt weigh mine eyelids down*
*And steep my senses in forgetfulness?*

**William Shakespeare,** *King Henry IV, Part II*

Insomnia, a major cause of distress, is present when a patient perceives that inadequate sleep has been achieved. Despite trying sometimes for hours, patients with insomnia cannot get sufficient sleep, in many cases leading to adverse daytime consequences.

## CLASSIFICATION OF INSOMNIA

Classifying insomnia has been challenging because of all the possible causes and subtypes. The definition of insomnia is particularly important for research purposes, because observations concerning epidemiology, etiology, natural history and treatment response may apply only to patients with similar characteristics.

Insomnia can be most easily divided in terms of duration of the condition (Table 10.1). This approach has clinical relevance because the treatment selected for transient insomnia often differs from that recommended for chronic insomnia. The classification of transient, short-term and chronic insomnia was used in a large American epidemiological study of the disorder funded by the National Sleep Foundation. In the USA, approximately 30% of adults report transient insomnia once a month and 10% describe chronic insomnia[1]. This study reported adverse consequences of untreated insomnia, including impaired concentration, decreased memory, reduced ability to fulfill roles and decreased enjoyment of interpersonal relationships. Although widely used, classifying by duration of symptoms does have significant limitations, as it does not adequately describe patients with recurrent bouts of insomnia or provide information about possible etiologies.

The International Classification of Sleep Disorders (ICSD) as revised in 1997 adopted a markedly different perspective, grouping insomnia by pathophysiology and etiology[2]. Insomnia was subdivided into primary and secondary forms. Primary insomnia was further subdivided into intrinsic (endogenous) or extrinsic (reactive to the setting or a specific trigger). A slightly different

**Table 10.1** Classification of insomnia

Transient insomnia: several days' duration

Short-term insomnia: up to 3 weeks' duration

Chronic insomnia: longer than 3 weeks' duration

classification is planned for the 2004 revised ICSD-2, but most categories will remain the same or similar (see Table 2.3). The ICSD offers more details about the diverse etiologies of insomnia than classification by duration of the illness allows. As a result, Table 10.2, modified from the 1997 ICSD, provides a useful perspective on the complexities of insomnia. However, because of the relative lack of knowledge about some of the entities, using these ICSD diagnostic categories may be difficult in the clinical setting.

For the purposes of this chapter, the intrinsic and extrinsic types of insomnia are considered together as primary insomnia. High-altitude insomnia is primarily related to a respiratory mechanism, and is discussed in Chapter 8. Insufficient sleep syndrome is discussed elsewhere (Chapter 6), as it results from a deliberate curtailment of sleep, whereas insomnia is an inability to sleep despite the desire to do so.

**Table 10.2** Classification of insomnia

*Primary insomnia*

Intrinsic sleep disorders

    psychophysiological insomnia

    Paradoxical insomnia (sleep state misperception)

    idiopathic insomnia

Extrinsic sleep disorders

    inadequate sleep hygiene

    environmental sleep disorder (discussed in Chapter 5)

    altitude insomnia (discussed in Chapter 8)

    adjustment sleep disorder

    insufficient sleep syndrome (discussed in Chapter 6)

    limit-setting sleep disorder

    sleep-onset sleep disorder

    food allergy insomnia

    hypnotic-dependent insomnia

    stimulant dependent insomnia

    alcohol-dependent insomnia

    toxin-induced insomnia

*Secondary insomnia*

Sleep disorders associated with mental, neurological or other medical disorders

## MECHANISMS OF INSOMNIA

Four major factors can contribute to insomnia (Table 10.3). In clinical practice multiple issues typically coexist.

### Homeostatic factors

Disturbances of sleep homeostasis may be an important factor in the pathogenesis of insomnia. Homeostasis must always be viewed in the context of the sleep–wake circadian rhythm. When the intensity of the homeostatic pressure is reduced, this may produce an unsatisfactory sleep latency or duration, identified as insomnia. However, when homeostatic and circadian signals

**Table 10.3** Four important potential mechanisms of insomnia

Homeostatic factors (weak sleep drive or debt)

Inhospitable environment

Maladaptive coping mechanisms or behaviors

Stress response

are of sufficient strength but their synchronization is the prominent concern, the sleep disorder is classified as a circadian rhythm problem (Chapter 13).

One possible explanation of primary insomnia is an absent or underdeveloped drive to sleep or ability to accumulate a sleep debt. This may be due to either a deficiency of inhibitory or an excess of stimulating neurotransmitters, thus impairing the brain's ability to initiate sleep. Chapter 1 provides an overview of the neuromodulators that are known to control sleep and wake, including the monoamines, acetylcholine and adenosine. Despite this hypothesis of a chemical imbalance being especially attractive in explaining the sleep difficulties of childhood-onset insomnia, to date no evidence supports this theory. However, the discovery of hypocretin (orexin) deficiency as a cause of narcolepsy with cataplexy makes the possibility of a neurochemical derangement being responsible for some types of insomnia more conceivable. So far no analogous findings have been reported for insomnia, but there may be many unidentified neurotransmitters and neuropeptides. Such investigations of insomnia will not be easy to conduct, as none of the subtypes have a phenotype as specific as narcolepsy with cataplexy. Lacking an animal model of insomnia further limits research avenues into potential neurochemical associations.

### Inhospitable environment

Falling and staying asleep is difficult if any of a large number of adverse environmental factors are present (Table 10.4). Although the adverse nature of a particular sleep environment may be obvious to a clinician, it is important to explore the degree to which the patient has awareness that the sleep environment is suboptimal. Some patients recognize the disruptive nature of their sleeping environment but do not believe they can modify it. An example is a woman sleeping next to a man with dream enactment behavior involving kicking and shouting. The bed partner may not be aware that treatment is available for her spouse's problem.

### Case 10.1

A 37-year-old hospital maintenance employee presented because of fatigue and sleepiness. The patient described decreased energy ever since he agreed to switch from the evening to the night shift. He welcomed this change because he was given more authority on the job and received an attractive increase in pay. He denied snoring, restless legs and any other specific sleep complaint. Typically he went to bed at 8 a.m., soon after returning home from work. He described falling asleep with moderate difficulty, and on average slept for 7 h. He did not feel refreshed upon arising at 4 p.m. He mentioned that his wife did not accompany him because she had to work. When asked specifically, he explained that she ran a day-care center in their home. He confirmed that he slept in a bedroom of their small bungalow while the 12 preschoolers were elsewhere in the house. His wife had started the day-care at about the same time as he switched to the night shift. At times he would awaken during the day because of the noise but he did not think this was significant because he quickly fell asleep again. He could see no easy way for him to sleep elsewhere or for his wife to relocate her business. After a

**Table 10.4** Environmental causes of insomnia

| | |
|---|---|
| Loud noises | snoring, coughing, sleep-talking by bed partner |
| | music |
| | television |
| | traffic |
| | pager and telephone |
| | burglar, car and other alarms |
| | mechanical sounds (such as elevator shaft) |
| | barking or other pet sounds |
| Extreme temperature | heat (such as no air conditioning) |
| | cold (such as insufficient bedcovers) |
| Bedding materials | uncomfortable bed, pillow and bedclothes |
| | allergy to laundry soap or feather pillow |
| Light | bright light (such as sunlight during the summer at high latitudes, shift worker sleeping during the day) |
| Body positioning | seated position (such as airplane, car or train) |
| | cramped bed (such as significantly obese patient in a twin bed) |
| Movement | vibration or turbulence (such as airplane, car or train) |
| | body movement (leg kicks or thrashing by bed partner) |

long discussion, further testing and pharmacological treatment were deferred until the patient managed to change his sleep environment.

This patient had a combination of shift work and environmental sleep disorder. He had not tried to hide the circumstances related to his daytime sleep, but did not realize that noise was probably compromising the quality of his sleep. This problem can be particularly challenging for shift workers who are trying to sleep when most of the community is awake. Clearly, some patients lack adequate understanding that an environmental factor, such as a television playing in the bedroom, may contribute to their difficulties falling and staying asleep.

## Maladaptive coping mechanisms and behaviors

Patients can adopt behaviors or habits that interfere with initiating or maintaining sleep (Table 10.5). In our society many people with demanding schedules stay busy right up to the time that they desire to fall asleep, continuing to tackle work or non-work activities well into the night. As a result, the body and mind are not in the relaxed state necessary for initiating sleep. Some people may need considerable time before they can relax sufficiently to fall asleep[3]. However, as they wait, they may become increasingly frustrated with their inability to sleep at the desired time, ironically causing more muscle tension and alertness which further distance them from sleep onset.

**Table 10.5** Maladaptive behaviors that can compromise sleep

Engaging in stimulating activities up to bedtime

Using the bedroom for activities other than sleep

Inconsistent sleep–wake rhythm

Checking the clock during the night

Consuming foods that promote heartburn

Inappropriate caffeine use

Using alcohol habitually as a sleep aid

Relying long term on benzodiazepines for sleep

Inadequate exercise

Patients can lose confidence that they can fall asleep in their own bed. Insomnia can also develop when people no longer associate their bed or bedroom with sleep, often caused by using their bed for other activities, such as studying or paying bills. They have developed negative conditioning because they have pursued activities associated with arousal in bed and do not expect to fall asleep there. Patients with this type of conditioned insomnia typically fall asleep more readily in an unfamiliar bed where these expectations do not apply[4].

Insomnia has been associated with a sedentary life-style. If a patient seldom exercises or spends most of the day inactive, this can contribute to poor sleep at night. The patient does not expend energy in a way that enhances the building of the homeostatic pressure to sleep. Furthermore, some sedentary patients may find themselves taking unplanned naps at their desk or on the couch, which further reduces their ability to fall asleep promptly at bedtime. Spending large amounts of time in bed during the day is an issue closely related to a sedentary life-style. Because of fatigue, some patients with insomnia stay in bed for much of the following day. Under these circumstances they may experience intermittent sleep during the day and therefore do not readily fall asleep that evening. Patients can become trapped in a vicious cycle whereby their attempts to compensate for poor night-time sleep and daytime fatigue actually aggravate the sleep initiation problems that are the root cause of their sleep complaint.

Patients who do not keep a regular sleep–wake cycle are at risk of being unable to fall asleep at a predictable time. Their homeostatic and circadian cues may no longer be co-ordinated with one another, or may both be delayed relative to the patient's desired bedtime. This situation can be voluntary, for example the young adult staying up late at the weekend but wishing to fall asleep earlier during the week, or related to work schedules as is seen with rotating shift workers.

Some patients remain acutely aware of the passage of time as they endeavor to fall asleep. Alternatively, when they awake they may check the clock. As morning nears, they become more fearful that they will have difficulty in fulfilling their daytime responsibilities and irritated that they cannot drift off to sleep. These distressing thoughts lead to muscle tension and increased alertness.

Caffeine is one of the most widely used stimulants, appearing in a growing number of beverages and foods. Recently, caffeine has been added to some brands of water and mints, which are then marketed as products that promote alertness. Injudicious use of caffeine later in the day, for example more than 300 mg or three cups of regular coffee, can lead to insomnia[5]. Studies have shown increased arousals from sleep throughout the night even when 200 mg of caffeine is consumed in the morning[6]. There is tremendous variability from person to person in the effects that small amounts of caffeine can have on sleep[5]. Poor-quality sleep at night can then lead to daytime fatigue, and patients may then further increase their consumption of caffeine, unaware that they are aggravating the situation[7]. Daily caffeine use quickly leads to a physical dependence, and if caffeine is abruptly discontinued, a headache of varying intensity can develop. Patients with a history of cardiac arrhythmia, tachycardia, palpitations or anxiety are typically advised to avoid caffeine use altogether. In stimulant-dependent insomnia, stimulants other than caffeine, including over-the-counter medications (OTC) for upper respiratory infections or prescription agents for asthma, weight loss or attention deficit disorder, lead to inability to sleep.

In a study that explored both self-medication with alcohol and OTC medications, a random group of 1324 people from metropolitan Detroit were asked what substances they used to fall asleep. Ten per cent used alcohol exclusively, 10% OTC medications, 8% prescription medication and 5% both alcohol and OTC medications[8]. Alcohol has several detrimental effects on sleep that outweigh the benefits. The initial sedation is short-lived, and within hours alcohol is metabolized. Use of alcohol at bedtime contributes to sleep maintenance difficulties with increased awakenings later in the night[9]. This condition is known as alcohol-dependent insomnia. The decreased quality of sleep in the second half of the night has been associated with excessive daytime sleepiness[10]. Long-term alcohol use, as well as chronic usage of benzodiazepines, can lead to a reduction in the time spent in slow-wave sleep. Sometimes alcohol use becomes more habitual because of a mistaken belief that alcohol would prevent insomnia. Frequent self-medication for insomnia has been identified as a risk factor for alcohol abuse (Chapter 14). An estimated 28% of patients presenting with insomnia also have substance abuse disorders[1].

When long-term benzodiazepine use evolves to become a perpetuating factor in insomnia, hypnotic-dependent insomnia can be diagnosed. After discontinuing benzodiazepines, patients can experience rebound insomnia that can lead them to resume the hypnotic medication. With continued use of benzodiazepines, tolerance can develop, with the patient needing to increase the dose to achieve the same response. After months or years of continuous usage, some patients develop insomnia not only with discontinuation but even with a dose reduction. Patients can become convinced that they cannot sleep without the medication.

## Case 10.2

A 52-year-old woman working the day shift as a waitress in a truck stop presented with worsening insomnia and fatigue. When she went to bed it often took her 90–180 min to fall asleep. During this time she would stay in bed listening to late-night talk shows. Some nights she would turn on the citizens' band radio near her bed and converse with her truck-driver friends. As the time passed, she would become increasingly frustrated with her increasing inability to sleep. Because she never felt refreshed, she started her morning with a large cup of coffee, which she refilled countless times during the day at work.

Many factors contributed to this patient's worsening insomnia. It is likely that the problem started when she was not consistent about the timing of bedtime or the activities she engaged in immediately before sleep onset. Listening to television and the citizens' band radio is not conducive to entering the relaxed state of sleep. Gradually, she no longer had the assumption that when she went to bed she would promptly fall asleep. To compound the problem further she tried to self-medicate her daytime fatigue with an undetermined but presumably large quantity of caffeinated beverages. Her efforts to cope were actually another reason why the insomnia steadily worsened.

### Stress response

Many people experience difficulty in relaxing and falling asleep when their coping skills are overwhelmed by the stress in their lives. Everyone faces stressful circumstances from time to time, whether negative, such as a possible bankruptcy, or positive, such as a wedding in the family. There is tremendous individual variability in the type of stressful situation that may lead to psychological and physical distress. Some individuals cope better with stress than others, and may deliberately seek out demanding professional roles, such as air-traffic controller, because they find this to be invigorating. The issues at play are the person's attitude and coping mechanisms as well as the intensity, duration and frequency of stressful circumstances. In a recent study, good and poor sleepers reported similar numbers of minor stressful events, but the poor sleepers regarded these events as more intense and having a greater impact upon them. Those who reported more difficulty in falling asleep erroneously perceived themselves as leading a more stressful life[11]. Patients with diagnosed anxiety or mood disorders would generally be expected to have considerably more difficulty in managing stressful circumstances with a resulting adverse effect on sleep (Chapter 14).

### PRIMARY INSOMNIA

### Psychophysiological insomnia

Psychophysiological insomnia has been extensively studied, with a clear understanding of the pivotal role that maladaptive attitudes and behaviors play. The name of this type of insomnia suggests an interplay of the mind and body. Psychophysiological insomnia represents a chronic disorder in which patients are unable to sleep at night and consequently function poorly during the day. Their difficulties are related to the interaction of anxious thoughts and tense muscles. Over time, they develop attitudes and practices that perpetuate their inability to sleep as desired.

### Case 10.3

A 48-year-old woman, working part-time in a retail store, was referred because of insomnia. One event stood out as exacerbating her pre-existing sleep problems, which up to that time had been intermittent and present only to a mild degree.

She took mefloquine as malaria prophylaxis while on an overseas trip, which markedly worsened her insomnia, leaving her awake all night. Even after discontinuing this medication, she continued to have great difficulty in falling asleep. She denied that she experienced chronically depressed mood or anxiety. As she remained wide-awake at night, she became increasingly irritated as time passed, and felt as if her muscles were tied in knots as she struggled to fall asleep. She was aware that she sometimes slept better when staying in a hotel or camping. Over the years she had tried many methods to fall asleep, including wine, diphenhydramine, aromatherapy and self-help books, without any sustained benefit. She had become disgusted with the time and effort that she had invested into her search for a solution. She asked whether she had a hopeless case of insomnia.

This is an example of a classic case of psychophysiological insomnia, with onset at the time of an episode of acute insomnia but persistent symptoms perpetuated by muscle tension and negative thinking.

Psychophysiological insomnia can start after an event or condition disrupts sleep. Once the vicious cycle is established, the insomnia may persist even though the initial trigger has disappeared. Over the ensuing months and years, patients can become preoccupied with their insomnia to the degree that their poor sleep dominates their existence. Affected patients develop muscle tension and negative associations that further hamper their ability to sleep. These two factors can create a self-perpetuating cycle with the insomnia leading to increased anxiety, more muscle tension and more conviction that sleep will not occur in a particular setting. This type of primary insomnia can only be diagnosed in the absence of any other disorder that might be causative, for example psychiatric disorders.

Patients with psychophysiological insomnia not only have poor sleep but also have impaired daytime functioning. They can experience daytime fatigue, poor attention and increased subjective physical complaints. When a multiple sleep latency test is conducted, no sign of objective sleepiness is documented. Patients at risk often have been poor sleepers since childhood, and as a result presumably lack confidence in their ability to fall asleep. The prevalence of this condition is unknown in the general population but women are more commonly affected than men. This is a chronic disorder with most patients experiencing insomnia for months, years or even decades.

### Idiopathic insomnia

When patients have a lifelong inability to sleep, idiopathic insomnia should be considered. This is a potentially debilitating sleep disorder that can start as early as childhood and typically persists throughout life. This is the type of insomnia most likely to be associated with impaired sleep debt or drive, leading to inadequate homeostatic pressure to sleep. Patients experience high levels of distress. As a result of their inadequate sleep, they complain of daytime fatigue, poor motivation, depressed mood and decreased attention. This condition rarely exists in isolation, because over time maladaptive sleep attitudes and behaviors typically evolve to complicate the picture. A patient may also seek relief by using caffeine, hypnotics or even stimulants that further add to the complex nature of the condition. Little is known about the pathogenesis, epidemiology or course of this disorder.

## Paradoxical insomnia (sleep state misperception)

Paradoxical insomnia, until recently known as sleep state misperception, is a rare type of primary insomnia. Patients with this disorder complain of subjective sleep disturbances that are not consistent with objective data. The patient is not exaggerating the severity of their insomnia or the consequences, but is genuinely distressed. In order to meet criteria for this diagnosis, some objective data need to be collected to compare with the patient's subjective complaint. The ICSD suggests polysomnography as the means to demonstrate normal duration and quality of sleep. Because polysomnography is often difficult to obtain owing to reimbursement issues when the patient's chief complaint is insomnia, actigraphy or reports of hospital nurses or even a family member must often suffice.

As the understanding of this sleep disorder and the sophistication of sleep diagnostic technology increase, some of these patients may eventually be diagnosed with more specific sleep disorders. The prevalence and natural course of this sleep disorder are not understood. An association has been suspected between paradoxical insomnia and anxiety disorders, but little evidence of this exists to date.

## Inadequate sleep hygiene

Inadequate sleep hygiene refers to insomnia owing to daily living activities inconsistent with the maintenance of good-quality sleep. Many of the factors discussed above under mechanisms of insomnia (inhospitable environment and maladaptive coping mechanisms or behavior) are responsible. Poor sleep hygiene practices are commonly seen in almost all causes of insomnia, and this diagnosis should be reserved for patients in whom these practices are the predominant cause of the problem.

## Adjustment sleep disorder

An adjustment sleep disorder should be diagnosed when insomnia is temporally related to acute stress or other emotional disturbances. These include marriage, divorce, loss of a job, bereavement and other major positive or negative life events. The insomnia usually runs a short course. If it is still present by 6 months, consideration should be given to an associated psychiatric disorder such as depression, or the start of psychophysiological insomnia.

### SECONDARY INSOMNIA

Multiple medical, neurological and psychiatric conditions can cause insomnia (Table 10.6). Some of the primary sleep disorders, most notably sleep apnea syndromes and restless legs syndrome, can present with insomnia rather than excessive daytime sleepiness. These conditions are discussed in detail elsewhere in this book.

## Medical disorders associated with insomnia

In addition to the respiratory disorders discussed in Chapters 8 and 9, several other medical disorders can create difficulty with sleep initiation and maintenance. Gastroesophageal reflux disorder (GERD) is a well-known cause of insomnia.

**Table 10.6** Selected causes of secondary insomnia

*Medical causes*

Obstructive sleep apnea syndrome (Chapter 8)

Chronic obstructive pulmonary disease (Chapter 9)

Asthma (Chapter 9)

Gastroesophageal reflux disorder

Hyperthyroidism

Benign prostatic hypertrophy

Acute and chronic pain

Fibromyalgia

*Psychiatric causes (Chapter 14)*

Medication-induced (psychostimulants, stimulating antidepressants, etc.)

Withdrawal-related (alcohol, benzodiazepines, etc.)

Anxiety disorders

Mood disorders (depression, mania)

*Neurological causes*

Restless legs syndrome (Chapter 15)

Parkinson's disease (Chapter 16)

Dementia (Chapter 16)

CNS Whipple's disease

Morvan's syndrome

Fatal familial insomnia

CNS, central nervous system

### Gastroesophageal reflux disorder

Some foods may be detrimental to sleep for susceptible individuals. Any dietary factor that enhances the dilatation of the lower esophageal sphincter, such as spicy foods, can contribute to GERD. The patient typically experiences chest tightness or pain and regurgitation of acidic fluids. When one lies flat in bed, the acidic stomach contents more readily enter the esophagus, which explains why this condition can worsen when a patient tries to sleep. Reflux and dyspepsia are well known to delay sleep initiation and trigger arousals from sleep[12]. GERD, like obstructive sleep apnea, is associated with obesity. Without polysomnography it can be difficult to determine whether the secondary insomnia is due to GERD or sleep-disordered breathing[13]. Monitoring gastric acidity by means of a pH probe can also clarify the role that reflux may play in patients with disturbances of sleep initiation and maintenance.

### Pain

Any patient experiencing pain at night is likely to have disturbed sleep. With acute pain or chronic pain due to cancer, adequate treatment is expected to improve both the unpleasant sensory experience of pain as well as decrease the associated sleep disturbance. Chronic non-malignant pain is a noteworthy cause of secondary insomnia and proves challenging to treat because it often has an indiscernible etiology and a prolonged course.

*Fibromyalgia*

Fibromyalgia is a diffuse and chronic musculoskeletal syndrome that causes significant distress, psychosocial impairment and decreased quality of life. A specific cause has not been identified. Patients complain of poor quality of sleep, and wake feeling unrefreshed. Fibromyalgia has been linked with alpha rhythm superimposed on non-rapid eye movment (NREM) sleep[14], and it has been hypothesized that this phenomenon may be responsible for the patients' sense of non-restorative sleep. Alpha intrusion is non-specific, and has also been found in other rheumatic pain syndromes as well as in subjects repeatedly woken during the night (see Chapter 4). Pain complaints are thought to worsen when sleep in fibromyalgia is more abnormal, and improve when the patients obtain better-quality sleep. Multiple sleep latency tests do not document objective excessive daytime sleepiness.

## Neurological disorders associated with insomnia

*Fatal familial insomnia*

Several extremely rare neurological disorders are closely linked with insomnia and provide insights into its pathogenesis. The most discussed entity in this group is fatal familial insomnia, a prion disease that affects a small number of families. This rapidly progressive neurodegenerative disease, which is related to Creutzfeld–Jakob disease, causes an extremely severe insomnia that has been documented with polysomnography. The insomnia develops in the setting of other neurological problems including cerebellar ataxia, dysarthria and dysautono-

mia. New diagnostic techniques include molecular genetic analysis of the prion protein gene on chromosome 20. Patients with the disorder show a mutation on codon 178 in combination with a specific polymorphism on codon 129[15]. Neuropathological examination of the brain reveals severe neuronal loss in the anterior and dorsomedial thalamic nuclei[16].

*CNS Whipple's disease*

Another extremely rare infectious cause of insomnia is central nervous system (CNS) Whipple's disease, a disorder better known for its gastrointestinal manifestations. Over time the disease can involve the CNS and can cause extremely severe insomnia, although the pathophysiology is unknown. The diagnosis is unusual in the absence of a history of gastrointestinal symptoms. The diagnosis is confirmed when polymerase chain reaction demonstrates the presence of the Whipple bacillus in the cerebrospinal fluid[17]. Antibiotics have been reported to improve sleep duration.

*Morvan's syndrome*

Morvan's syndrome is a rare disorder combining hyperexcitability of peripheral nerves with CNS symptoms. The patient presents with severe insomnia, usually in the setting of an encephalopathy and sometimes muscle cramping and stiffness[18]. An electromyogram (EMG) reveals fasciculations and neuromyotonic discharges. Polysomnography shows severe and sometimes total insomnia. Abnormally increased muscle tone in rapid eye movement (REM) sleep may be present during recovery. Morvan's syndrome is believed to be an immune-mediated disorder, with laboratory studies indicating the presence of antibodies to voltage-gated potassium channels. An idiopathic autoimmune form occurs as well as a paraneoplastic variety, often related to a thymoma. This disorder can remit spontaneously or respond to immunosuppression or plasmapheresis. The pathogenesis of the sleep disturbances is uncertain, but the similar phenotype to fatal familial insomnia has led to the hypothesis that thalamic dysfunction may be responsible.

## INSOMNIA DURING CHILDHOOD

### Colic

Colic is a common condition in which an infant cries for an extended time (more than 3 h/day several times a week) for unclear reasons. If a specific problem such as physical pain or food intolerance can be identified, then the term colic should not be used. Colic usually begins soon after birth and remits spontaneously by the end of the third month. A colicky child is difficult to parent, because holding them does not provide comfort. Medications and devices are also largely ineffective. Parents need assistance in learning how to cope with this difficult situation until it remits. Becoming informed about the ultradian rhythm of a developing child's sleep–wake cycle and learning how to take full advantage of this is helpful. Parents should be encouraged to try various interventions to soothe their baby, with the hope that a particular infant may respond for example to swaddling or vibration. Since some parents become distressed by inexplicable crying, they may need to be reminded

that their baby's crying does not reflect poor parenting skills.

### Food allergy insomnia

Occasionally a child, most commonly less than 4 months of age, may be unable to sleep because of a food allergy, for example to lactose. Until the allergy is identified, the child may be suspected to have colic, but once identified, alternative foods can be substituted. If the child's sleep improves, the suspicion of food allergy is confirmed and treatment involves avoiding the implicated food. The existence of this sleep disorder means that parents and clinicians faced with a sleepless child need to consider the possibility of food intolerance. Trials of alternative nutritional options, including soy-based products, should then be considered.

### Limit-setting sleep disorder

Learning to go to bed and fall asleep at an appropriate time is an important part of human development. Not surprisingly, many children at one time or another struggle with going to sleep at an appropriate time. Questions about how to assist a child to fall asleep are among the most frequent posed by parents to pediatricians.

### Case 10.4

A 4-year-old boy was brought to the pediatrician's office by his mother because of sleep problems. She described him as resisting bedtime night after night. This problem became evident when he first learned to speak at about age 2. He typically had a series of requests which included trips to the bathroom, snacks, drinks and specific toys. His parents would comply with some of his demands, because of a desire to prevent bedwetting or awakenings at night due to thirst or hunger. Even though his planned bedtime was 7:30 p.m., rarely would he be in bed by 9 p.m. The parents knew that they needed to enforce bedtime more strictly, but had not reached agreement on which requests were reasonable and which were frivolous.

The pediatrician met with the child's mother at several well-child visits. Eventually, both parents came in to discuss their son's sleep problem, which the pediatrician identified as limit-setting sleep disorder. The pediatrician helped both parents agree on a specific bedtime and to start to prepare their child for bed 45 min earlier. The bedtime rituals were revised always to include the boy emptying his bladder, having one specific toy and listening to one story. The boy was told that neither parent would respond to his requests after his lights were out. The child was able to settle down and fall asleep more readily within weeks when this new routine was implemented.

Preschool and school-aged children sometimes hesitate to go to sleep at a conventional bedtime or, for younger children, naptime. Occasionally these children will also refuse to return to sleep after awakening during the night, especially if they awoke because of a nightmare. Children will make unnecessary requests, such as asking for something to drink or to visit the bathroom, to delay lights out. Children may describe fears of ghosts or monsters, but instead of being genuinely afraid, they are seeking a reason to stay awake. If parents or care-givers do not place strict limits on bedtime, patients can be awake for a prolonged time at night.

Some parents do not appreciate the importance of a regular sleep–wake schedule, and make no effort to determine a consistent bedtime. Because of their own life-style, especially if they have psychiatric or chemical-dependency problems, parents can find it difficult to insist upon a specific bedtime. If a child has medical problems, some parents, in an attempt to compensate, may become unreasonably lenient. Limit-setting sleep disorder often produces tension around bedtime that causes distress to both the patient and the parents. This problem can be both a cause and the result of a strained parent–child relationship. If the child succeeds in staying up late, an irregular sleep–wake cycle and insufficient sleep can result. As the child grows into adolescence, limit-setting sleep disorder can evolve into delayed sleep phase disorder where the sleep problem is no longer the result of inadequate limits placed by the parents, but due to a circadian change in the sleep pacemaker.

### Sleep-onset association disorder

In sleep-onset association disorder, a child, typically an infant or preschooler, is unable to sleep unless a certain condition is present. When the child is in the accustomed setting, for example being held by a parent, sleep comes easily. If the parents remove the comforting condition, for example by placing the child in his crib, the child awakens and has difficulty in returning to sleep. Sleep-onset association disorder can occur both at the beginning and in the middle of the night. Children typically awaken during the night, and if left undisturbed fall asleep again. However, if the parents routinely intervene, the child can become dependent on their presence. Children at risk for this sleep disorder may have experienced disruptions in their normal schedule because of social problems, such as parental divorce. If a child develops a medical illness requiring parental attention throughout the night, sleep-onset association disorder can emerge, with the sleep disorder persisting after the medical illness resolves.

## REFERENCES

1. Ancoli-Israel S, Roth T. Characteristics of insomnia in the United States: results of the 1991 National Sleep Foundation Survey. *Sleep* 1999;22:S347–53

2. American Academy of Sleep Medicine. *International Classification of Sleep Disorders, Revised*. Rochester, MN: American Academy of Sleep Medicine, 1997:32

3. Nowell P, Buysse D, Reynolds C III, *et al*. Clinical factors contributing to the differential diagnosis of primary insomnia and insomnia related to mental disorders. *Am J Psychiatry* 1997;154:1412–16

4. Hauri P, Linde S. *No More Sleepless Nights*. New York: John Wiley & Sons, 1996

5. Smith A. Effects of caffeine on human behavior. *Food Chem Toxicol* 2002;40: 1243–55

6. Landolt H, Werth E, Borbely A, Dijk D. Caffeine intake (200 mg) in the morning affects human sleep and EEG power spectra at night. *Brain Res* 1995;675:67–74

7. Brown S, Salive M, Pahor M, *et al*. Occult caffeine as a source of sleep problems in an older population. *J Am Geriatr Soc* 1995;43:860–4

8. Roehrs T, Hollebeek E, Drake C, Roth T. Substance use for insomnia in Metropolitan Detroit. *J Psychosom Res* 2002;53:571–6

9. Rosenthal L. The Sleep Wake Inventory: a self report measure of daytime sleepiness. *Biol Psychiatry* 1993;34:810-820

10. Roehrs T, Roth T. Sleep, sleepiness and alcohol use. *Alcohol Res Health* 2001;25: 101–9

11. Morin C, Rodrigue S, Ivers H. Role of stress, arousal and coping skills in primary insomnia. *Psychosom Med* 2003;65:259–67

12. Suganuma N, Shigedo Y, Adachi H, *et al*. Association of gastroesophageal reflux disease with weight gain and apnea, and their disturbance of sleep. *Psychiatry Clin Neurosci* 2001;55:255–6

13. Salin-Pascual R, Roehrs T, Merlotti L, Zorick F, Roth T. Long-term study of the sleep of insomnia patients with sleep state misperception and other insomnia patients. *Am J Psychiatr* 1992;149:904–8

14. Moldofsky H, Tullis C, Lue F, Quance G, Davidson J. Sleep related myoclonus in rheumatic pain modulation disorder (fibrositis syndrome) and in excessive daytime somnolence. *Psychosom Med* 1984; 46:145–51

15. Goldfarb LG, Petersen RB, Tabaton M. Fatal familial insomnia and familial Creutzfeldt–Jakob disease: a disease phenotype determined by a DNA polymorphism. *Science* 1992;258:806–8

16. Manetto V, Medori R, Cortelli P, *et al*. Fatal familial insomnia: pathological study of five new cases. *Neurology* 1992;42:312–19

17. Voderholzer U, Riemann D, Gann H, *et al*. Transient total sleep loss in cerebral Whipple's disease: a longitudinal study. *J Sleep Res* 2002;11:321–9

18. Barber P, Anderson N, Vincent A. Morvan's syndrome associated with voltage-gated potassium channel antibodies. *Neurology* 2000;54:771–3

# Chapter 11

# Approach to the patient who cannot sleep

*A ruffled mind is a restless pillow*

**Charlotte Brontë,** *The Professor*

## CLINICAL APPROACH

The approach to the patient who cannot sleep starts with a comprehensive sleep history as outlined in Chapter 3. In many cases, the diagnosis of insomnia does not require additional testing. Figure 11.1 provides an algorithm for the diagnosis of chronic insomnia. However, as with excessive daytime sleepiness, each patient should be assessed individually. Clinicians should also keep in mind that many patients have more than one contributing factor. The clinician must first identify all of the possible factors and then determine the relevance of each one for the patient's presenting complaint.

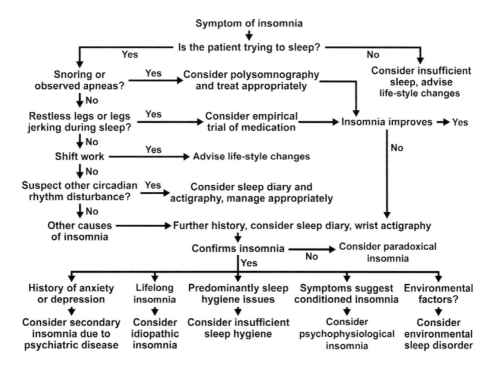

**Figure 11.1**   Algorithmic approach to the patient who cannot sleep

First, it is essential to determine whether the patient is trying sufficiently to fall asleep. Some patients present with insomnia (sometimes to appease concerned family members who worry about wakefulness during the night), only for the clinician to realize that the patient is not making an adequate effort to sleep. Instead of trying to sleep, patients may stay up late into the night surfing the Internet or doing household chores. These patients probably have insufficient sleep syndrome rather than insomnia. On the other hand, if they are trying to sleep but are unable to initiate or sustain sleep, wakefulness may be consistent with insomnia. Second, the clinician should carefully search for another primary sleep disorder that may present with the symptom of insomnia, such as obstructive sleep apnea or restless legs syndrome. Because insomnia has a dual role as a symptom and a primary sleep disorder, the need to exclude carefully other sleep disorders by following a step-by-step diagnostic process is of the utmost importance. Likewise, it is vital to determine whether the patient's inability to sleep is related to an altered sleep–wake cycle due to jet lag, shift work or other circadian rhythm disorders.

Once these issues have been considered, an attempt should be made to reach a diagnosis of one or more primary types of insomnia. Often this can be achieved with the history alone, but sleep diaries and wrist actigraphy may be very helpful adjunctive techniques. In particular, for a diagnosis of paradoxical insomnia (sleep state misperception), an objective measure of sleep (actigraphy or polysomnography) is essential. Insomnia due to psychiatric disorders always needs to be considered in the presence of diagnosed depression or anxiety disorder, but may not be the correct diagnosis, especially if the psychiatric disorder is in remission. A history of lifelong sleep disturbances from childhood suggests idiopathic insomnia. Insomnia commencing acutely and persisting despite alleviation of the initial cause is typical of psychophysiological insomnia. Noise in the bedroom disturbing sleep suggests environmental sleep disorder.

Insomnia as a primary sleep disorder can coexist with other sleep disorders. An example would be a patient with longstanding insomnia that began in childhood who later in life developed snoring and decreased quality of sleep after gaining considerable weight. In this case the patient probably first had insomnia, which more recently has been complicated by obstructive sleep apnea. The diagnostic approach in these cases is first to diagnose and treat the sleep disorders other than insomnia. If the insomnia persists after a reasonable treatment trial, then it is probably not a symptom of the other condition but a separate disorder that merits targeted treatment.

## Case 11.1

A 56-year-old woman presented to the sleep disorder center accompanied by her husband. Her chief complaint was that it took her 3–4 h nightly to fall asleep, lying in bed thinking about her plans for the next day. Once asleep she slept fitfully until her alarm went off in the morning. She did not complain about daytime fatigue or excessive daytime sleepiness, her concerns being primarily centered on her wakefulness at night. She acknowledged that she had a tendency to worry. Her husband reported that she snored loudly but he had never observed any apneic spells. The evaluation included polysomnography in view of the possibility of sleep-disordered breathing. In the questionnaire completed the morning after the study, the patient reported that she slept poorly in the laboratory and perceived that it took her 2–3 h to fall asleep, similar to her experiences at home. However, the sleep study indicated an initial sleep latency of only 19 min. When advised of these findings the patient was surprised and disbelieving. The physician discussed the discrepancy with the patient and her husband at length, striving to take an optimistic approach. While he did not challenge the patient's perspective directly, he emphasized that the sleep study indicated the absence of obstructive sleep apnea. He reassured her that she appeared to function fairly well during the day despite her sleep concerns. He encouraged the patient to pursue behavioral and pharmacological treatment for her worrying and anxiety, commenting that this may improve her sleep. After the appointment, the patient's husband spoke privately to the physician in the hallway. He revealed that he often went to bed an hour later than his wife and that she was typically asleep by then. However, he had been unable to reassure his wife that she was getting adequate sleep. He appreciated the physician's efforts to assist his wife with her significant anxiety.

Paradoxical insomnia (sleep state misperception) entails a comparison of the patient's subjective report with objective data by polysomnography or actigraphy. Asking the patient to complete a questionnaire about their experience in the sleep laboratory can be helpful. Often, patients are not easily convinced that their sleep is not as disturbed as they thought, and the supportive and non-confrontational approach taken here is often useful. Patients are often reassured about the absence of a specific sleep disorder as well as daytime consequences. As in this case, the focus should shift to management of associated conditions such as anxiety disorders.

## TESTS IN THE ASSESSMENT OF INSOMNIA

### Sleep diary

Understanding the patient's sleep–wake schedule is especially important in the evaluation of insomnia. At the time of a clinical interview, patients often have difficulty recalling the details of their bedtime, sleep time and awakening time over the preceding weeks. Patients must agree to fill out their sleep diary on a prospective basis. Completing a 7- or 14-day diary in the waiting room is not much more useful than retrospectively trying to answer interview questions. The diary should be as simple and easy to use as possible, as long as it still provides the clinician, with sufficient information about the patient's sleep–wake cycle[1] (Figure 11.2). Many advocate using a graphic format to depict periods of sleep throughout the 24-h day. Data from the sleep diary help to uncover circadian sleep disorders as well as poor sleep hygiene. The diary can assist in understanding subjective complaints and be used over time to monitor the response to intervention.

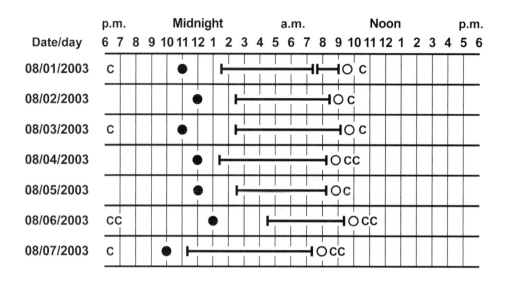

**Figure 11.2** Example of a sleep log. This figure shows an example of a sleep log completed by a patient. The solid circles indicate the time that the patient went to bed. The open circles indicate the time that the patient got out of bed. The lines are the patient's estimated time asleep. C, cup of coffee

## Wrist actigraphy

A wrist actigraph is a compact portable device that generates a voltage each time it is moved, and measures acceleration (see Chapter 4). Worn on an extremity, most typically a wrist, the actigraph is programmed and downloaded using a computer and proprietary software. The device registers movement collected during a specified and adjustable time interval. The recording period can be as long as 4 weeks before the memory capacity is full or the battery must be recharged, but data are typically collected for 1 week at a time.

The use of wrist actigraphy in the assessment of insomnia has been examined in studies and practice parameters[2–4]. Its advantage is that it can collect longitudinal data while patients are pursuing routine activities in their home environment. However, actigraphic information should be interpreted carefully, because the absence of electroencephalogram (EEG) data precludes definitely identifying sleep. Clearly, patients can have increased movement during sleep, or alternatively lie still for prolonged times when awake[3]. Wrist actigraphy is most useful in identifying patterns of sleep–wake schedules, and is most effective when paired with a sleep diary completed simultaneously by the patient. Comparing the lights-out and lights-on periods of the sleep diary with the wrist actigraphic information improves the reliability of the recorded data[4]. Although the proprietary software programs typically provide a myriad of sleep variables, a wrist actigraph is less reliable when used to estimate total sleep time, wakefulness after sleep onset and sleep efficiency. If these data are desired, polysomnography provides a more valid measure.

## Physiological assessment

High levels of physiological arousal prevent sleep. Although not in widespread use, some specialists perform measurements of several physiological variables, including a surface electromyogram (EMG) of the forehead muscles and skin temperature in the relaxed and tensed states. This tool has been used for assessment and to evaluate treatment outcome[5]. Factors limiting the use of this technology are the absence of consistent objective standards, lack of clinician training and inadequate time to conduct this testing during a consultation. If skin temperature and EMG remain relatively high in the relaxed state, compared with the tense one, this may be an indication of somatized tension. This condition has been associated with psychophysiological insomnia, and such patients may particularly benefit from learning and practicing relaxation techniques.

## Polysomnography

In research studies, polysomnography has shown that patients with insomnia underestimate their total sleep time and overestimate their sleep efficiency when self-report is compared with polysomnographic data[6]. However, insomnia is not defined by the presence or absence of any particular events measured by polysomnography. As a result, polysomnography does not provide informa-

tion in clinical practice that confirms the diagnosis or aids in the development of a specific treatment plan. Polysomnography has also not been demonstrated to be useful in differentiating different subtypes of insomnia. Polysomnography is of value when there are additional concerns such as snoring or observed apneas associated with insomnia.

Furthermore, significant difficulties can arise when polysomnography is used for the assessment of insomnia. Many patients with insomnia experience increased anxiety and muscle tension when hooked up to multiple monitors in a sleep laboratory. As a result, some patients sleep very poorly while being studied. In addition to having a miserable night, no specific information about the cause of their sleeplessness in the home setting will be obtained. A smaller number of patients with insomnia may report better sleep in the sleep laboratory than at home, and comment that the polysomnographic data are not representative of their sleep at home. These patients have typically learned to associate their bed with an inability to sleep, and have improved sleep when sleeping away from home whether at a hotel or even in the sleep laboratory[7].

## REFERENCES

1. Spielman AJ, Nunes J, Glovinsky P. Insomnia. In Aldrich M, ed. *Neurologic Clinics*. Philadelphia: WB Saunders, 1996; 14:513–54

2. Hauri P, Wisbey J. Wrist actigraphy in insomnia. *Sleep* 1994;15:293-301

3. Sadeh A, Hauri P, Kripke D, Lavie P. The role of actigraphy in the evaluation of sleep disorders. *Sleep* 1995;18:288-302

4. Littner M, Kushida C, Anderson W, *et al.* Standards of Practice Committee of the American Academy of Sleep Medicine. Practice parameters for the role of actigraphy in the study of sleep and circadian rhythms: an update for 2002. *Sleep* 2003;26:337–41

5. Hauri P, Percy L, Hellekson C, Hartmann E, Russ D. The treatment of psychophysiologic insomnia with biofeedback: a replication study. *Biofeedback Self Regul* 1982;7:223–35

6. Carskaden M, Dement W, Mitler M, Guilleminault C, Zarcone V, Spiegel R. Self-reports versus sleep laboratory findings in 122 drug-free subjects with complaints of chronic insomnia. *Am J Psychiatry* 1976;133:1382

7. Hauri P, Olmstead E. Reverse first night effect in insomnia. *Sleep* 1989;12:97–105

# Chapter 12

# Management of insomnia

*A bower quiet for us, and a sleep*
*Full of sweet dreams, and health, and quiet breathing*

**John Keats,** *Endymion*

In view of the multiple factors that can cause insomnia (Chapter 10), it is not surprising that a variety of treatment approaches have been developed. All patients, irrespective of whether their insomnia is primary or secondary, should strive for excellent sleep hygiene. The treatment options identified for primary insomnia apply equally well for secondary insomnia, but are typically not sufficient (Table 12.1). When insomnia can be attributed to another disorder, for example major depression, treating the underlying condition is beneficial, as discussed in Chapter 14. For selected patients, behavioral techniques (relaxation strategies including tapes, self-hypnosis and music) and hypnotic medications are adjuvant therapeutic options[1].

## SLEEP HYGIENE

The term 'sleep hygiene' is frequently used to describe optimal sleep conditions, but relatively few patients or physicians have a complete understanding of all of the factors involved. Sleep is a sensitive and dynamic state that can be perturbed by a multitude of avoidable factors. Sleep hygiene can be subdivided into two components: optimizing the sleep environment and improving routines and attitudes conducive to sleep.

## Optimizing the sleep environment

Easily falling and staying asleep are dependent on a conducive environment. As discussed in Chapter 10, many factors including loud noise, movement, extreme temperature, body position, pillow choice and uncomfortable bedding can make it difficult to sleep. Surprisingly, some people consistently attempt to sleep in adverse circumstances, for example a woman sleeping next to a husband who snores loudly, without fully appreciating the impact upon her sleep. Circumstances may make it necessary to tolerate suboptimal sleeping conditions for a short stretch of time, for example while traveling or camping. Despite having inadequate sleep for several days, people can generally adapt and continue to function. Trying to sleep in an uncomfortable setting for longer stretches of time significantly contributes to chronic partial sleep deprivation. Affected persons need to be willing to modify their sleep environment to promote high-quality sleep.

**Table 12.1** Overview of treatment options for insomnia

| Sleep issue | Technique |
|---|---|
| *Primary insomnia* | |
| Optimizing the sleep environment | eliminate a disruptive sleep environment |
| Altering routines and attitudes related to sleep | relaxing bedtime rituals |
| | associating the bed with sleep |
| | consistent sleep–wake schedule |
| | limiting caffeine use |
| | avoiding gastroesophageal reflux |
| | avoiding exercise near bedtime |
| | avoid clock-watching |
| | avoid daytime naps |
| Improving relaxation skills | relaxation techniques |
| Applying behavioral techniques | scheduling worry time |
| | sleep restriction |
| Considering hypnotic medications | benzodiazepines |
| and nutritional supplements | benzodiazepine receptor agonists |
| | sedating antidepressants |
| | antihistamines |
| | alternative therapies |
| *Secondary insomnia* | treatment of psychiatric disorders, such as depression and anxiety disorders |
| | treatment of medical disorders, such as chronic pain, nausea, gastroesophageal reflux |

## Improving routines and attitudes conducive to sleep

The patient's life-style choices may compromise sleep quality. The 30–60 min before desired sleep onset should ideally be treated as a transitional time from the demanding activities of the day to the relaxed state of sleep. Many individuals with hectic schedules and multiple responsibilities continue engaging in activities that are mentally or physically stressful, right up to bedtime.

Work-related activities such as preparing for the next day's work by reading professional materials or planning for upcoming events can contribute to heightened anxiety. Stressful non-professional activities, for example preparing taxes or planning a social event, can be equally invigorating. When a person pursues cognitively demanding tasks, muscle tension increases, which is incompatible with the generalized muscle relaxation that is the prerequisite for sleep onset. For some people it can take considerable time to cease thinking about these matters and subsequently relax their mind and body[2]. Although relaxation techniques may be helpful ways to unwind in many cases, refraining from these stimulating activities prior to bedtime is the preferable approach. More suitable pastimes for this period prior to sleep onset include personal hygiene practices, watching relaxing television, reading for pleasure and romantic activities[3].

Different measures have been recommended for conditioned insomnia. Prevention of this maladaptive conditioned state is more desirable than later attempting to restore the patient's confidence in their ability to fall asleep in their own bed. Once this state has developed, patients are advised to limit the use of their beds to sleep and sexual activity. Gradually, a patient's confidence in their ability to fall asleep readily increases. Stimulus control techniques have been used to help patients with conditioned insomnia who find that they are sleepy near bedtime, but as soon as they enter the sleeping environment become aroused and unable to sleep[4]. This conditioned association between sleeplessness and the bedroom may need to be interrupted by instructing patients to avoid 'trying to sleep'. If they find that they are hyperaroused while lying in bed, they should not try to sleep. They are advised instead to get up and go to a different setting, engage in a different activity (read a book, watch relaxing television, listen to music) until they become sleepy again and return to bed. Patients need to be cautious not to walk too far from their bedroom, since the process of returning to bed when sleepy may cause them to become fully awake again. Patients should repeat this process of not trying to sleep as long as is needed to extinguish the arousal state conditioned to the bedroom. Some patients find that rather than getting out of bed or leaving the bedroom, the same results can be achieved by reading or watching a monotonous video in the bedroom with the video recorder set to turn off automatically[5].

A consistent sleep–wake cycle is important. Sleep is optimized when circadian rhythms are harnessed in promoting sleep. Sleep comes more easily when patients attempt to sleep at the same time. Establishing a regular waking time, 7 days a week, optimizes the circadian rhythms. Patients with insomnia should preferably avoid daytime naps. Self-discipline is important. Improving the consistency of sleep–wake schedules in college undergraduate students by recommending a minimum of 7.5 h sleep a night on a regular schedule increased daytime alertness and decreased subjective daytime sleepiness[6].

Many people when awakened check the time. Avoiding 'clock watching' can reduce the arousal effects of becoming annoyed or fearful when tracking the slow passage of time through the night. Most people recall only the periods of wakefulness at night, so clock-watching can reinforce the perception that no sleep has occurred. The clock can be kept from view, yet close at hand, so that the alarm can be heard in the morning.

Persons with insomnia need to be fully aware of the quantity and timing of their consumption of stimulating agents. Patients who realize that they are using excessive caffeine can readily avoid this situation by partially or totally substituting decaffeinated products later in the day, and restricting their intake of caffeinated products to the morning. A gradual taper of caffeine may be initially necessary for patients consuming excessive quantities. Patients should be warned not to rely on alcohol to facilitate sleep, since this substance can lead to increased snoring and sleep fragmentation. Use of nicotine close to bedtime is not advised because of nicotine's stimulatory properties, and after long-term use the possibility that nicotine withdrawal will delay sleep onset.

The relationship between sleep and diet is of interest to many patients, but has not been extensively studied. Each year, around the Thanksgiving holiday, television talk-shows discuss the possibility that turkey, rich in tryptophan, will promote sleep. Although tryptophan is thought to enhance sleep, few studies have been conducted of tryptophan-rich foods such as poultry and milk, resulting in a paucity of evidence demonstrating its benefits[7]. Patients particularly prone to gastroesophageal reflux (GERD) should not sleep on a full stomach. For patients with GERD, over-the-counter or prescription medication as well as elevating the head of the bed may be necessary to reduce gastrointestinal distress and promote sleep.

Recent studies have demonstrated the positive impact of regular moderate exercise on sleep initiation, duration and quality[8]. A reduced risk of sleep problems was noted with physical activity at least once a week by walking at a brisk pace for at least six city blocks[9]. Extremely prolonged strenuous exercise, however, may be detrimental for sleep, possibly because of physical discomfort. The timing of exercise should be carefully considered. A vigorous physical work-out within several hours of bedtime increases body temperature and muscle tension and can promote a stimulated state of mind. These conditions take time to fade, and can interfere with sleep onset. To avoid delaying sleep onset, exercise should preferably be performed at least 4 h before the desired bedtime, such as in the late afternoon. One postulated mechanism is that falling body temperature is associated with sleep, and body temperature decreases approximately 4 h after exercise[8]. Regular physical exercise taking place at a consistent time of day for as little as 2 weeks has been reported to increase slow-wave sleep. An association between exercise and increased slow-wave sleep has been reported in both middle-aged and aging adults[10].

## RELAXATION TECHNIQUES

Given enough psychological stress, everyone has a threshold above which they feel anxious and physically tense. Everyone can benefit if under stress they are able consciously to relax the body and mind. Some people intuitively learn and practice relaxation techniques, but most can benefit from instruction and practice. For example,

Table 12.2  Relaxation strategies

| |
| --- |
| Reading |
| Listening to music |
| Watching television |
| Following a relaxation tape |
| Progressive muscle relaxation |
| Diaphragmatic breathing |
| Guided visual imagery |

elite athletes vying to perform under extreme stress almost invariably seek out the coaching of a sports psychologist. Having a toolbox of cognitive or behavioral techniques allows a person to adapt to stressful circumstances (Table 12.2). These tools can be applied to minimize insomnia, and their effectiveness has been repeatedly demonstrated in well-designed clinical trials overseen by expert sleep psychologists[11,12] examining both young and aging populations. The value of behavioral techniques outside research settings prescribed in routine clinical practice has not been as well studied.

## Case 12.1

A 54-year-old woman experienced regular difficulty in falling asleep. This problem dated back many years and had not changed over time. She did not snore or have unpleasant feelings in her legs. The patient had never mentioned her sleep problem to her physician, feeling that the limited time available during her primary-care appointments should be devoted to other issues such as cancer surveillance, given her family history of malignancy. Over time she had tried several techniques to hasten sleep onset. She had sampled several health food-store supplements, including melatonin and valerian root, without being convinced that the effect justified the cost. She had also read several books on insomnia, trying to identify effective coping strategies. Gradually she developed a nightly routine that was beneficial. She typically spent time early each evening preparing lists of what she needed to accomplish the next day. She then spent the half-hour before going to bed engaged in monotonous activities such as brushing her teeth and removing her make-up. Each night she read for approximately 30 min in bed. She deliberately selected a book with short chapters that she could easily put down once her eyelids felt heavy. At times she would consciously take deep breaths, concentrating on the breathing process. As long as she followed these steps, despite her longstanding insomnia, she was able to fall asleep without undue difficulty.

This case illustrates how a self-help program aimed at improving sleep hygiene can sometimes be highly effective in combating even chronic insomnia. However, many patients require ongoing counseling from health-care providers to achieve similar results.

Limitations to behavioral techniques being used widely include physicians' lack of awareness of the patient's sleep concerns, their inadequate knowledge of the techniques and their lack of adequate time to teach the interventions. Inadequate follow-up to reinforce the teaching, as well as problems with patient acceptance and adherence, can also contribute to less than optimal results. For these reasons, hypnotic medications are more often provided for the management of insomnia in primary-care practice than relaxation training.

Several relaxation techniques are known to be beneficial for hastening sleep onset, allowing selection of those with which the patient feels most comfortable. Some people are able to relax consciously by simply listening to music, watching television or reading. Others need to start by using a relaxation tape, with cues designed to encourage peaceful thoughts and release of muscle tension[5]. Other practices include progressive muscle relaxation, a technique similar to yoga, in which the patient sequentially contracts and then slowly relaxes each muscle group[13]. This approach should be used cautiously by patients with pre-existing chronic pain, since it may cause them to remain preoccupied with their physical state. An alternative relaxation exercise is diaphragmatic breathing, encouraging the patient to concentrate on slow deep breathing. Other relaxation practices focus more specifically on thoughts. In guided visual imagery, a person spends an extended time, for example 15 min, imagining being in a serene setting. Depending on the person's life experience, the patient may conjure up images of an Alpine lake, tropical beach, shady hammock or other scene. The image is elaborated to encompass all the senses, including vision, hearing, touch and smell[14].

## BEHAVIORAL THERAPIES

Two techniques which aim to alter maladaptive behaviors that interfere with sleep have become widely used for insomnia. 'Worry time' is a technique recommended to those who find that they spend inordinate amounts of time worrying when awake at night. Patients are recommended to take 15–30 min in the late afternoon or early evening (not near sleep onset) during which there is time to devote attention to worries. Patients are expected to use this scheduled time to list and examine their concerns. When patients awaken at night and begin to worry about a 'new' problem, this is added to the list, to be included in the next day's session. Eventually, the energy and time spent worrying at night diminishes, and

wakefulness is not perpetuated by anxious thought content[15].

For patients with severe persistent insomnia, a sleep restriction management method may be helpful (Table 12.3). Patients are instructed to allow no more hours in bed than they estimated they slept the previous night. Initially, this may be considerably less than 7.5 h. When they are able to sleep for

**Table 12.3** Sleep restriction intervention guidelines for insomnia

Patients estimate their total sleep time (TST) using a sleep diary

Time in bed (TIB) is reduced until it equals estimated TST but not less than 4 h (some clinicians advocate that this is done abruptly while others suggest a gradual reduction in TIB)

Clinicians may wish to specify bedtime and arising time initially

Patients monitor their quality and quantity of sleep nightly by estimating sleep efficiency

Once a patient has a sleep efficiency of 90% or better, after a week TIB is increased by 15 or 30 min (some clinicians require a lower sleep efficiency of 80–85%)

This process is continued over several weeks until the patient is getting 7.5 h of good-quality sleep nightly

The patient may experience some excessive daytime sleepiness initially and daytime napping should be discouraged

TST, sleep efficiency and patient subjective report of satisfactory sleep are expected to improve over time, while initial sleep latency and wakefulness after sleep onset decrease essentially all the time in bed for several nights, they are advised to increase their time in bed by small increments until they achieve optimal sleep time and sleep efficiency. Although pharmacological and behavioral treatments are both effective for insomnia management over the initial weeks of treatment, a recent randomized controlled trial of these treatments in the elderly suggests that behavioral therapy is associated with more sustained improvement than is pharmacological therapy[11].

## MEDICATIONS

### General principles

Sedative-hypnotic medications are widely used. Over time, several new medications have been specifically developed to improve the quality of sleep, and have obtained US Food and Drug Administration (FDA) approval for this indication. Many medications developed to treat other symptoms, primarily depression and allergies, have been prescribed to address sleep complaints, despite not being FDA-approved for this purpose.

The clinician should not prescribe a hypnotic without first performing a comprehensive evaluation of the patient's sleep problem and exploring sleep hygiene issues. The goal of hypnotics should be to improve subjective sleep quality, decrease daytime fatigue, improve concentration and enhance overall improved daytime functioning. Using the lowest effective dose for the shortest amount of time is good medical practice. The prescriber should be aware of several characteristics of hypnotics listed in Table 12.4. The rate of absorption and time for

**Table 12.4** Relevant characteristics of a hypnotic medication

Rate of absorption

Rapidity of distribution to the central nervous system

Action on specific neurotransmitters

Duration of the elimination half-life

Site of metabolism

Rate of metabolism

Presence of an active metabolite

Likelihood of tolerance

Risk of dependence

distribution to the central nervous system determine the time of administration in the evening, so that patients experience sedation shortly after they have gone to bed. The duration of the elimination half-life and rate of metabolism are most pertinent when a hypnotic is used on an ongoing rather than intermittent basis, since these characteristics will influence the effect of the medication over time. For aging patients or those with liver disease, prolonged elimination can put them at risk for excessive sedation that in turn can lead to cognitive impairment and falls.

In general, hypnotics need to be used cautiously because of the possibility, especially for those agents with long half-lives, that there will be residual sedation in the morning. Some patients interpret this morning sedation as a need for more sleep, and increase the dose of the hypnotic. Long-acting medications have also been associated with cognitive problems, including slowed performance, compromised learning of new information, less efficient recall of previously learned material and reduced visuomotor speed. Hypnotics with short half-lives raise a different set of concerns. These agents can wear off before morning, contributing to early-morning awakening or rebound insomnia. In particular, triazolam has been associated with amnesia, probably because this rapidly eliminated medication leads to a state of abrupt drug withdrawal.

Another clinically relevant general principle in the pharmacology of sedative medications is the tendency for a patient to develop tolerance to a hypnotic medication. If, over time, the medication ceases to induce sleep, the patient may increase the dosage to experience sedation once again. Many of the newer sleeping medications have been developed with the specific objective of avoiding tolerance. Physical dependence is another undesirable pharmacological property, whereby over time patients experience adverse physical or psychological consequences when they discontinue the medication. When the barbiturates were the

only sedatives available, the issues of tolerance and physical dependence were of critical importance because of the high risk of addiction and withdrawal.

## Benzodiazepines

When benzodiazepines were first developed, they were viewed as a significant therapeutic breakthrough because of their safety with regards to overdose and chemical dependency compared with the barbiturates. Chlordiazepoxide received FDA approval in 1960, followed over the years by 30 different agents in this class.

All benzodiazepines are sedating, but only five have specifically received FDA approval as sedative hypnotics (Table 12.5). Clonazepam is also included since it has been widely used to manage sleep disorders, although it is not FDA-approved for this purpose. They also all have anxiolytic, anticonvulsant and muscle relaxant properties. These medications differ in terms of half-life and route of elimination. Three ben-

**Table 12.5** Selected benzodiazepines used as sedative hypnotics

| Benzodiazepine | Half-life | Absorption | Comments |
| --- | --- | --- | --- |
| Triazolam | 2 h | fast | short-acting, associated with amnesia |
| Temazepam | 11 h | moderate | intermediate-acting, no active metabolites |
| Estazolam | 16 h | moderate | intermediate-acting |
| Quazepam | 50 h | fast | long-acting due to active metabolite |
| Flurazepam | 50 h | fast | long-acting due to active metabolite |
| Clonazepam | 35 h | fast | long-acting, FDA-approved for seizures and panic disorder, not approved as a sedative hypnotic |

FDA, Food and Drug Administration

zodiazepines, lorazepam, temazepam and oxazepam, are eliminated by conjugation instead of oxidation, and therefore lack active metabolites. As a result these medications are preferred for patients with liver failure.

The benzodiazepines act by binding to the benzodiazepine–γ-aminobutyric acid (GABA) receptor complex. Activation of this complex produces neuronal inhibition by increasing chloride flux. Their effect on sleep architecture includes increasing the duration of stage 2 sleep and probably decreasing the amount of slow-wave sleep. They have also been described to delay or slightly suppress REM sleep[16]. Total sleep time increases with their use.

The benzodiazepines, despite their low cost, have some notable disadvantages, including the possibility of respiratory depression, gait instability, impaired cognition and rebound insomnia on discontinuation. These possible effects need to be carefully considered, especially in aging patients. The safety of benzodiazepines in pregnancy has not been established. The hypnotic-dependent sleep disorder is discussed in Chapter 14.

The published literature about the benzodiazepines is extensive for short-term use (approximately 1 week), and reveals these medications to be effective and well-tolerated. However, clinicians face a dilemma in treating chronic insomnia in the absence of clinical trials indicating long-term safety and efficacy. Until recently, pharmaceutical companies had not conducted studies lasting weeks or months because of the expense, and awareness that clinicians often opt to use the sedative agents for longer durations than the label specifies. In the coming years, more published studies are expected to fill this void of evidence on managing chronic insomnia with the benzodiazepines. Despite this paucity of data, many experienced clinicians have favorable anecdotal reports of carefully prescribing benzodiazepines over years for selected patients. In general, there is little evidence that benzodiazepines cause tolerance or dependence in patients without chemical dependency issues. When benzodiazepines are prescribed continuously for months, years or decades, ongoing monitoring is important to identify possible dose escalation, sleep-disordered breathing, cognitive impairment and risk of falls.

In order to prevent a withdrawal phase when a patient has been using a benzodiazepine for several months or longer, the medication should not be abruptly discontinued. The dosage needs to be gradually reduced step-wise, with longer tapers when patients have used large quantities of medication. Tapers of benzodiazepines with short half-lives are often better tolerated when the patient is first switched to an equivalent dose of a longer-acting one that is then progressively reduced. The dose reduction can be more rapid initially, for example decreased by 50% the first day, and then more gradually thereafter. Patients taking extremely large doses of benzodiazepines or with coexisting chemical dependency issues may require an inpatient chemical dependency program as described in Chapter 14.

## Benzodiazepine receptor agonists

Three non-benzodiazepine agonists specifically developed as hypnotics are now available. These medications act on the benzodiazepine–GABA-A receptor and therefore

**Table 12.6** Benzodiazepine receptor agonists

| Agent | Half-life | Absorption | Side-effects | Comments |
|---|---|---|---|---|
| Zolpidem | 3 h | fast | amnesia, sleepwalking, sleep-eating | FDA-approved for 7–10 days of use |
| Zaleplon | 1 h | fast | ? | FDA-approved for 7–10 days of use |
| Zopiclone | 6 h | fast | ? | not approved in the USA |

FDA, Food and Drug Administration

also open the chloride ion channel. These newer hypnotics, zolpidem, zopiclone and zaleplon, have short half-lives that reduce the morning 'hangover' effect (Table 12.6). Patients have been shown to have alertness adequate for driving and other activities that require sustained vigilance[17]. Zaleplon, which has the shortest half-life of those currently available, can be administered in the middle of the night to reduce middle insomnia or sleep maintenance difficulties. They selectively cause sedation without respiratory depression, muscle relaxation or reducing anxiety. Their effect on sleep architecture is subtle, with possibly a slight increase in slow-wave sleep[16].

Physical dependence has not been reported with the short-term usage approved by the FDA. A long-term placebo-controlled trial of eszopiclone, an isomer of racemic zopiclone, has shown no evidence of tolerance and continued control of insomnia over a 6-month period[18]. The safety of these medications in pregnancy has not been established. There have been several case reports over the past 8 years of transient amnesia, sleepwalking and sleep-eating associated with recommended doses of zolpidem. Reports of patients who after taking 5 or 10 mg of the sedative have been unable to recall telephone calls have led to warnings that patients should avoid making major decisions on nights when they use zolpidem[19]. Following discontinuation, these agents are less likely than traditional benzodiazepines to cause rebound insomnia or anxiety. Since these agents are all currently produced under patent protection, they are more expensive than the benzodiazepines.

## Case 12.2

A 40-year-old lawyer experienced intermittent difficulty in sleeping. Apart from her recurrent insomnia, she was in good health without any physical or psychiatric disorders. She was aware that her insomnia would predictably worsen at times when she faced challenges at work. As she worked on major briefs or prepared for trials, she had more issues on her mind which she could not put aside as she lay in bed trying to sleep. Some nights she would lie awake for 3 h. At other times she would fall asleep initially, but awaken 2–3 h later and not be able to fall back to sleep. During these bouts of insomnia she tried to relax her muscles, practice deep breathing, read novels and imagine herself in relaxing places, without succeeding in falling asleep. She had eliminated caffeine and tried to maintain regular exercise during these episodes. At the time of a preventive medicine visit, she mentioned her insomnia to her primary-care physician. After checking that she was making an adequate effort to sleep and did not have symptoms of any other primary sleep disorder, he prescribed zaleplon 5 mg to take at bedtime when needed. On nights when she awoke at least 4 h before dawn, she could also use this agent. She found the zaleplon to be effective and did not experience any side-effects. She used it intermittently, with a 30-tablet prescription typically lasting 5–6 months. The patient reported that she no longer dreaded major assignments at work since now she knew that she had access to a reliable method to manage her insomnia.

This case illustrates how, in the correct setting, intermittent use of a hypnotic may continue to be effective in the long term. Clinicians should feel comfortable with this approach in selected patients with chronic insomnia after non-pharmacological methods have failed.

## Sedating antidepressants

Several of the antidepressants with prominent sedative side-effects, such as mirtazepine and trazodone, are valuable therapeutic options especially if the patient has a coexisting mood or anxiety disorder. For patients with depression and insomnia, subjective and objective sleep as measured by polysomnography improve after treatment with an antidepressant. Mirtazepine has prominent antihistaminergic side-effects at doses of 15 mg or less; however, this drug can result in undesirable weight gain[20]. Because of cardiac and anticholinergic side-effects, the tricyclic antidepressants are now seldom used expressly because of insomnia. Trazodone is rarely used alone for patients with depression and insomnia because most practitioners do not regard it as a reliable antidepressant. Patients generally have unacceptable daytime sedation when treated with the doses (400–600 mg) recommended for depression, but lower doses may help sleep. The selective serotonin reuptake inhibitors (SSRIs) are more stimulating and generally more useful for depression than insomnia. Combining a morning SSRI with an evening dose of trazodone may be a useful strategy in some patients.

Sedating antidepressants are also widely used for primary insomnia, but little evidence has been collected regarding their usefulness. In part this is because pharmaceutical companies with an FDA indication for depression are not compelled to make the substantial investment in clinical trials examining their role in primary insomnia. Trazodone has been studied and observed to reduce sleep latency, improve sleep continuity and suppress rapid eye movement (REM) sleep[21]. It is less clear whether this benefit is sustained after 2 weeks of administration. Trazodone used to target insomnia is typically prescribed at a low dose of 25–100 mg. At these doses side-effects are less common, but can include orthostatic hypotension and sedation. Priapism, which is not a dose-related side-effect, has been reported in

1 out of 6–10 000 patients. Paroxetine has been studied in primary insomnia and has been observed after 6 weeks of treatment to improve subjective sleep quality. Polysomnographic markers of sleep did not change[22].

## Antihistamines

Sedating antihistamines are readily available without a prescription. Many preparations, including diphenhydramine, hydroxyzine and doxylamine, are used for insomnia. Despite their widespread use, relatively few data are available showing their efficacy. These agents are probably most useful when used for no more than several days and targeted for sleep-onset insomnia. The common side-effects include dry mouth and residual morning sedation. Some children and aging patients can develop paradoxical agitation or confusion[23].

## Alternative modalities

Many complementary and alternative modalities have been used for insomnia. Apart from relaxation techniques (described earlier in this chapter), alternative therapies include herbal preparations, massage, chiropractic treatment, megavitamins, energy healing, homeopathy, acupuncture, naturopathy and aromatherapy. Large numbers of patients try these interventions, spending impressive sums of money, although to date little evidence is available demonstrating the benefits of any of these approaches. In particular, patients are increasingly opting to take herbal medications for insomnia. (Table 12.7). Apparently they view these preparations as safe, effective and less expensive than conventional medical care, although

few research data support these beliefs. Melatonin's usefulness strictly as a hypnotic agent appears limited because it lacks potent sedating properties. As a result, melatonin has more value as a means to shift the timing of the sleep–wake rhythm for patients with circadian rhythm disorders. Melatonin is discussed in more detail in Chapters 1 and 13.

## SPECIAL ISSUES

### Combining medications and behavioral therapies

If possible, behavioral techniques ought to be tried without concomitant hypnotic medications, because patients treated with both appear to have a less good outcome[24]. Potentially, the availability of medication reduces their motivation and confidence in the behavioral techniques. In clinical practice, behavioral techniques may be introduced to patients starting or already on hypnotic medications. Combining medications and behavioral approaches is especially necessary for patients with more severe insomnia. In these circumstances the clinician needs to educate the patient about the value of behavioral therapy. It may be desirable to reduce the dosage of medication gradually in order to produce some mild insomnia, which the patient can then address with the behavioral techniques. Once patients observe that this mild insomnia will respond, they develop more confidence in the effectiveness of behavioral techniques. Ideally, over time, the hypnotic medication can be gradually discontinued.

**Table 12.7** Commonly used nutritional supplements in insomnia

| Preparation | Targeted sleep issue | Efficacy | Concerns |
|---|---|---|---|
| Melatonin | irregular circadian rhythms<br>insomnia | better established<br>less established | vasoconstriction,<br>impurities,<br>source of origin |
| Kava kava | insomnia | poorly established | dermatitis,<br>hallucinations,<br>dyspnea, excessive<br>sedation when used<br>with other hypnotics |
| Valerian root | insomnia | poorly established | excessive sedation when<br>used with opiates |
| Black cohosh | hot flushes,<br>secondary insomnia | poorly established | nausea/vomiting |
| Hops | insomnia | poorly established | possible action on<br>estrogen receptors |
| L-Tryptophan | insomnia | poorly established | contamination during<br>production in the 1980s<br>linked to eosinophilia–<br>myalgia syndrome |

## Treating paradoxical insomnia (sleep state misperception)

This condition is addressed separately because the physician and the patient may have markedly different impressions of the need for treatment. Management involves discussing the discrepancy in subjective and objective data with the patient, but the symptoms should be treated in a similar manner to insomnia confirmed objectively. All the modalities discussed in this chapter are potentially applicable, and both behavioral techniques and hypnotic medications have been successfully used. Since recent studies have suggested that patients with sleep state misperception have a high rate of anxiety disorders, treatment targeting anxiety may be of particular value.

## Treating insomnia in children

The treatment of insomnia in children emphasizes the role of sleep hygiene and behavioral techniques over medications, except for children with insomnia secondary to anxiety or depression. For preschool children, daytime naps need to be carefully scheduled, with attention to the nap not becoming so prolonged that it reduces the pressure to sleep at night. Children need to spend the time prior to bedtime winding down. Parents need to teach them how to prepare for sleep by spending the time just before going to bed brushing their teeth or listening to a story. Sticking to a predictable bedtime is important[25], especially for children with limit-setting sleep disorder who benefit from a consistent sleep–wake schedule. Parents should encourage routines that are comforting to their child, such as providing a stuffed animal for the child to clutch. Having a beloved toy or blanket may be very reassuring to a fearful or anxious child. However, they should avoid rituals such as having the child fall asleep while being held, as this leads to the need for the parent's presence during every night awakening. In problematic cases of limit-setting sleep disorder, a single or double gate may need to be placed in the doorway to the child's room at least initially. Parents should be taught to enforce all these limits strictly but kindly. For children over the age of 3 years, a reward system using a star chart may also be effective.

If the child awakens at night, parents should initially pause, listening from a distance to understand whether the child has a specific problem, and giving a chance for returning to sleep without assistance. Going to help the child should not be the automatic response, and is necessary only in situations when it becomes clear that the child has a specific concern that needs attention. When the child has learned to be dependent on the presence of a parent to return to sleep on waking during the night, a progressive behavioral program needs to be instituted. This involves allowing the child to remain alone for increasingly longer intervals, start-

ing with minutes only, interspersed with brief calm reassurances. Again, consistent but compassionate behavior from the parents is essential, however distressing the child's initial response to the plan may be.

## REFERENCES

1.  Toney G, Ereshefsky L. Sleep disorders: assisting patients to a good night's sleep. *J Am Pharm Assoc* 2000;40:S46–7

2.  Nowell P, Buysse D, Reynolds C III, *et al.* Clinical factors contributing to the differential diagnosis of primary insomnia and insomnia related to mental disorders. *Am J Psychiatry* 1997;154:1412–16

3.  Ellis C, Lemmens G, Parkes D. Pre-sleep behaviour in normal subjects. *J Sleep Res* 1995;4:199–201

4.  Bootzin R, Perlis M. Nonpharmacologic treatments of insomnia. *J Clin Psychiatry* 1992;53:37–41

5.  Pallesen S, Nordhus I, Kvale G, *et al.* Behavioral treatment of insomnia in older adults: an open clinical trial comparing two interventions. *Behav Res Ther* 2003;41:31–48

6.  Manber R, Bootzin R, Acebo C, Carskadon M. The effects of regularizing sleep–wake schedules on daytime sleepiness. *Sleep* 1996;19:432–41

7.  Regestein Q. Postprandial drowsiness. *J Am Med Assoc* 1972;221:601–2

8.  Montgomery P, Dennis J. Physical exercise for sleep problems in adults aged 60+. *Cochrane Database Syst Rev* 2002;4: CD003404

9.  Sherrill D, Kotchou K, Quan S. Association of physical activity and human sleep disorders. *Arch Int Med* 1998;158:1894–8

10. Kubitz KA, Landers DM, Petruzzello SJ, Han M. The effects of acute and chronic exercise on sleep. A meta-analytic review. *Sports Med* 1996;21:277–91

11. Morin C, Hauri P, Espie C, Spielman A, Buysse D, Bootzin R. Nonpharmacologic treatment of chronic insomnia. An American Academy of Sleep Medicine review. *Sleep* 1999;22:1134–56

12. Rybarczyk B, Lopez M, Benson R, Alsten C, Stepanski E. Efficacy of two behavioral treatment programs for comorbid geriatric insomnia. *Psychol Aging* 2002;17:288–8

13. Viens M, De Koninck J, Mercier P, St-Onge M, Lorrain D. Trait anxiety and sleep-onset insomnia. Evaluation of treatment using anxiety management training. *J Psychosom Res* 2003;54:31–7

14. Hauri P, Linde S. *No More Sleepless Nights*. New York: John Wiley & Sons, 1996

15. Hauri P, Esther M. Insomnia. *Mayo Clin Proc* 1990;65:869–82

16. Nishino S, Mignot E, Dement W. Sedative–hypnotics. In Schatzberg A, Nemeroff C, eds. *Essentials of Clinical Psychopharmacology*. Washington DC: APPI, 2001:283–301

17. Richardson G, Roth T, Hajak G, Ustun T. Consensus for the pharmacological management of insomnia in the new millennium. *Intern J Clin Pract* 2001;55: 42–52

18. Krystal AD, Walsh JK, Laska E *et al.* Sustained efficacy of eszopiclone over 6 months of nightly treatment: results of a randomized, double-blind, placebo-controlled study in adults with chronic insomnia. *Sleep* 2003; 26:793–9

19. Canaday B. Amnesia possibly associated with zolpidem administration. *Pharmacotherapy* 1996;16:687–9

20. Artigas F, Nutt D, Shelton R. Mechanism of action of antidepressants. *Psychopharmacol Bull* 2002;36:123–32

21. Montgomery I, Oswald I, Morgan K, Adam K. Trazodone enhances sleep in subjective quality but not in objective duration. *Br J Clin Pharm* 1983;16:139–44

22. Nowell P, Reynold C, Buysse D, Dew M, Kupfer D. Paroxetine in the treatment of primary insomnia: preliminary clinical and electroencephalogram sleep data. *J Clin Psychiatry* 1999;60:795

23. Basu R, Dodge H, Stoehr G, Ganguli M. Sedative–hypnotic use of diphenhydramine in a rural, older adult community-based cohort: effects on cognition. *Am J Geriatr Psychiatry* 2003;11:205–13

24. Hauri P. Can we mix behavioral therapy with hypnotics when treating insomniacs? *Sleep* 1997;20:1111–18

25. Ferber R. *Solve Your Child's Sleep Problem*. New York: Simon and Shuster, 1985:55–80

# Chapter 13

# Circadian rhythm disorders

*What hath night to do with sleep?*

**John Milton,** *Comus*

The term 'circadian' refers to a circuit or period that is about 24 h long. Many physiological, biochemical and behavioral activities have a circadian rhythm, with the sleep–wake cycle being the most easily recognized. The sleep–wake cycle is related to other circadian rhythms, such as core body temperature and concentrations of melatonin or cortisol, through a complex interaction of afferent and efferent signals (Figure 13.1).

Patients with a circadian rhythm disorder have adequate quality and quantity of sleep

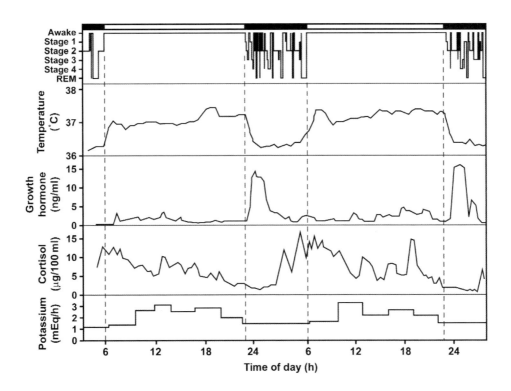

**Figure 13.1** Circadian rhythms. This figure illustrates a number of human circadian rhythms, including the sleep–wake cycle, the core body temperature rhythm, the growth hormone and cortisol rhythms, and the urinary excretion of potassium. The time frame is 48 h. REM, rapid eye movement. Reproduced with permission from reference 1

**Table 13.1** Classification of the circadian rhythm disorders

Delayed sleep phase disorder

Advanced sleep phase disorder

Non-24-h sleep–wake disorder

Irregular sleep–wake disorder

Jet lag sleep disorder

Shift work sleep disorder

but are unable to sleep at the desired or expected time (Table 13.1). As a consequence, they may be awake or asleep at inappropriate times, possibly experiencing both insomnia and excessive daytime sleepiness. Circadian rhythm disorders can be conceptualized according to which component of the sleep–wake cycle is aberrant: the ability to develop periodicity (non-24-h sleep–wake disorder), the motivation to perpetuate periodicity (irregular sleep–wake disorder) or timing relative to the community in which the person lives (delayed and advanced sleep phase disorders, shift work and jet lag sleep disorders).

## CIRCADIAN INFLUENCES ON SLEEP–WAKE ACTIVITY

The sleep–wake rhythm is determined by several important factors. Two major processes, circadian rhythmicity (process C) and sleep homeostasis (process S), were initially recognized during temporal isolation studies which allowed the sleep–wake schedule to become dissociated from the body's temperature cycle (see Chapter 5). Sleep homeostasis represents the time elapsed since the last episode of sleep. As time passes, the pressure to sleep builds up, and eventually reaches a point where sleep is irresistible owing to the accumulated sleep debt. Once this debt has been satisfied, the pressure to sleep decreases but with time again progressively increases. Circadian rhythmicity, which determines time points when sleep is more likely to occur based on the sleep–wake pacemaker, is the other important factor. The interplay of homeostatic and circadian factors determines sleep in rigorously controlled conditions such as a temporal isolation chamber. In a community setting many other factors, including personal choice, work schedules, family responsibilities, physical activities and exogenous substances, such as hypnotics or caffeine, play a contributory role to setting sleep onset and awakening.

Circadian rhythmicity is primarily determined by a group of cells in the suprachiasmatic nuclei (SCN) located in the hypothalamus, often called the biological clock (Figure 13.2). This pacemaker produces the circadian rhythm of sleep for the adult (one major sleep period per 24 h) that replaces the daytime and night-time sleep in infants. Isolation of these nuclei from the rest of the brain results in an abolition of circadian rhythms outside the small hypothalamic island, but persistence of neural circadian rhythm within the nuclei themselves. Uptake of 2-deoxyglucose within the nuclei follows a circadian rhythm, as does their neuronal electrical activity. Although in more primitive animals, such as the fruit fly, a variety of body regions such as the limbs appear to be capable of setting the circadian

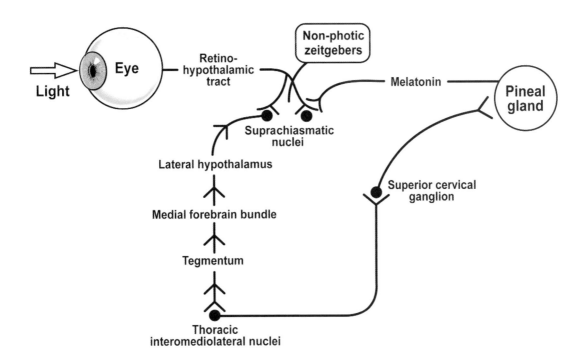

**Figure 13.2** Physiology of circadian rhythms. This schematic diagram indicates inputs into the suprachiasmatic nuclei and the control of melatonin synthesis by the pineal gland. Light on the retina results in afferent neural stimuli via the retinohypothalamic tract to the suprachiasmatic nuclei. The signal is also transmitted via the thoracic spinal cord and superior cervical ganglion to the pineal gland, resulting in melatonin synthesis. Melatonin receptors are present on the suprachiasmatic nuclei, completing the feedback loop

rhythm, in mammals the circadian pacemaker is restricted to the suprachiasmatic nuclei. Intriguing reports that a region on the human lower extremity can respond to light stimuli and determine circadian rhythms have not been replicated[2].

The periodicity of the biological clock has been studied by means of temporal isolation experiments in which subjects are placed in an environment totally without time cues. Early experiments indicated that, in such an environment, the sleep–wake cycle would free-run, with subjects electively

going to sleep and waking approximately 1 h later every day. This suggested that the human biological pacemaker has an intrinsic periodicity of 24.9 h, compared with the environmental cycle of 24 h (Figure 13.3). However, more recent work with rigorously controlled light conditions has shown that the actual periodicity of the human pacemaker is 24 h 11 min ± 8 min, with the earlier erroneous figure caused by the masking effects of low level illumination used in the experiments[4]. Over time, even this small mismatch between the periodicity of the

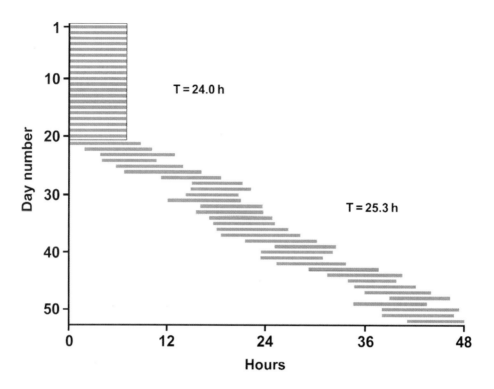

**Figure 13.3** Human sleep–wake cycle in a temporal isolation environment. This figure shows a 55-day recording of sleep–wake cycles in a normal volunteer. The first 20 days were recorded under entrained conditions, while the remainder of the study took place in an environment devoid of time cues. A free-running cycle (T) of about 25.3 h developed. In more recent experiments without the masking effect of light, the true duration of the intrinsic circadian cycle has been shown to be about 24.2 h. Reproduced with permission from reference 3

environmental 24-h clock and the intrinsic human sleep–wake cycle can still result in some people's internal sleep–wake phase becoming desynchronized from the community's predominant schedule. This potential desynchronization may underlie delayed sleep phase disorder (DSPD).

Intensive efforts have been made to understand the molecular mechanism of circadian rhythms and genetic influences on these influential cells. Several genes have been identified, although their exact role is still to be determined. In essence, protein gene products feed back to the nucleus, temporarily inhibiting their own genetic synthesis, thus establishing a biological rhythm with fixed periodicity. In the mouse, a gene (Clock) which controls the circadian sleep–wake rhythm has been identified[5]. When the Clock gene is mutated, the circadian rhythm of sleep, and in particular the ultradian rhythm of rapid eye movement (REM) sleep, is altered. In humans, a mutation has been reported in another circadian gene (Per), with the finding that the hPer2 gene is dysfunctional in families with advanced sleep phase syndrome[6].

The process of adapting the biological clock's intrinsic periodicity to the geosynchronous cycle of 24 h is called entrainment. This is an adaptable and dynamic system, with several factors being able to alter the sleep–wake circadian rhythm. Such factors leading to entrainment are called 'zeitgebers', a German neologism meaning 'time givers' (Figure 13.4). Bright light is indisputably the predominant zeitgeber, although social cues and food play a role. Whether a person's eyes are open or closed, light enters the eye and excites photoreceptor cells in the retina. Melanopsin, discovered in 2000, is a light-sensitive pigment found in those retinal ganglion cells that project to the SCN. Studies in mice with absent melanopsin show that this novel pigment is required for normal circadian phase setting[7]. The signal from the retinal ganglion cells is transmitted along the retinohypothalamic tract to the SCN in the anterior hypothalamus, thus

directly causing entrainment. In addition, the signal is then transmitted down brainstem sympathetic pathways to the intermediolateral cell column of the upper thoracic spinal cord and from there to the superior cervical ganglion, which provides sympathetic input to the pineal gland (Figure 13.2). The degree to which exposure to light affects the sleep–wake rhythm depends on the timing, intensity and duration of light exposure. In general, light exposure in the morning delays sleep onset while evening light does the reverse.

When a person is in the dark, or dim light, at night, the pineal gland secretes the hormone melatonin. Melatonin receptors are present in the SCN and thus the hormone may be involved in humoral feedback regulation of the pacemaker. When a person is exposed to bright natural or artificial light (10 000 lux, which is the intensity of unfiltered light from the sun), regardless of the time of day or night, melatonin secretion is promptly suppressed. The reverse situation,

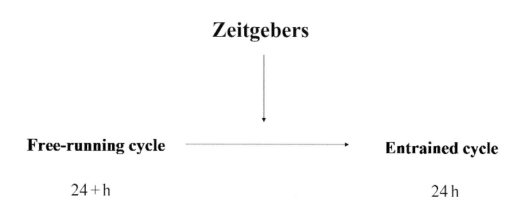

**Figure 13.4** Entrainment of a free-running cycle to an entrained cycle

the absence of bright light, does not lead to melatonin release unless the darkness corresponds to the appropriate point on the circadian rhythm of melatonin, approximately 16 h after cessation of the previous cycle's secretion. In healthy persons, melatonin is secreted from about 10 p.m. until 6 a.m., depending on the timing of bedtime and light exposure. Since people with a normal sleep–wake circadian rhythm typically sleep during the night, by extension melatonin is often used as a marker of the circadian rhythm of sleep–wake activity. However, melatonin data must be interpreted carefully with awareness of the light conditions and medication use ($\beta_1$-adrenergic antagonists block the noradrenergic innervation of the pineal gland). Because of these factors, the initial rise of melatonin concentration at night in blood, saliva or urine should be referred to as dim-light melatonin onset (DLMO).

## DIAGNOSTIC CONSIDERATIONS

Circadian rhythm disorders can be diagnosed based on a careful history of the patient's sleep–wake schedule. A detailed sleep diary covering several weeks can be helpful. Because many patients struggle to complete a sleep diary accurately, wrist actigraphy can be an extremely useful supplemental procedure (see Chapters 6 and 11). Poor recall, misperception or deliberate distortion may be factors that cause the sleep diary data to differ markedly from the information collected with the actigraph. In these cases, the actigraphic data may be more reliable than the patient self-report.

## DELAYED SLEEP PHASE DISORDER

### Demographics

Patients with DSPD fall asleep later and awaken later than expected or desired. This disorder is suspected to be common, although in-depth epidemiological studies are lacking. In one study of 10 000 Scandinavians followed with sleep logs, a prevalence of 0.72% was reported[8]. This number is suspected to be an underestimate because of the limitations of survey research. In this dataset the mean age of onset was during adolescence at 15.4 years, and the disorder was chronic with a mean duration of 19.2 years. The condition rarely starts after age 30 years. The gender mix is uncertain, but some studies note a male predominance. There are no reports of a familial predisposition.

### Case 13.1

A 16-year-old boy presented to the sleep clinic after his high school administration required him to have home tutoring because he had missed 3 months of school. Prior to the previous year, the boy had done well academically, although he had frequently missed the first class or two of the day. The patient explained that he could not make it to school because he could not awaken even when he set multiple alarms. He tried to have adequate sleep. Typically he would go to bed at approximately midnight, but had difficulty in falling asleep. After several hours lying awake he would watch TV or listen to music, intending this to help him fall asleep. He was unsure, but suspected that

## Time of day

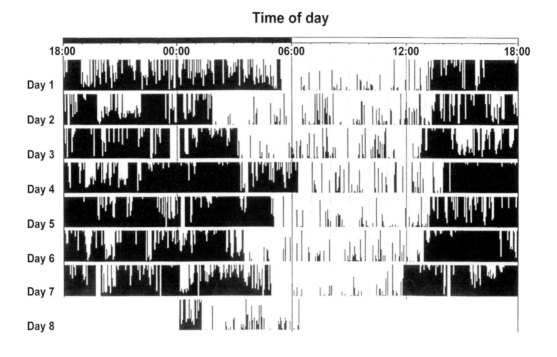

**Figure 13.5** Wrist actigraphy in delayed sleep phase disorder (case 13.1). Wrist actigraphy demonstrates a going-to-bed time ranging from 2 to 6:30 a.m. and a rise time from 11:45 to 2 p.m. (see Figure 4.9 for more details)

he was often awake until 4 a.m. When his alarm went off at 6 a.m., he did not awaken. His parents had tried to rouse him but ceased to intervene after he became very angry at being disturbed. He would often sleep without any awakenings until noon or even 2 p.m., at which time he would arise without significant difficulty. The patient would meet his friends to socialize and play basketball for several hours. He denied any sleepiness between 2 p.m. and midnight. Over time, he started to feel that his future was bleak because he was failing all his subjects, and he also missed being part of the school social activities. He feared that if he did

not get up earlier then he would fail to graduate, and be unable to fulfil his goal of attending college on an athletic scholarship.

Psychiatric evaluation revealed depressed mood, excessive guilt, poor self-esteem and hopelessness. The patient's sleep diary had little detail, but reported a bedtime of midnight with prolonged initial sleep latency. Wrist actigraphy (Figure 13.5) confirmed that he typically fell asleep at 4 a.m. Neither a polysomnogram (PSG) nor a multiple sleep latency test (MSLT) were performed. The patient was advised to start using bright-light therapy each morning, and also advised to pursue psychotherapy to examine his adjustment issues. The patient's sleep–wake rhythm gradually improved to the point that he was able to return to school with an hour later start-time than his classmates. The patient appeared to be more interested in being involved in school-related activities. A future goal was for him to start school at a conventional time.

DSPD is relatively common in adolescents. Getting up late interferes greatly with school attendance and academic success. Over time, patients often develop poor self-esteem because they are struggling with not only the academic but also the social components of school. The high association of delayed sleep phase disorder and depression is probably explained by the combination of sleep difficulties with a frustrating school experience. As a result, treatment should involve both phototherapy and psychotherapy to ensure that both sleep and psychosocial issues are targeted.

### Clinical features

DSPD is characterized by initial sleep and awake times that are consistently later than desired. The total sleep time over the 24-h period is normal. Many patients note that this problem arises after a stretch of late-night studying or social activities. If the patient manages to arise at a socially acceptable hour, excessive daytime sleepiness is usually present during the morning hours. On vacation, when the patient is not trying to conform to any specified schedule, wake time will be delayed. Patients with DSPD often recognize that they have the long-standing trait of being 'night owls' who feel most alert and perform best late at night. Some individuals cope by selecting careers that involve evenings and avoid mornings, such as restaurant work. Students may compensate by going to night school.

DSPD is often associated with psychiatric disorders, specifically depression. It is unclear whether the adolescent first has psychiatric symptoms and then develops delayed sleep phase or whether the circadian rhythm disorder leads to absenteeism which in turn results in psychiatric, academic and social problems. Patients and their families are often intensely frustrated by the condition. Because hypnotics are not usually effective, most patients do not use them long term, and dependence issues are therefore rare.

### Differential diagnosis

The differential diagnosis includes major depression with patients having an increased need to sleep, sometimes coexisting with an initial insomnia. If a patient pursues treatment for the mood disorder, with improvement in mood and other symptoms but persisting delayed sleep phase, then a coexisting circadian rhythm disorder should be suspected. Some patients with avoidant or schizoid personality disorder will seek out the solitude of night. A careful history should not only explore the person's sleep–wake schedule but also look for signs of deliberate avoidance of daytime interactions. Some people who are on vacation, disabled or unemployed may voluntarily select a late night schedule. Determining the motivation and effort expended to conform to the more conventional timetable is of value in differentiating them from true DSPD patients.

Occasionally, patients will appear to have a disorder of excessive daytime sleepiness such as narcolepsy or idiopathic hypersomnia. The assessment should include careful exploration of the presence of excessive sleepiness during the evening and night, with normal alertness during these times more likely to indicate DSPD. Patients with DSPD may have sleep-onset REM periods during the first or second naps of the MSLT, especially if the MSLT start time was not delayed in accordance with the patient's phase shift. This does not reflect REM sleep intruding into daytime alertness but rather the patient's final REM sleep of their major sleep period. Initial sleep latencies usually increase with successive naps in DSPD. In all the circadian rhythm disorders, polysomnography may be indicated if there is suspicion that a coexisting sleep disorder such as obstructive sleep apnea may be present. When polysomnography is employed, the start time of the sleep study might need to be adjusted.

## Management

Patients must strive towards a consistent sleep–wake schedule, since staying up late deliberately during weekends and holidays may interfere with falling asleep as desired on week nights. Patient motivation is an essential component in a successful treatment plan. If the patient does not actively embrace the practices necessary to correct their circadian rhythm disorder, treatment is unlikely to be effective. In some cases, patients espouse an intention to strive towards a phase shift, but actually maintain a passive aggressive attitude that can contribute significantly to family strain. In many cases, psychotherapy may be essential in giving a patient an opportunity to understand and modify the factors that may be contributing to late night activity. Family as well as individual therapy may be useful in finding solutions to complex family and school problems.

The most commonly recommended treatment is to have the patient use bright-light therapy in the morning from 6 to 9 a.m. to adjust their sleep–wake cycle. When patients are adherent, this has been demonstrated to be effective[9]. Patients typically start at a later time, for example 9 a.m., and as their ability to awake earlier improves, they advance the time of light exposure earlier in 30-min increments. However, despite this, many patients have difficulty in awakening to undertake the light exposure from a light box or the sun. Adherence is often inconsistent, with patients complaining that they cannot find the necessary 30 min each morning for the treatment.

The recommended light intensity is 10 000 lux. Several different light units are available, and the manufacturer's specifications should be followed concerning the distance that the patient should sit from the light box. This varies depending on whether the unit has a single central light or two smaller units on either side of the patient. Patients should make light exposure their priority, and engage in activities such as reading, applying make-up or eating breakfast only as long as their eyes are positioned adequately in front of the box. Many patients prefer to combine exposure to natural sunshine with exercise by jogging, cycling or running outside in clear weather. Patients should be reminded not to look directly at the sun, to prevent eye damage. Potential side-effects of light boxes include retinal burns, which are more likely to develop if the patient is taking anticholinergic medications that increase the pupillary diameter. Patients taking photosensitizing medications should not be advised to use phototherapy.

Patients should also be advised to avoid bright light, possibly by wearing sunglasses, from 4 p.m. to dark. Other treatment options have included melatonin which has been beneficial in several controlled trials[10–12]. Melatonin is given 1–3 h (depending on the severity of the phase delay) before the desired bedtime, and is used on an ongoing basis. The dose of melatonin is typically low at 3 mg. Melatonin has not been as rigorously tested for side-effects as hypnotic agents. Since it is not considered a pharmaceutical agent by the US Food and Drug Administration, but rather is classified as a nutritional supplement available in health-food stores, patients may have difficulty verifying the purity of the product available for purchase. Safety data regarding chronic usage have not appeared in the medical literature, although no anecdotal reports of serious side-effects have surfaced to date. In general, melatonin is only weakly sedating. Some preliminary studies have combined melatonin with phototherapy. This combined approach may be desirable when patients are suspected to have poor adherence with phototherapy and be more likely to take a tablet. Apart from the increased cost there are no known disadvantages of combining melatonin with light therapy.

Most treatment plans for DSPD no longer emphasize the role of chronotherapy. This approach involved patients sequentially delaying their bedtime by 1–2 h a night around the clock until they fell asleep at the desired time. Outcomes were poor because of the understandable difficulty in conforming to this complex regimen, and the tendency for many patients to slip back into a delayed sleep phase pattern over time. Hypnotics and psychostimulants have not been found to be useful, since the patient fundamentally has adequate sleep but is not synchronized with their community. If the patient has coexisting major depression, antidepressant medications may be appropriate. Some clinicians opt to prescribe sedating antidepressants such as mirtazapine, although these have not been demonstrated to be preferable to others.

## ADVANCED SLEEP PHASE DISORDER

Patients with this condition fall asleep and awaken at times earlier than desired. Patients may inappropriately fall asleep during evening activities and experience loneliness or boredom when awake in the early morning. This condition is rare, especially when compared with DSPD. A survey of 10 000 Scandinavians did not find a single case of advanced sleep phase disorder[8]. This striking difference in prevalence between advanced and delayed sleep phase disorder is likely because the human sleep–wake circadian period of slightly more than 24 h promotes phase delay. The condition probably becomes more common with age. In nursing homes and assisted living facilities, the institutional routines frequently encourage bedtime in the early evening, sometimes because of reduced staffing at those times. The differential diagnosis includes major depression, since both conditions can be characterized by insomnia in the early morn-

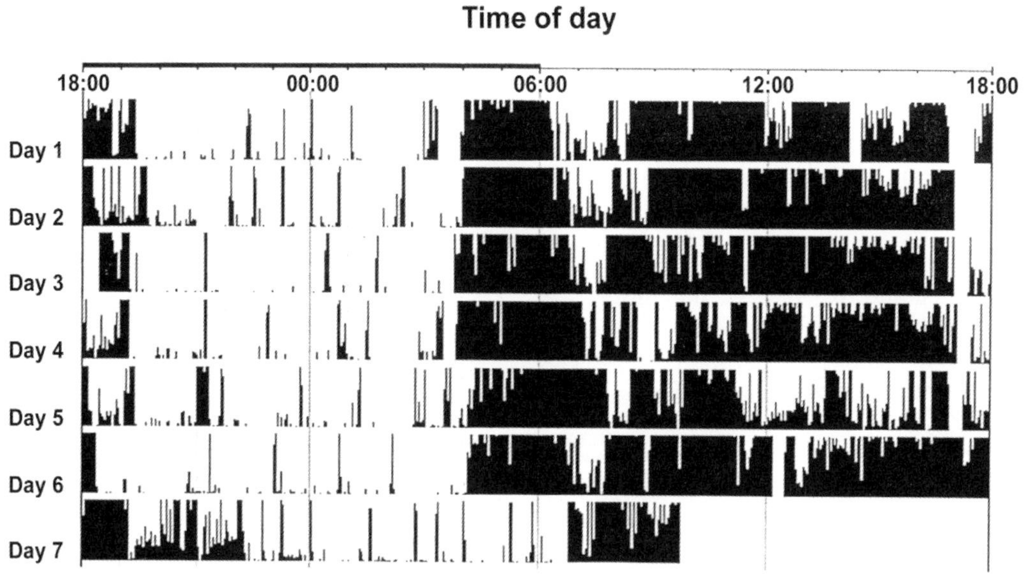

**Time of day**

**Figure 13.6** Wrist actigraphy in advanced sleep phase disorder. Wrist actigraphy demonstrates a going-to-bed time ranging from 6:30 to 7:30 p.m. and a rise time of about 4 a.m. (see Figure 4.9 for more details)

ing. The evaluation should include a sleep diary (completed by the patient or facility staff) and wrist actigraphy (Figure 13.6).

An autosomal dominant familial form of advanced sleep phase disorder has been reported in three families. All affected patients fell asleep and wakened 4 h earlier than expected, and had melatonin and temperature rhythms that were also advanced by 3–4 h. The circadian sleep–wake period was shortened to 23.3 h. The genetic defect was traced to a mutation in the period (per) gene named hPer2. Affected individuals have a mutation in the casein kinase 1-binding region of the hPer2 gene with a serine to glycine mutation. This mutation interferes with the functioning of the clock component, causing a significant advance in the circadian period consistent with advanced sleep phase disorder[6].

Treatment involves avoidance of morning bright-light and a daytime schedule that encourages entrainment to a conventional sleep–wake schedule. Evening light therapy has also been successfully used in short-term studies[13,14]. Progressive earlier shifting of bedtime by 3 h every 2 days has been reported as having short-term utility in one case report[15]. One recent study examined therapy of advanced phase sleep disorder in a group of children with Smith–Magenis syndrome, a complex genetic disease caused by a deletion in chromosome 17p. Sleep, as well as melatonin phase, was delayed with the combined administration in the evening of controlled-release melatonin and in the morning a $\beta_1$ adrenergic antagonist, blocking the noradrenergic neurotransmission to the pineal gland that releases melatonin[16].

## NON-24-h SLEEP–WAKE DISORDER

Non-24-h sleep–wake disorder, otherwise known as hypernychthemeral disorder, is a rare condition usually limited to visually impaired people, some of whom are also mentally handicapped. These patients develop sleep patterns similar to those observed in subjects living without environmental time cues. They cannot benefit from the powerful entraining effect of light on the suprachiasmatic nucleus, experiencing a free-running rhythm without a consistent phase. Clinically these patients may present with intermittent insomnia and excessive daytime sleepiness. For a brief time their sleep–wake activity may be synchronized with the community, but after several days it will again drift out of phase. In addition to idiosyncratic sleep–wake patterns, they may develop other unpredictable circadian rhythms, for example melatonin secretion. Patients complain of undesired daytime sleep corresponding to diurnal melatonin that in the absence of light perception is not suppressed. The sleep–wake rhythm may also dissociate from the body's other circadian rhythms, such as temperature (internal desynchronization). Sleep initiation difficulties may worsen at times when the free-running circadian rhythm for sleep–wake activity corresponds to points of the temperature rhythm other than the nadir. Because many affected patients try to conform to a socially acceptable sleep–wake schedule, they awaken earlier than appropriate, resulting in insufficient sleep. However, even on vacation, when they are less likely to arise at a specified time, they do not develop a consistent sleep schedule.

## Case 13.2

A 35-year-old man with congenital blindness due to bilateral optic nerve hypoplasia presented with intermittent insomnia and excessive daytime sleepiness. His visual impairment prevented him from recognizing whether his environment was light or dark. The patient also had short stature and lifelong anosmia. He wished to avoid an unconventional sleep–wake schedule so he could be awake during the day to interact with his family and to work in his pottery studio. Using a clock to determine time, he went to bed at 10 p.m. and arose at 6 a.m. However, his sleep pattern was highly variable. For several days he slept at the desired time but thereafter he reported initial insomnia lasting from 1–5 h. At these times he also took daytime naps, despite his preference to be awake. A magnetic resonance imaging (MRI) scan of the brain revealed a small pituitary stalk and no optic chiasm.

This case illustrates typical non-24-h sleep–wake disorder in a blind patient. His circadian rhythm was managed primarily by social cues. He was strongly motivated to be awake at the same time as other people because he valued the social interaction. At times he would struggle to maintain a consistent schedule and drift by an hour or two. By using an alarm and asking family members to awaken him he kept a relatively consistent sleep–wake schedule. His keen desire to have a specific sleep–wake schedule was sufficient to keep him entrained, despite his neurological condition. However, many similar patients find it extremely difficult to entrain in the absence of light cues.

In one recent study using polysomnography, actigraphy and Braille sleep logs, sleep was studied in 26 totally blind patients and matched controls[17]. These patients were living in the community but were still observed to have multiple sleep complaints, presumably due to a free-running cycle. Patients who were employed had a longer major sleep period than those who were retired or unemployed. Patients who have mental handicap or multiple disabilities may cope more poorly because of increased difficulty in conforming to social routines.

This condition should be suspected in any patient without light perception who has sleep complaints. Non 24-h sleep–wake disorder should be differentiated from the other circadian rhythm disorders, including DSPD. In DSPD, patients have initial insomnia and force themselves to arise at an inappropriately early time because of social obligations. In contrast to non-24-h sleep–wake rhythm disorder, DSPD patients experience a stable sleep–wake cycle on vacation, albeit delayed. Another diagnostic consideration is the irregular sleep–wake disorder, in which patients with an inconsistent schedule are capable of entrainment but disregard the cues. A detailed sleep diary recording several weeks of functioning accompanied by wrist actigraphy can assist in distinguishing

these syndromes. The medical and social consequences of a non-24-h sleep–wake rhythm have not been well studied, but would be expected to include professional and family difficulties.

Few therapeutic options have been studied. Melatonin has been explored as a means to entrain circadian rhythms. Low-dose melatonin is typically administered at 8 p.m. (expected to be near the time of the dim-light melatonin onset) to achieve an 11 p.m. effect[18]. A sleep diary should be used before starting melatonin, allowing the treatment to begin only after the major sleep period shifts to night. Assessing whether bright light suppresses melatonin may be worthwhile in some blind persons, as occasionally the retinohypothalamic pathway remains intact, despite the absence of sight. In such cases, bright light may be used for entrainment purposes. Other schedule cues such as social activities and exercise have therapeutic value in this lifelong disorder.

## IRREGULAR SLEEP–WAKE DISORDER

Irregular sleep–wake disorder is a state in which patients permit their sleep–wake rhythms to become desynchronized. Patients voluntarily disregard the day–night transitions in their community and override their internal sleep–wake rhythm.

Irregular sleep–wake rhythms are most common in adolescents and young adults. In most cases the state develops in the second decade, and the duration is highly variable. The incidence and prevalence of the disorder is unknown.

## Clinical features

In this condition, patients have an average amount of sleep tallied over a 24-h period, but there is marked day-to-day variability in length and timing of the major sleep period. Patients can have insomnia and excessive daytime sleepiness because of their extremely variable sleep schedule. Unlike patients with non-24-h sleep–wake disorder, these patients are capable of entraining to a regular sleep–wake rhythm. Reasons for the unconventional sleep–wake schedule can include social activities, hobbies (including Internet usage), schoolwork and absence of sleep–wake discipline.

Irregular sleep–wake cycles are associated with psychiatric disorders which may either predispose to the circadian dysfunction or occur as a result of it. The condition may also occur in patients with neurological disorders such as dementia, delirium, head injury and coma emergence, where cognitive, behavioral or environmental issues, such as a supervised care-facility's erratic bathing schedule, promote irregular sleep–wake rhythms. Patients with chemical dependency states including intoxication, dependence and withdrawal may similarly be unwilling or, as long as they are influenced by the exogenous substance, unable to sustain sleep–wake rhythmicity.

The consequences of this condition depend on its severity. A pattern of staying up late on weekend nights may cause no impairment beyond some mild sleep deprivation. For people with a flexible occupation, such as writing or Internet-based pursuits, fewer adverse consequences may arise from their choice to have irregular hours. However, for individuals who have family or occupational responsibilities, an irregular sleep–wake rhythm may seriously interfere with their functioning. Excessive daytime sleepiness and insomnia develop because of timing issues. Inattention or irritability due to sleep deprivation can impair work and school performance and can result in motor vehicle accidents.

### Case 13.3

A 17-year-old high-school student presented for a second opinion regarding insomnia. Her mother reported a highly variable sleep–wake cycle since age 14 years. The patient typically went to bed between midnight and 1 a.m. but did not fall asleep until hours after her intended bedtime. She then slept through most of the next day, arising in the evening. At times she would stay awake for 30 h at a stretch and fall asleep whenever she was exhausted. When unable to sleep, she typically surfed the Internet or sent email messages. Gradually her ability to function during the day became compromised by fatigue, and she had not attended school in 2 years. Major depression had been suspected, based primarily on her fatigue, but trials of five different antidepressant medications had been ineffective.

Wrist actigraphy (Figure 13.7a) revealed a very irregular sleep–wake schedule. Polysomnography was not conducted. The treatment plan included establishing a regular sleep–wake cycle by setting a consistent awakening time, but she experienced limited improvement. Melatonin 3 mg was then added at 10 p.m. She gradually worked towards a consistent bedtime 8 h prior to awakening. She was advised to put her computer

## Time of day

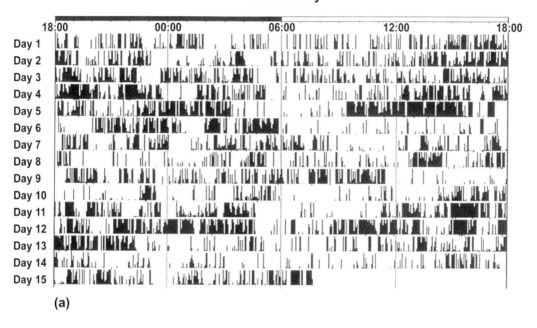

**(a)**

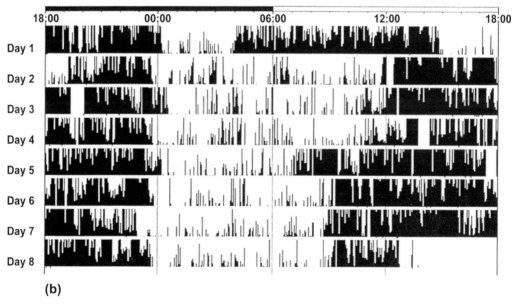

**(b)**

**Figure 13.7** Wrist actigraphy in irregular sleep–wake disorder (case 13.3). Wrist actigraphy (a) demonstrates a highly irregular sleep–wake cycle with sleep periods scattered throughout the day and night without discernible pattern. Repeat actigraphy (b) shows a far more regular pattern with a consistent bed time of 12 midnight and less variable rise time (see Figure 4.9 for more details)

usage on a regular schedule. Wrist actigraphy was repeated 3 months later (Figure 13.7b). The first night of the recording showed a short major sleep episode because of a camping trip, but overall her sleep–wake schedule was markedly less erratic.

In this case the patient was not making an adequate effort to maintain a consistent sleep–wake schedule, placing a higher priority on other pleasurable pursuits. Treatment involves patient education to emphasize the importance of structure, and a discussion about the undesirable consequences of missing school and other activities. Once the patient is more motivated to conform to a specific schedule, melatonin may be of benefit. Wrist actigraphy can be repeated as a measure to provide more objective outcome data to the patient, her family and the clinician.

### Assessment and management

Obtaining an accurate history of the patient's actual sleep–wake cycle can be difficult owing to poor recall, distortion or denial. Recognizing the irregular schedule is necessary to avoid an inappropriate and misleading diagnosis of a chronic fatigue state. Assessment involves careful tracking of the sleep–wake schedule using a sleep diary, completed each day. Wrist actigraphy can be very useful to obtain more objective observations from patients who may be unable or unwilling to describe their schedule accurately.

The patient's motivation to change is a major determinant of treatment outcome. Psychotherapy may be important to help a patient appreciate the adverse consequences of this life-style, and to examine reasons why she might resist change. The first step is to have a consistent schedule even if it has a pronounced abnormal phase. Over time, a sleep–wake schedule with an abnormal phase can be shifted using the modalities and cues described earlier in this chapter, including phototherapy and social cues. Melatonin has not been extensively studied, but has potential to be beneficial in this circadian rhythm disorder.

## JET LAG SYNDROME

### Clinical features

With the development of long-distance transmeridian travel, a new sleep disorder has emerged. Jet lag (otherwise known as time zone change syndrome) represents an acute problem in which travelers' sleep–wake circadian rhythms become out of phase with the light–dark cycle at their destination. The magnitude of the problem increases as travelers cross more time zones. In general, without measures to accelerate adjustment, 1 day is required to adjust to every hour of time zone change. Longitudinal (north–south) travel may result in sleep debt related to obtaining quality sleep on board a plane, but does not challenge a traveller with adapting to a new time zone.

In contrast to shift workers, the entrainment process is facilitated for travelers with jet lag, as they are attempting to adapt to the sleep–wake cycle of the destination community. Most people can more readily phase delay than phase advance the timing of their major sleep period, probably because of the longer than 24-h periodicity of the human circadian pacemaker. Thus, east to west travel is typically easier to adjust to than the equivalent travel west to east. Travelers who make frequent long-distance trips can develop a more chronic condition because they have not adequately adapted before a further change in sleep–wake schedule occurs. When people such as airline personnel face frequent circadian adjustments because of work schedules, jet lag overlaps with shift work sleep disorder.

The consequences of jet lag are similar to other sleep–wake rhythm disorders, with excessive daytime sleepiness, insomnia, disturbed nocturnal sleep and occupational problems due to inadequate alertness. The effect of jet lag on other circadian rhythms is less well known. Some travelers tolerate transmeridian travel without significant jet lag, but the reasons for individual variations are not well understood. No gender differences exist for jet lag, but the ability to adapt sleep–wake rhythms decreases with age.

## Treatment

Treatment options are controversial, and no one strategy is clearly preferred. Numerous research studies have been conducted, but most have significant limitations, primarily due to study design issues, including controlling light exposure and ensuring subject adherence with the protocol. Few experimental models exist for jet lag that account for all of the variables encountered in the real world of travel. For example, a protocol might call for three successive days of bright-light exposure at a consistent time after arrival at one's destination, steps that would be inconvenient for most tourists or business travelers.

The most commonly used strategies are optimizing sleep hygiene, manipulating one's sleep–wake schedule, using melatonin, phototherapy and cautious use of hypnotics. The traveler should be urged to obtain sleep of sufficient quality and quantity. A daytime flight eliminates the need for adequate sleep in an uncomfortable setting. Helpful measures include using a bedroom at the destination that is dark, quiet and at a comfortable temperature. Relaxation techniques may hasten sleep onset at an unfamiliar hour. Alcohol use is not recommended. Dietary measures have been proposed, such as a pre-sleep tryptophan-rich carbohydrate diet (promoting sedation mediated by serotonin and therefore melatonin production) and protein intake upon awakening (increasing alertness by means of tyrosine), but these programs are not supported by convincing evidence. Herbal remedies, other than melatonin, have limited usefulness.

One helpful approach is to try to adapt the time of the major sleep period as quickly as possible to the new schedule. For example, if a traveler arrives at 6 a.m. in Europe after a west to east transatlantic flight, the person is phase delayed as much as 6–7 h behind the time at the destination. The traveler's sleep–wake rhythm may be at 1 or 2 a.m., while he has arrived in time for morning activities in Europe. The traveler needs to phase advance, and should avoid sleeping until as close to the desired bedtime as possible. For westward flights, the circadian challenge is the opposite. The person needs to adapt to their advanced sleep phase by phase delaying their sleep–wake schedule in order to conform to their destination's time.

Meals and exercise at the destination should be timed carefully to serve as social cues that encourage and reinforce an appropriate sleep–wake cycle. Some experts advocate naps before, during and after transmeridian travel to prevent developing a significant sleep debt. These naps should be timed carefully, to allow sufficient sleep pressure to build up so that the traveler can still initiate sleep at the desired bedtime at their destination. Caffeine use should be carefully tracked, to minimize caffeine-related insomnia.

Hypnotics, traditionally the short-acting benzodiazepines such as triazolam, have been shown to be of some benefit in jet lag. These compounds decrease sleep latency, reduce awakenings and increase total sleep time. A more recently available but less studied option are the non-benzodiazepine agents with short half-lives such as zolpidem, zaleplon and zolpiclone. The half-life of any hypnotic should be short, to avoid a hangover effect. Potential side-effects of both these classes of hypnotics include amnesia, while cognitive impairment may occur with the benzodiazepines (see Chapter 12).

Since bright light is known to exert the strongest influence on the suprachiasmatic nuclei, this modality has clear potential for resetting the sleep–wake circadian rhythm to match the schedule of the destination. Numerous studies have led to jet lag algorithms. The intention is to obtain light exposure before the concurrent melatonin peak and temperature nadir if a phase advance is desired. The light exposure should come after these circadian markers if a phase delay is sought. Use of carefully timed light exposure may accelerate phase adjustments from 1 h to 3 h change per day. This strategy,

while scientifically based on the physiology of the suprachiasmatic nuclei, is difficult to implement in real-life travel. There are no simple tools for determining the melatonin peak or measuring core body temperature. The duration of an episode of phototherapy, the number of successive daily sessions, the light spectrum and the effects of age and individual differences are unknown. Nonetheless, awareness of the effects of light on circadian rhythms is important, because at a minimum travelers should avoid bright-light exposure at critical times. If phase advance is desired, morning bright-light exposure should be minimized (potentially by using wrap-around sunglasses), and bright light should be avoided in the evening for a desired phase delay.

Melatonin has been the subject of intense interest as a tool for the prevention or treatment of jet lag. Some, but not all, studies show the value of this compound as a chronotherapeutic agent for improving jet lag subjectively[19,20]. Melatonin should be administered at a 12-h phase difference from light therapy. If provided before the nadir of the core body temperature, melatonin will advance the sleep–wake circadian rhythm. If administered after this pivotal point, rhythms will delay. Experts advise travelers to start using melatonin during the early evening before departure for eastward trips and thereafter at the desired bedtime at the destination. For westward travel, after arrival at the destination, melatonin should be administered at 11 p.m. or even later to promote a phase delay.

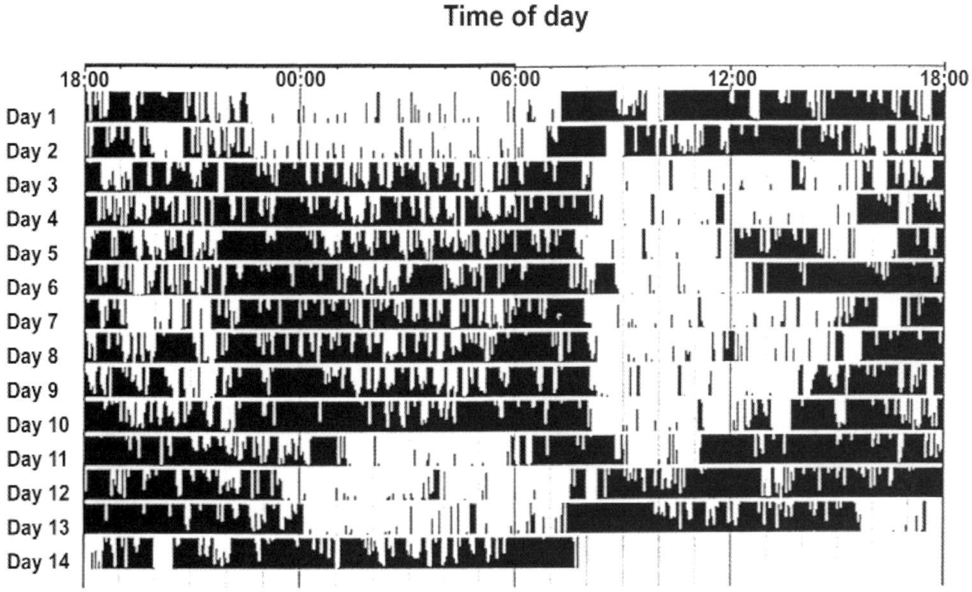

**Figure 13.8** Wrist actigraphy in shift work (case 13.4). Wrist actigraphy demonstrates sleep cycles in a shift worker. Night shift work is being performed on days 3–10. Note the variable and sometimes very short day sleep time during this period as well as the reduced amplitude activity between midnight and 6 a.m., suggesting inactivity or sleepiness while at work. Days 1–2 and 11–14 represent days off work (see Figure 4.9 for more details)

## SHIFT WORK SLEEP DISORDER

### Clinical features

An increasing number of people are employed in jobs that involve working shifts. The type of shift varies, but can encompass early morning start times, evening shifts, night work, split 24-h schedules and on-call responsibilities. Workers with rotating schedules as opposed to straight second (evening) or third (night) shifts are at higher risk for complications because their sleep–wake circadian rhythm is constantly adapting to a new timetable. In general, older persons find it harder to adapt to shift changes than younger ones.

### Case 13.4

A 58-year-old registered nurse presented with excessive daytime sleepiness. She had worked the night shift at the hospital for 37 years. Overall she had adjusted well, as long as she was assigned to the night shift consistently. She tried to sleep during the day on days when she did not work unless she had a long series of days off. She typically slept all morning and into the early afternoon. She was known to snore, but had never been observed to have apneas. She denied insomnia and restless legs symptoms. She rated herself a 14 on the Epworth sleepiness scale. She drank four cups of coffee daily and consumed a small amount of alcohol weekly.

Wrist actigraphy showed her daytime sleep and night-time activity to be consistent with her work schedule (Figure 13.8). The analyses reported a median time in bed of 459 min and a median total sleep time of 412 min, with a sleep efficiency of 89%. Her recording showed an abrupt switch from night-time to daytime activity. She was attending a family reunion, but tried to get as much sleep as possible before arising during the day for the event. In general she tried to limit daytime activities in order to sleep during the day, but for an important family occasion like this she had to sacrifice her daytime sleep. She later had polysomnography conducted during the day, which demonstrated an apnea–hypopnea index of 21/h. The treatment plan consisted of a recommendation to increase her total sleep time, and use nasal continuous positive airway pressure (CPAP) at 11 cmH$_2$O pressure for her obstructive sleep apnea syndrome. Her adherence was excellent, and her excessive daytime sleepiness decreased.

This case illustrates the challenges faced by shift workers. One could debate whether this patient had shift work sleep disorder or not. She certainly worked the night shift and made consistent daytime sleep a high priority. However, at times, special events make daytime sleep impossible, even for a determined patient. Among sleep experts there is controversy about whether any shift worker working the night shift is completely free of shift work sleep disorder. In our society, is it possible for anyone to switch completely away from daytime to nocturnal activities, 7 days a week, 52 weeks a year? Certainly, some shift workers fare better than others. As illustrated in this case, stable sleepiness in a shift worker may worsen when a new sleep disorder such as obstructive sleep apnea syndrome later develops.

Shift workers have high rates of both insomnia and excessive daytime sleepiness. Because of environmental factors, such as neighborhood noise or sunlight, initiating or maintaining sleep during the day can be difficult. Many shift workers have 2–4 h insufficient sleep nightly, because they sacrifice daytime sleep to spend time with family, pursue leisure activities or run errands. Having a coexisting sleep disorder, such as obstructive sleep apnea, increases the probability of excessive daytime sleepiness. Shift work puts individuals at high risk for several problems. Working when not fully alert poses the risk of performance difficulties owing to inadequate vigilance. Research into fatigue reveals that patients can experience cognitive or motor impairment[21].

Many industrial or transportation incidents, including the Exxon Valdez and the Three Mile Island accidents, have occurred at night, suggesting that worker fatigue may have been contributing factors. Missing opportunities to interact with family or friends because of shift work or recovery sleep can lead to social problems and family strain. Young children in particular may have difficulty understanding that a parent must be allowed to get adequate sleep after returning home from work. A recent study has found an increase in common respiratory infections and gastroenteritis in shift workers, third shift more than second, with the hypothesis that fatigue renders employees vulnerable to infection[22].

## Treatment

Several strategies have been identified to assist workers who must incorporate shift work into their life-style. Some people have an affinity for functioning well at certain times; for example, people with a tendency towards a delayed sleep phase may actually cope satisfactorily with an evening work schedule providing they can sleep late the following morning. Meals should be timed to promote sleep. Hunger, or foods that cause dyspepsia, may fragment sleep. The

workplace environment should be carefully planned to take into account workers' safety and sleep needs. Bright lights and a slightly cool air temperature may improve alertness. Ideally, attention should be given to the type of tasks undertaken by employees, especially on the night shift, with monotonous duties interspersed with more stimulating activities.

The sleeping environment at home may need to be modified. A person may wish to wear wrap-around dark glasses as he drives home at dawn from work. A quiet and dark bedroom is more important to a shift worker than others. Special window coverings may be required. The telephone should be switched off and messages collected with an answering machine. Family members should be urged not to awaken someone in the

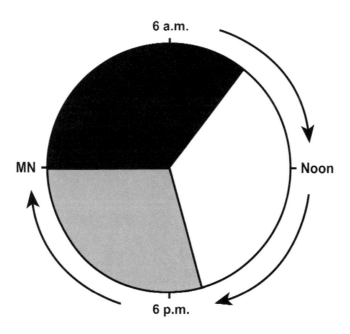

**Figure 13.9** Clockwise rotating shifts. Phase delay is preferable to phase advance for shift changes. MN, midnight

midst of their major sleep period. Sleep hygiene should be optimized.

Studies have shown that workers cope better when switching from one shift to another if they delay, rather than advance, their work and sleep time. For instance, if they move from evening to night shift, most individuals adjust more easily to the change (Figure 13.9). Preparing for an approaching shift change by gradually shifting bedtime and wake time back by 2 h, starting several days before the switch, has been found to be beneficial. However, family responsibilities often complicate careful sleep schedule adjustments of this type. Other effective coping strategies include taking a break during work hours. Recent work has focused on the transportation industry, specifically airline personnel, where a 30-min nap part way through the shift increases productivity, reduces fatigue and improves employee satisfaction. Long-haul aircraft have now been designed to include bunks or reclining seats for scheduled naps[23].

Some employers and employees prefer work schedules that use permanent shift assignments. Night shift workers should endeavor to keep to a consistent sleep–wake schedule, even on days when they do not work. Reverting to night-time sleep over a weekend or even a single day off presents adjustment problems similar to those faced by workers assigned to rotating shifts. Again, family and social responsibilities make it difficult for people to follow an exclusive night activity schedule. Workers with on-call schedules present a slightly different problem, as they cannot predict when they will be required to perform a task. Typically, the time block for on-call workers is longer than for most other shift workers (for example

24 h), and they cannot plan their sleep–wake schedule in advance. Naps may be especially important in these circumstances. Although in general people are urged to have a major sleep period each day as opposed to several shorter stretches of sleep, naps are reasonable if that is the only means by which adequate sleep can be obtained.

Medications to help shift workers initiate sleep at the desired time have been examined. Regular use of benzodiazepines creates the risk of physical dependence, as well as a hangover effect, especially with the longer-acting agents. Short-term use of a newer non-benzodiazepine hypnotic such as zaleplon or zolpidem is preferable to a benzodiazepine. Caution must be exercised even with these agents, since they have not been studied or approved for long-term use. Shift workers should first fully explore ways of obtaining adequate sleep by means of careful schedule changes, making sufficient sleep a priority and taking naps if indicated. The hypnotics provide symptomatic relief without addressing the underlying circadian rhythm disturbance inherent in shift work. Alcohol should be avoided as a means of inducing sleep, because of its detrimental effects on the patency of the upper airway and tendency to reduce the quality of non-rapid eye movement (NREM) sleep. Caffeine may be useful to boost alertness, but should be avoided close to bedtime in order not to interfere with sleep onset. In general, there is agreement that prescribing methylphenidate and the amphetamines is not an appropriate means to assist shift workers. However, modafanil was recently approved by the US Food and Drug Administration for shift work sleep disorder, following studies showing modest benefit in increasing alertness with this condition. Patients who choose to use this medication must make every effort to get adequate sleep and not attempt to function with voluntary reduced sleep time. As with the hypnotics, patients should be discouraged from what might become long-term use of a habituating medication, and instead be encouraged to rely on scheduling issues and naps. As in jet lag, bright-light therapy delivered at precise times may be a useful option. Melatonin has been explored as a possible chronotherapeutic agent, although it is not currently widely used. Very recently, melatonin agonists have been synthesized and show promise in pilot studies[24].

## REFERENCES

1. Moore-Ede MC, Czeisler CA, Richardson GS. Circadian timekeeping in health and disease. Part 1. Basic properties of circadian pacemakers. *N Engl J Med* 1983;309:469–76

2. Campbell S, Murphy P. Extraocular circadian phototransduction in humans. *Science* 1998;279:396–9

3. Czeisler CA, Richardson GS, Coleman RM, *et al.* Chronotherapy: resetting the circadian clocks of patients with delayed sleep phase insomnia. *Sleep* 1981;4:1–21

4. Czeisler C, Duffy J, Shanahan T, *et al.* Stability, precision, and near-24-hour period of the human circadian pacemaker. *Science* 1999;284:2177–81

5. Naylor E, Bergmann B, Krauski K, *et al.* The circadian clock mutation alters sleep homeostasis in the mouse. *J Neurosci* 2000; 20:8138–43

6. Toh K, Jones C, He Y, *et al.* An hPer2 phosphorylation site mutation in familial advanced sleep phase syndrome. *Science* 2001;291:1040–3

7. Hattar S, Lucas RJ, Mrosovsky N, *et al.* Melanopsin and rod–cone photoreceptive systems account for all major accessory visual functions in mice. *Nature (London)* 2003;424:75–81

8. Schrader H, Bovim G, Sand T. The prevalence of delayed and advanced sleep phase syndromes. *J Sleep Res* 1993;2:51–5

9. Cole R, Smith J, Alcala Y, Elliott J, Kripke D. Bright-light mask treatment of delayed sleep phase syndrome. *J Biol Rhythms* 2002; 17:89–101

10. Arendt J, Deacon S, English J, Hampton S, Morgan L. Melatonin and adjustment to phase shift. *J Sleep Res* 1995;4:74–9

11. Kayumov L, Brown G, Jindal R, Buttoo K, Shapiro C. A randomized, double-blind, placebo-controlled crossover study of the effect of exogenous melatonin on delayed sleep phase syndrome. *Psychosom Med* 2001; 63:40–8

12. Nagtegaal JE, Kerkhof GA, Smits MG, Swart AC, Van Der Meer YG. Delayed sleep phase syndrome: a placebo-controlled cross-over study on the effects of melatonin administered five hours before the individual dim light melatonin onset. *J Sleep Res* 1998;7:135–43

13. Campbell S, Dawson D, Anderson MW. Alleviation of sleep maintenance insomnia with timed exposure to bright light. *J Am Geriatr Soc* 1993;41:829–36

14. Murphy P, Campbell S. Enhanced performance in elderly subjects following bright light treatment of sleep maintenance insomnia. *J Sleep Res* 1996;5:165–72

15. Moldofsky H, Musisi S, Phillipson E. Treatment of a case of advanced sleep phase syndrome by phase advance chronotherapy. *Sleep* 1986;9:61–5

16. De Leersnyder H, Bresson J, de Blois M, *et al.* β1-Adrenergic antagonists and melatonin reset the clock and restore sleep in a circa-

dian disorder, Smith–Magenis syndrome. *J Med Genet* 2003;40:74–78

17. Leger D, Guilleminault C, Santos C, Paillard M. Sleep/wake cycles in the dark: sleep recorded by polysomnography in 26 totally blind subjects compared to controls. *Clin Neurophysiol* 2002;113:1607–14

18. Lewy A, Bauer V, Hasler B, Kendall A, Pires M, Sack R. Capturing the circadian rhythms of free-running blind people with 0.5 mg melatonin. *Brain Res* 2001;918:96–100

19. Petrie K, Dawson AG, Thompson L, Brook R. A double-blind trial of melatonin as a treatment for jet lag in international cabin crew. *Biol Psychiatry* 1993;33:526–30

20. Spitzer RL, Terman M, Williams JB, *et al.* Jet lag: clinical features, validation of a new syndrome-specific scale, and lack of response to melatonin in a randomized, double-blind trial. *Am J Psychiatry* 1999; 156:1392–6

21. Wright S, Lawrence L, Wrenn K, Haynes M, Welch L, Schlack H. Randomized clinical trial of melatonin after night-shift work: efficacy and neuropsychologic effects. *Ann Emerg Med* 1998;32:334–40

22. Moran D, Jansen K, Kant I, Galana J, van der Brandt P, Sween G. Prevalence of common infections in employees on different work shifts. *J Occup Employee Med* 2002; 44:1003–11

23. Rosekind M, Smith R, Miller D, *et al.* Alertness management: strategic naps in operational settings. *J Sleep Res* 1995;4:62–6

24. Nickelsen T, Samel A, Vejvoda M, Wenzel J, Smith B, R G. Chronobiotic effects of the melatonin agonist LY 156735 following a simulated 9 h time shift: results of a placebo-controlled trial. *Chronobiol Int* 2002;19:915–36

# Chapter 14

# Sleep in the patient with psychiatric disorders

*Thy spirit within thee hath been so at war,*
*And thus hath so bestirred thee in thy sleep,*
*That beads of sweat have stood upon thy brow,*
*Like bubbles in a late-disturbed stream*

**William Shakespeare,** *King Henry IV, Part I*

Many psychiatric disorders are associated with prominent sleep disturbance, most often with insomnia but sometimes with excessive daytime sleepiness or parasomnias. Sleep can be disrupted by the symptoms associated with the psychiatric disorder or by the treatment employed. The psychiatric disorders most likely to coexist with sleep disturbance are identified in Table 14.1.

## MOOD DISORDERS

For decades psychiatrists and neuroscientists have examined the association between mood and sleep. Depressed patients often seek out medical care because of changes in the quantity or quality of their sleep, and physicians often select specific antidepressant medications based on a desire to modify these symptoms. The relationship between sleep architecture, specifically initial rapid eye movement (REM) latency, and major depression has the potential to promote greater understanding of the pathophysiology of the condition.

### Major depression

Major depression is a common medical problem, with a lifetime prevalence in the

**Table 14.1** Psychiatric disorders coexisting with sleep disturbances

---

*Insomnia*
Major depression
Dysthymia
Bipolar disorder, manic phase
Generalized anxiety disorder
Panic disorder
Post-traumatic stress disorder
Psychotic disorders
Alcohol dependence
Stimulant intoxication
Hypnotic withdrawal
Opioid withdrawal

*Excessive daytime sleepiness*
Major depression, atypical type
Dysthymia
Drug dependence
Stimulant withdrawal
Alcohol intoxication
Hypnotic dependence
Opioid dependence

*Parasomnias*
Alcohol intoxication
Post-traumatic stress disorder

---

**Table 14.2** Features of major depression: the diagnosis of major depression requires the presence of at least five of these symptoms for 2 weeks or longer in the absence of any medical disorder that could be the cause

| |
|---|
| Depressed mood |
| Sleep disturbance nearly every day |
| Weight loss or gain of 5% or disturbed appetite |
| Restlessness or psychomotor slowing |
| Decreased interests |
| Decreased energy |
| Decreased concentration or indecisiveness |
| Increased guilt |
| Thoughts of death |

USA of 20%. According to the *Diagnostic and Statistical Manual* (DSM)-IV[1], major depression involves a constellation of at least five symptoms (Table 14.2). More than 90% of patients with major depression have sleep disturbances[2]. Insomnia, encompassing initial insomnia, sleep maintenance difficulties, non-refreshing sleep and early morning awakenings, is the most common sleep symptom.

## Case 14.1

A 56-year-old retired registered nurse presented with an inability to fall asleep as well as frequent awakenings during the night. She estimated that she obtained less than 4 h sleep nightly. Her insomnia had begun approximately 3 months previously, without any specific trigger. She had a history of major depression 20 years before, lasting several months, that occurred when her teenage daughter died of leukemia. Insomnia was a feature of this previous depressive episode. At that time she pursued individual psychotherapy and was prescribed a tricyclic antidepressant, doxepin, which she continued to use for several years. She had recently seen her primary-care physician who prescribed a selective serotonin reuptake inhibitor (SSRI), fluoxetine. The concern was that the patient was having a recurrence of her depression, based on her insomnia, depressed mood, hopelessness, fatigue and inability to experience pleasure. A new psychosocial problem had been the patient and her husband realizing that they had not saved enough money for a comfortable retirement. The patient had been taking fluoxetine for about 2 months but had not seen any improvement in her sleep or mood. She did not wish to resume doxepin because of the dry mouth that she had experienced in the past. The patient was not known to snore, have leg kicks or strange behaviors at night. She was not interested in a sleep study because she predicted that she would be unable to sleep in a strange place. The impression was that her insomnia was related to a recurrent episode of major depression. She was advised to try a novel antidepressant, mirtazepine, which is sedating without causing dry mouth. She was also encouraged to undergo training in relaxation techniques and obtain some time-limited exploratory psychotherapy to examine the retirement issues. Over time her insomnia and mood improved.

This case illustrates the classic situation where insomnia is a symptom of depression. Two months of fluoxetine treatment should be a long enough time to produce a favorable response, and use

**Table 14.3** Effects of representative antidepressants on sleep

| Antidepressant | Class* |
|---|---|
| *Significantly sedating* | |
| Mirtazepine | novel |
| Trazodone | novel |
| Nortriptyline | TCA |
| Amitriptyline | TCA |
| | |
| *Neutral* | |
| Paroxetine | SSRI |
| Citalopram | SSRI |
| Escitalopram | SSRI |
| | |
| *Significantly stimulating* | |
| Bupropion | novel |
| Fluoxetine | SSRI |
| Sertraline | SSRI |
| Protriptyline | TCA |
| Atomoxetine | SNRI |
| Venlafaxine | novel |
| Phenelzine | MAOI |

*Novel, atypical mechanism of action; TCA, tricyclic antidepressant; SSRI, selective serotonin reuptake inhibitor; SNRI, selective norepinephrine reuptake inhibitor; MAOI, monoamine oxidase inhibitor

of a medication from a different class of antidepressants is highly recommended after such a failed medication trial (Table 14.3). In this case mirtazepine, a highly sedating agent, at doses up to 15 mg was employed, with success. At doses higher than 15 mg, mirtazepine is less antihistaminergic and less likely to yield the sedation desired by this patient.

Insomnia is very common in depression, with approximately 20% of patients with insomnia also having major depression[3]. The presence of insomnia appears to be a useful risk factor for prediction of the development of major depression within the following year[4]. For unknown reasons, women with depression are more likely to experience insomnia than men. Patients with major depression classically awaken 2–4 h earlier than desired, with an inability to fall back to sleep[5]. During the day, depressed patients report fatigue, but without objective excessive daytime sleepiness. In atypical major depression, patients may have hypersomnia and increased appetite in place of insomnia and anorexia. SSRIs are known sometimes to cause insomnia in the first week of treatment, generally resolving within a week. Low-dose trazodone or non-benzodiazepine hypnotics such as zolpidem 5–10 mg a day can be used to treat this phenomenon.

Polysomnography in major depression has consistently showed decreased initial REM sleep latency that persists even after effective treatment of the depressive symptoms. REM latency is not as short as is seen in narcolepsy. Reduced REM latency has also been reported in unaffected first-degree relatives of patients with major depression raising the possibility that this is a trait rather than a state marker[6]. Reduced REM latency in major depression has been used as a predictor of response to antidepressant medications and psychotherapy[7]. Other abnormalities of REM sleep in major depression include a shortened initial REM period and increased REM density. Possible explanations are that REM sleep is phase advanced in major depression, or associated with increased cholinergic activity relative to monoaminergic neurotransmission. Other non-specific polysomnographic findings in major depression include decreased sleep continuity and reduced slow-wave sleep.

### Dysthymia

Dysthymia is a milder but more chronic form of depression, with two or more depressive symptoms lasting at least 2 years. If a patient meets criteria for major depression in the first 2 years of dysthymia, the diagnosis is revised to major depression. After 2 years of a milder depressed state, episodes of major depression can be superimposed on dysthymia. Patients with dysthymia report significant fatigue in addition to their other depressive symptoms. A study of multiple sleep latency tests in apparently sleepy patients with dysthymia did not reveal any abnormal findings, suggesting the absence of actual sleepiness and rather the presence of fatigue or lethargy[8].

### Bipolar disorder, manic phase

Bipolar patients in the manic phase are in a hyperaroused state, classically with pressured speech, elevated mood, distractibility, agitation, inflated self-esteem and excessive involvement in pleasurable abilities. They characteristically have a decreased need to sleep, despite their high energy levels. Often patients have poor insight into their disorder, and do not recognize the extent of their elevated mood state. Because of this poor insight, bipolar patients sometimes seek assistance specifically for their unsatisfying sleep, without awareness that it is a component of a mood disorder. By means of a history-taking and a mental status examination, clinicians need to screen patients

with insomnia for a possible evolving manic state. Patients with chronic bipolar disorder, who can experience mixed mood states with coexisting depressive and manic symptoms, can also present requesting intervention for their inability to sleep. Taking a careful history of past mood states and swings can aid in the identification of these patients. Appropriate treatment includes discontinuing antidepressant medications and starting mood stabilizers such as lithium or valproic acid. In some cases, short-term usage of benzodiazepines may be helpful for insomnia and daytime agitation.

### Major depression, seasonal type

A seasonal variant of major depression has been described that affects up to 5% of North Americans[9]. This condition is more common in higher latitudes where there is less daylight during the winter months. Affected patients have depressed mood that occurs exclusively during the winter months, characteristically experiencing an increased need for sleep, increased appetite and weight gain. This form of depression responds to antidepressant medications, particularly the SSRIs. Phototherapy with bright-light exposure in the morning has been demonstrated to be efficacious, and lends support to the theory that this condition is linked to excessive production of melatonin. Bright-light putatively improves the depression by suppressing melatonin secretion

### ANXIETY DISORDERS

Anxiety, defined as a subjective sense of unease, dread or anticipation, can indicate a primary psychiatric condition. Anxiety is of great relevance in sleep medicine because it can easily interfere with the relaxed state necessary for sleep initiation. Anxiety disorders, the most prevalent psychiatric illnesses in the general community, are present in 15–20% of patients seeking health care. Insomnia, described in 38% of patients, is frequently a feature of anxiety disorders[10]. This section reviews the effect of the most common anxiety disorders upon sleep.

It is important to recognize that anxiety can develop in the absence of a primary psychiatric disorder. For example, patients with respiratory diseases such as chronic obstructive pulmonary disease can experience fear if they are unable to breathe readily. In this situation, optimizing pulmonary function is the most immediate way to reduce the patient's anxiety. In another situation highly relevant to sleep medicine, some patients respond to the use of a nasal continuous positive airway pressure (CPAP) mask with anxiety because of unfamiliarity or a sensation of being smothered. Patient education with gradual and ongoing exposure is often sufficient to decrease this discomfort. If the problem persists, behavioral techniques and medications employed for the primary anxiety disorders may be required.

### Generalized anxiety disorder

Generalized anxiety disorder, present in approximately 4% of the US population[11], is the presence of daily worrying or anxiety over 6 months or longer (Table 14.4). The patient's worries are relentless, and do not markedly fluctuate in intensity as seen in panic disorder. Experiencing stressful life events only complicates matters, since susceptible individuals have more issues to pre-

**Table 14.4** Features of generalized anxiety disorder

| |
| --- |
| Worry or anxiety at least every other day |
| A variety of issues that cause worry |
| Patient cannot control the anxiety |
| At least three of |
|     restlessness |
|     fatigue |
|     difficulty concentrating |
|     irritability |
|     muscle tension |
|     sleep disturbance |

occupy them, thus perpetuating the anxiety. Patients often have increased tension in their muscles, which they are unable consciously to relax.

### Case 14.2

A 66-year-old physician presented with an inability to fall sleep and a desire to find better treatment. His insomnia had been present for over 20 years. At the urging of the patient, his primary physician prescribed lorazepam on a nightly basis. The dose had gradually increased over time from 0.5 to 4 mg a night, but the patient denied any other indicators of substance abuse. He claimed to have no adverse consequences related to benzodiazepine use, and only used the medication at bedtime. The patient realized that the dose of lorazepam was now relatively high, and that it should not be used indefinitely, especially as its use had not resulted in satisfactory sleep. The patient described lying in bed for hours unable to sleep. During these times his muscles felt as if tied in a knot. As a result of inadequate sleep, he had intermittent distressing daytime fatigue, but denied that this compromised his ability to function at work. He also described fairly unrelenting anxiety during the day and night, with his work being a notable and important escape. He had ongoing anxiety that occurred while at home and on vacation. The patient indicated that he had been trying to plan his retirement, and knew that this decision had been a source of stress for years. He enjoyed tremendously his medical career that consumed most of his time, and had no leisure skills or interests to fill his retirement years.

Treatment included a 2-month taper of the lorazepam that proceeded as planned. He had a slight increase in his level of anxiety. The patient underwent trials of mirtazepine, trazodone and nortriptyline therapy that he did not tolerate well. He responded well to paroxetine, which was gradually increased from 5 to 60 mg a day. He agreed to obtain relaxation training from a local psychologist that included several techniques, including progressive muscle relaxation, guided visual imagery and hypnosis. The patient attended all the recommended psychological sessions but did not find this approach to be particularly effective for his anxiety or sleep. The patient's persisting anxiety abated as he examined his retirement issues in psychotherapy. He decided to take a part-time position for several years, consciously taking advantage of his flexible schedule to develop new interests. The patient was eventually permitted to use intermittent doses of lorazepam for sleep, not to exceed 1 mg nightly. The dose did not escalate over time and the usage was, as instructed, on an infrequent basis. The patient felt very reassured that he had access to a small supply of the drug, even though he rarely used it.

This case illustrates how insomnia can be a prominent symptom of a more pervasive psychiatric disorder, in this example generalized anxiety disorder. In addition to insomnia often presenting because of anxiety, generalized anxiety disorder frequently presents with insomnia. In a large epidemiological study, generalized anxiety disorder was identified as the psychiatric condition most often associated with insomnia[12]. In this case, the patient was initially using excessive doses of benzodiazepines but did not appear to have a coexisting benzodiazepine dependence because of his ability to taper off the medication without difficulty. Often in these clinical situations it can be difficult to determine whether benzodiazepine dependence has developed as a separate disorder.

Many patients find psychotherapy, antidepressant medications or a combination of the two modalities effective for generalized anxiety disorder. These treatment modalities are the standard of care for patients with and without prominent sleep complaints. Cognitive therapy aiming at the reduction of distorted perceptions (such as anticipating possible but improbable outcomes), usually in conjunction with relaxation training (discussed in Chapter 12), is a mainstay of treatment (Table 14.5). Numerous studies have shown that essentially all antidepressants

**Table 14.5** Basic elements of cognitive therapy

Strive towards a realistic view of the present and the future

Collaborate with a therapist to gain insight

Identify perceived threats, catastrophic thoughts, reinforcing worries

Look for distorted or exaggerated thoughts

Learn to avoid thinking about the worst-case scenario in each situation

Keep records of worries including the topic, place and time

Employ logic and evidence

Create more realistic perceptions

Examine the actual outcome of events

(tricyclic antidepressants, SSRI, monoamine oxidase inhibitors as well as most atypical agents) are useful treatments. Benzodiazepines are a less preferred therapeutic option because of the risk of daytime sedation, cognitive impairment, falls and dependency issues. Some patients are fairly treatment resistant until the underlying issues are identified and explored. An in-depth assessment and careful consideration of treatment modalities are needed to reach a satisfactory resolution of the symptoms.

## Panic disorder

Panic disorder, another common psychiatric disease with a prevalence rate of 1–3%, is more common in women than in men[13]. This disorder is characterized by episodes of intense anxiety, which have two important components, fearful thoughts and the resulting physical symptoms, including tachycardia, tachypnea and diaphoresis (Table 14.6).

Many patients seek to identify what triggers these extremely unpleasant experiences and then avoid those situations. When this avoidance causes them to steer clear of crowded places, as is often the case, the patient is said to experience agoraphobia. Panic episodes arising from sleep are common, and may result in a sense of anxiety about falling or remaining asleep.

### Case 14.3

A 66-year-old woman presented for a general medical evaluation because of nocturnal episodes. For several years she had been able to fall asleep without difficulty, but had woken up several times a night. She would suddenly awaken from sleep

**Table 14.6** Features of panic disorder

Recurrent, unexpected panic attacks characterized by at least four of
    palpitations
    sweating
    trembling
    dyspnea
    feelings of choking
    chest pain
    nausea
    dizziness
    fear of losing control
    fear of dying

One of the following circumstances lasting at least 1 month
    persistent concern about future attacks
    worry about the consequence of a panic attack
    a change in behavior (avoiding certain activities)

feeling anxious, short of breath and tremulous. For some but not all of these episodes she would recall having a vivid, disturbing dream. It would take her an hour to relax and fall asleep again. She estimated that she obtained a total of 3 h sleep a night, and as a result experienced excessive daytime sleepiness. She had visited the emergency room several times during the night because of these episodes, but extensive medical evaluations had not found any cardiac cause, despite a diagnosis of long-standing hypertension. A psychiatric evaluation revealed that she experienced similar episodes during the day. Without warning, she would feel alarmed, and have associated physical symptoms. She had several complicated psychosocial problems that had preoccupied her over the preceding year. Most significant was the recent death of her daughter-in-law from cancer, leaving the patient responsible for the partial care of four school-age grandchildren. The psychiatrist diagnosed panic disorder without agoraphobia, with episodes both during the day and at night. He did not detect a co-existing depressive disorder. Treatment was recommended with an SSRI, citalopram, as well as cognitive behavioral therapy. The patient was also referred to a sleep-disorder center. Her sleep history was notable for obesity, snoring and rare observed respiratory pauses while asleep. A sleep study was arranged after she had been on citalopram 10 mg for 1 month, with the episodes decreasing in frequency. Polysomnography revealed moderate snoring, primarily in the supine position, with an apnea–hypopnea index of 12/h. A discrete episode did not occur. She was advised to use nasal CPAP for mild positional obstructive sleep apnea syndrome and to continue to take citalopram, gradually increasing the dose.

Based on her psychiatric history, this patient had panic disorder without agoraphobia. The majority of patients with panic disorder have both daytime and nocturnal events[14]. All patients with panic disorder need a comprehensive evaluation to screen for medical problems including cardiac, respiratory and neurological disease. Indeed in this case the patient had coexisting obstructive sleep apnea, but the relative contribution of upper airway obstruction versus anxiety as the initial trigger of her nocturnal episodes was difficult to determine. The prevalence of obstructive sleep apnea in panic disorder is unclear, but increased irregularity of tidal volume during REM and 'subclinical apneas' have been described in one controlled study of 14 patients[15]. Clinicians should take a careful history, looking for other causes of nocturnal episodes in panic disorder, although polysomnography is typically not indicated in the absence of specific symptoms such as snoring.

Panic attacks that arise exclusively from sleep appear to be rare, with relatively few cases in the literature[14,16]. Most panic attacks are not preceded by dreams, and occur in non-rapid eye movement (NREM) sleep at the transition from stage 2 to 3. In contrast to patients with sleep terrors who are not fully aware of their surroundings and return easily to sleep, nocturnal panic-attack patients are awake and hyperalert, often for a considerable time. Insomnia is the most common sleep complaint reported by patients with panic disorder. Treatment options include antidepressants, such as the SSRIs. For patients with predominantly nocturnal panic attacks, sedating antidepressants such as mirtazepine and nortriptyline may be particularly useful, despite not having specific Food and Drug Administration (FDA) approval for this purpose. Benzodiazepines may be useful in the acute management of severe panic disorder, but are generally not preferred in the long term because of the same issues as mentioned above for generalized anxiety disorder. Behavioral therapy utilizing exposure to anxiety-provoking situations as well as training in relaxation techniques has been repeatedly demonstrated to be effective for the motivated patient.

## Post-traumatic stress disorder

Post-traumatic stress disorder (PTSD) is characterized by chronic hyperarousal and anxiety (Table 14.7). Patients recall and re-experience severely distressing life events such as terrorist attacks, natural disasters and accidents. The most commonly reported sleep disturbances are insomnia and nightmares. Studies of PTSD using polysomnography show conflicting results, ranging from no objective abnormalities to increased wakefulness after sleep onset, frequent arousals and occasional awakenings from NREM sleep. The nightmares occur primarily during REM sleep. Many studies have reported a high prevalence of other primary sleep disorders, especially sleep-disordered breathing[17]. Whether PTSD places a pa-

**Table 14.7** Features of post-traumatic stress disorder

Exposure to a traumatic event which presented the risk of death or serious injury plus the patient responding with intense fear

One or more of

    recurring intrusive memories of the event

    recurrent distressing dreams

    re-experiencing the event through illusions or dissociative experiences

    intense psychological distress when any factors trigger recall of the initial trauma

    physiological response when recalling the event

Avoidance of any stimuli that serve as a reminder including

    avoiding thoughts

    avoiding activities

    inability to recall details of the trauma

    decreased ability to experience pleasure

    feeling of detachment

    restricted range of expressed emotions

    expecting a foreshortened future

Symptoms of increased arousal including

    sleep difficulties

    irritability

    poor concentration

    hypervigilance

    heightened startle response

tient at increased risk for parasomnias is controversial.

Treatment for PTSD includes careful use of exposure therapy to help patients reduce their arousal when confronted with circumstances that remind them of the original traumatic event. Individual and group supportive psychotherapy is often valuable. Medications include the SSRIs, of which the US FDA have specifically approved paroxetine and sertraline for the treatment of PTSD. A recent study indicated that nightmares and insomnia substantially improved in chronic PTSD after a 20-week trial of the centrally acting $\alpha_1$-adrenergic antagonist prazosin, which was added to previous psychotropic medication or psychotherapy[18].

## PSYCHOTIC DISORDERS

### Schizophrenia

Schizophrenia is a chronic disorder of thought and perception that affects 1% of the population. Schizophrenia is commonly associated with insomnia that may begin in the prodromal phase of the disorder, prior to the first episode of psychotic symptoms. Polysomnography has shown an increase in sleep fragmentation, shortened REM latency and decrease in slow-wave sleep. In contrast with major depression, treatment with antipsychotic medication lengthens REM latency, and thus its significance in the pathophysiology of the disorder is uncertain. Treatment also improves sleep continuity, but is associated with persisting reduction in slow-wave sleep[19].

Treatment of schizophrenia consists primarily of antipsychotic medications. These reduce the positive symptoms of schizophrenia (auditory hallucinations, delusions and unusual thought patterns) as well as negative symptoms (lack of motivation, inability to speak and affective flattening). The primary

mechanism of action of these medications is dopamine antagonism, with some of the newer ones also having significant serotonin receptor antagonism that reduces the frequency of extrapyramidal side-effects. Sedation is a feature of several of these newer medications, particularly quetiapine, olanzapine and clozapine. This can be beneficial for insomnia, but at times the dose must be titrated downwards because of excessive daytime sleepiness. Since many of the atypical antipsychotic medications approved in the mid- to late 1990s are associated with weight gain, the possibility of obstructive sleep apnea syndrome must be considered in schizophrenic patients using these drugs (Table 14.8).

### Case 14.4

A 35-year-old woman presented with excessive daytime sleepiness. After the onset of hallucinations and paranoia at age 21 years, she was diagnosed with chronic paranoid schizophrenia. Her insight into her mental illness and motivation to pursue treatment were poor. She was switched to a newer antipsychotic medication, clozapine 400 mg a day, with the objective of improving her response and decreasing her risk of worsening extrapyramidal side-effects. She gained 60 lb weight in the first 6 months of treatment. The staff members at her half-way house noted her to fall asleep periodically during the day, and polysomnography was ordered for probable obstructive sleep apnea syndrome. The patient received the standard patient education before her sleep study that included a video about obstructive sleep apnea, and mask sizing with an opportunity to wear the mask.

**Table 14.8**  Effects of antipsychotic agents on sleep and weight

| Agent | Effect on weight | Class |
|---|---|---|
| *Significantly sedating* | | |
| Quetiapine | promotes | atypical |
| Olanzapine | markedly promotes | atypical |
| Risperidone | promotes | atypical |
| Clozapine | markedly promotes | atypical |
| Haloperidol | promotes | typical |
| Chlorpromazine | promotes | typical |
| *Neutral* | | |
| Apiprazole | neutral | atypical |
| Ziprasidone | neutral | atypical |
| Molindone | neutral | typical |

The sleep study revealed an apnea–hypopnea index of 25/h, with a respiratory arousal index of 45/h. Using a split-night protocol, nasal CPAP was introduced after 2 h. The patient became very alarmed as soon as the mask was positioned over her nose, telling the technologists that she suspected that toxic gas was being delivered through the mask. She refused to continue the study and stayed awake for the remainder of the night. The next day the sleep specialist attempted to explain the rationale of nasal CPAP and discuss the significance of her study results. Although she agreed to try nasal CPAP again, she did not attend any subsequent appointments. Follow-up was available 3 years later when the patient was admitted to a psychiatric unit because of ongoing paranoia, excessive daytime sleepiness and poor functioning. She had continued on clozapine with ongoing weight gain. She had also developed adult-onset diabetes mellitus and hypertension. Overnight pulse oximetry showed oxyhemoglobin desaturations to as low as 60%. Except while in the hospital, her CPAP compliance remained very poor, despite the involvement of public-health nurses.

This case illustrates the relationship between atypical antipsychotics, weight gain and excessive daytime sleepiness most probably resulting from obstructive sleep apnea. Unfortunately, this patient's ongoing paranoia interfered with her compliance with nasal CPAP, and prevented her from getting optimal therapy. Ideally, new antipsychotic drugs will be developed in the future that are not associated with marked weight gain or sedation and, by extension, obstructive sleep apnea.

### Delusional disorder

Rare patients have an unshakeable belief that they cannot sleep. One patient seen in our center insisted that she had obtained absolutely no sleep in 3 years. The extreme nature of the belief and lack of any insight differentiate this condition from paradoxical insomnia (sleep state misperception) (Chapter 10). Family members may realize the extremely distorted nature of the perception, but have given up trying to reason with the patient. This disorder is a chronic psychotic disorder identified as delusional disorder, somatic type, in the DSM-IV, whereby the patient is absolutely convinced that a physical defect or medical problem exists despite evidence to the contrary. Unlike in schizophrenia, the patient may be fairly high-functioning in society, with delusions that are not bizarre and without hallucinations. Delusional disorders are challenging to manage effectively. Anti-psychotic medications, sedating ones in the case of patients who perceive themselves as being unable to sleep, are the mainstay of treatment.

### CHEMICAL DEPENDENCY

Alcohol and drugs are widely used because of their mood-altering effects. In most Western communities, 90% of people consume alcohol at some point in their lives and 30% develop transient alcohol-related difficulties[20]. Alcohol and drugs have many possible effects on sleep, including insomnia, excessive daytime sleepiness and parasomnias. When patients present with a sleep complaint, the clinical interview should always include questions about substance use. Many patients with chemical dependency problems presenting for detoxification and rehabilitation have prominent sleep issues. These must be addressed thoughtfully in order not to complicate the situation by prescribing hypnotics, specifically benzodiazepines, which because of cross-tolerance may interfere with the recovery process.

### Acute effects of alcohol intoxication

Alcohol is often consumed with the intent of inducing relaxation and sleep, leading to the common use of the term 'nightcap' to refer to a late-night drink. Acute alcohol use in a non-habitual user does lead to sedation. Alcohol is metabolized rapidly at a rate of 10–12 g or about one drink per hour, resulting in the sedating effects being short-lived. As a result, alcohol can lead to sleep maintenance insomnia in some people whose usage is limited to moderate amounts of alcohol used on infrequent social occasions. Alcohol intoxication has been linked to decreased REM sleep and increased stage shifting in NREM sleep, leading to sleep fragmentation.

Probably because of increased fragmentation of sleep, alcohol ingestion can induce NREM parasomnias primarily in adolescents and young adults (see Chapter 16). Within an hour or two of falling asleep, while in slow-wave sleep, the patient will sleepwalk. The patient is not awake during the activity, which must be differentiated from behaviors while intoxicated but awake or in an alcohol-related blackout. Many intoxicated patients are also sleep-deprived from partying, another well-known trigger for episodes of NREM parasomnia. Since serious injury is possible, susceptible persons should be told to avoid both alcohol intoxification and an irregular sleep–wake schedule.

Alcohol is a potent muscle relaxant, decreasing the neural input to the upper airway muscles, and is a well-known precipitant of snoring and obstructive sleep apneas[21]. In persons who do not typically snore, consuming a small amount of alcohol can relax the muscles of the upper airway leading to snoring, while patients with pre-existing snoring will be highly likely to experience obstructive breathing events. Similarly, patients with obstructive sleep apnea who consume intermittent or daily alcohol can have aggravation of their sleep-disordered breathing.

## Case 14.5

A 25-year-old man employed as a cook was referred because of disruptive snoring and observed apneic events. The patient was at high risk for cardiac disease because of family history, hypertension, obesity and hypertriglyceridemia. The patient also had a history of alcohol dependence treated 5 years ago in a 28-day rehabilitation program. The patient remained abstinent for 6 months and then resumed daily alcohol use. On the night of polysomnography, the patient told the technicians that he had visited the bar and consumed five beers in 2 h. Since this appeared to be his typical life-style, they proceeded with the sleep study. During the first hour the patient had an apnea–hypopnea index of 91/h, with oxyhemoglobin saturation falling below 50%. The staff intervened, introducing nasal CPAP, and the patient's sleep-disordered breathing was stabilized with 12 cmH$_2$O in the laboratory. The patient was advised to re-enter alcohol treatment, and warned that he had life-threatening hypoventilation and severe obstructive sleep apnea syndrome. He agreed to use nasal CPAP, but insisted that he could control his drinking on his own. Five years later the patient finally re-entered a program to address his relapse with alcohol. After becoming abstinent again several years after his sleep evaluation, he successfully lost weight and complied better with his medications and nasal CPAP therapy.

This case illustrates the risk of exacerbating obstructive sleep apnea with heavy alcohol use. The sedative properties of alcohol compound the problem by increasing the arousal threshold, thus prolonging the apneas and leading to more pronounced oxyhemoglobin desaturation. Because of the rapid rate of alcohol metabolism, the effect of alcohol on breathing is most pronounced at the beginning of the night soon after the patient's last drink.

## Alcohol-induced sleep disorder

For some patients, occasional alcohol use evolves into alcohol abuse and dependence. Because at lower levels of intoxication alcohol leads to some degree of euphoria, people develop a drive to continue drinking even in the face of adverse consequences. Daily alcohol use can lead to complex changes in the brain, mind and body. Alcohol abuse is defined in DSM-IV as alcohol use leading to repeated undesirable consequences. Alcohol dependence by DSM-IV criteria is impairment in at least three areas of functioning, including occupational, academic, social and recreational activities, for at least 12 months. The factors that make an individual vulnerable to alcohol dependence are unclear, but familial factors may play a significant contributing role. Previous editions of the DSM psychiatric classification required evidence of tolerance or withdrawal for alcohol dependence, but this was set aside in favor of a more inclusive concept of the disorder. Physical dependence on alcohol can occur with the presence of withdrawal symptoms when alcohol is abruptly discontinued.

Patients with alcohol abuse or dependence can have a wide variety of sleep complaints including insomnia, hypersomnia and parasomnias. Sometimes the patients start using alcohol frequently because of a belief that an evening drink will enhance sleep. Acute alcohol intoxication causes sedation that starts 30 min after consumption, with the duration depending on the amount consumed. One study indicated that 61% of patients with alcohol dependence had insomnia before entering chemical dependency treatment[22]. Polysomnography in patients using alcohol on a habitual basis revealed shorter initial sleep latency, decreased wakefulness after sleep onset for the first half of the night and decreased slow-wave sleep[23]. In the second half of the night patients experience more indeterminate arousals, stage changes and REM rebound, which may lead to nightmares.

Treatment typically includes the patient being advised to reduce alcohol consumption. If they are unable to do so without assistance, a referral to an out-patient or in-patient alcohol treatment program may be required. In these settings patients are generally advised to discontinue alcohol use abruptly, and a benzodiazepine on a tapering schedule is used to prevent withdrawal symptoms. If a patient has entered alcohol withdrawal, delirium tremens, severe restlessness, visual hallucinations, seizures and total absence of sleep can develop[24]. Polysomnography shows a marked reduction in slow-wave sleep, sleep fragmentation and increased REM sleep with loss of muscle atonia. Slow-wave sleep may take months to years to recover. Aggressive treatment with benzodiazepines and possibly anticonvulsants is mandated by this condition, which is associated with significant mortality.

In the absence of withdrawal, an acute adjustment phase occurs for the first 1–2 weeks when patients typically experience insomnia. Patients have predominantly light NREM sleep without slow-wave or REM sleep. If at all possible, other than benzodiazepines used for detoxification, behavioral measures should be employed to address the insomnia. Patient education should emphasize that sleep initiation and maintenance problems are a core component of the transition away from excessive drinking. Patients with persisting insomnia 5 months after stopping alcohol are at higher risk for relapse, probably because of a tendency to self-medicate the insomnia with alcohol[22]. Using a medication, especially a benzodiazepine but possibly a non-benzodiazepine such as zolpidem, zaleplon or zopiclone, reinforces the patient's perspective that exogenous substances are necessary for satisfactory sleep. If a patient is in a rehabilitation setting, sedating antidepressants such as trazodone are often preferred. Some patients experience distressing insomnia and daytime fatigue for up to 12 months after achieving sobriety[22]. Polysomnography demonstrates reduced total sleep time and slow-wave sleep. The physician should consider whether a coexisting mood or anxiety disorder is contributing to the sleep disturbance. By convention, these cannot be diagnosed for at least 4 weeks after alcohol cessation, although clinicians treating a visibly symptomatic patient sometimes cannot adhere rigidly to this guideline. Sedating antidepressants and mood stabilizers are strongly preferred over benzodiazepines that, owing to cross-tolerance, may trigger a craving for alcohol. The potential exists for the non-benzodiazepine receptor agonists to trigger a relapse with alcohol. Case reports indicate a risk of tolerance, dose escalation and relapse with alcohol related to zolpidem in particular, in this population of patients with demonstrated vulnerability for addiction[25].

## Sedative-, hypnotic- or anxiolytic-induced sleep disorder

The DSM-IV groups these agents together in the classification of chemical dependency-related sleep disorders. Because of related pharmacological actions and cross-tolerance, this cluster of sleep disorders is fairly similar to alcohol-induced sleep disorder. Benzodiazepines are commonly prescribed medications for insomnia and anxiety disorders. Although initially leading to desired sedation, over time they reduce the quality of sleep. Especially longer-acting agents (such

as clonazepam or flurazepam) can cause morning sedation due to a hangover effect. This can be misinterpreted by some patients as a sign of inadequate sleep, and may lead to an increase in benzodiazepine dosage. Clinicians should intervene by designing a gradual taper of the benzodiazepine and re-evaluating sleep once this is complete. Withdrawal or abstinence from these agents, especially after years of use, can contribute to insomnia similar to that seen after cessation of chronic alcohol use. When benzodiazepines are discontinued after long-term daily use, polysomnographic studies show a reduction in slow-wave sleep and increase in wakefulness after sleep onset[26].

## Opioid-induced sleep disorder

Sleep disruption related to opioid use can arise in the setting of prescribed and illicit use of these substances. Polysomnography shows reductions in total, slow-wave and REM sleep time, but tolerance to these effects can develop quickly. When patients initially use opioids they can experience a euphoria which can be followed at times by psychomotor agitation that precludes sleep. Insomnia is commonly experienced upon withdrawal after prolonged use. Users with a binge pattern of usage may have their sleep disrupted in a repeated fashion, alternating between poor-quality sleep due to opioid intoxication and insomnia related to withdrawal.

Treatment depends on the context of opioid usage. For patients being prescribed opioids for pain, use of a longer-acting formulation (such as methadone) with a consistent dosing schedule may reduce the sleep disruption. This approach will also provide better pain control and thus improve sleep quality. For opioid abusers, treatment in a chemical dependency program is typically necessary. These programs offer a controlled environment, group therapy and medically supervised detoxification.

### Stimulant-dependent sleep disorder

#### Case 14.6

A 30-year-old woman presented for a third opinion regarding her medically refractory narcolepsy. The patient developed excessive daytime sleepiness at age 23. She was referred to a sleep-disorder center because of falling asleep while operating a motor vehicle, with a resulting accident. She denied cataplexy, sleep paralysis and hypnogogic hallucinations. The polysomnogram was unremarkable, but the multiple sleep latency test (MSLT) revealed a mean initial sleep latency of 3 min and two sleep-onset REM periods (SOREMPs). After the patient was confronted with the results of a drug screen revealing the presence of amphetamine, she acknowledged free-basing methamphetamine frequently over the past year. She had been using drugs the day before the motor vehicle accident and getting very little sleep. The patient was diagnosed with stimulant-related sleep disorder and advised to pursue chemical dependency treatment. The patient did not obtain drug rehabilitation, but sought out a sleep consultation at another institution. After a repeat MSLT demonstrated two SOREMPs, she was diagnosed with narcolepsy. A drug screen was not performed and the patient did not reveal her history of ongoing drug use. Even when prescribed high-dose methylphenidate (200 mg/day), her excessive daytime sleepiness did not remit. She had repeated tardiness and absences from work that placed her secretarial job in jeopardy. Her sleep specialist became unwilling to continue the medication and requested an opinion from a third institution.

Actigraphy was conducted prior to the first appointment (Figure 14.1). The patient presented with severe excessive daytime sleepiness (Epworth sleepiness scale score of 24). She also complained of a sensation of bugs crawling over her skin, and had placed a plastic bag over her head trying to catch the insects. She indicated that she was so desperate for relief that she no longer cared whether she lived. She denied any history of illicit drug use and provided only limited outside records. A urine drug screen was positive for amphetamines. When confronted, the patient admitted that, in addition to the prescribed methylphenidate, she had used amphetamine pills purchased on the street. She agreed to a 1-week admission to a chemical dependency program, where the formication resolved 24 h after a psychostimulant taper was undertaken. She was advised to abstain from use of all stimulants for 1 month and then return for poly-somnography and an MSLT. However, she resumed using methylphenidate because overwhelming excessive daytime sleepiness left her fearful of driving, and the planned MSLT could be not performed. The patient claimed that she could not find anyone else to provide transportation. She was once again urged to have chemical

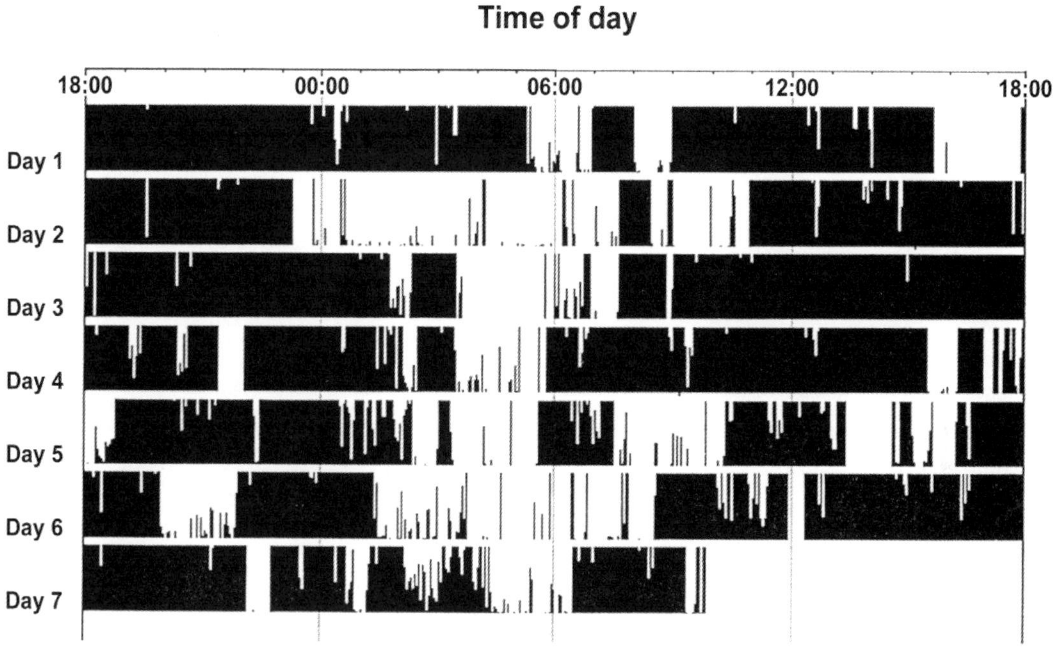

## Time of day

**Figure 14.1** Wrist actigraphy in stimulant abuse (case 14.6). This wrist actigraphy shows extremely short times in bed, with very high activity levels when awake. This combination suggests the possibility of stimulant abuse (see Figure 4.9 for more details)

dependency therapy, this time in a facility offering long-term treatment. She did not comply, and elected to go elsewhere for her medical care.

Whether this patient had narcolepsy remained unknown because a reliable MSLT could not be conducted. Her ongoing use of illicit and prescribed psychostimulants was a major concern, and greatly complicated her sleep assessment. In situations such as these, measuring cerebrospinal fluid levels of hypocretin-1 may in the future be the optimal means to establish the diagnosis of narcolepsy (see Chapter 7). Her actigraphic recording

showed severely inadequate sleep over a 7-day period, with high activity levels while awake. This degree of activity with extremely limited sleep strongly suggests an exogenous factor such as abuse of a stimulant medication. Tactile hallucinations are extremely rare in patients taking methyl-phenidate, but are more commonly des-cribed with the use of street drugs[27]. This case demonstrates both the importance of drug screening to detect covert drug use that can invalidate MSLT results, and the limitations of drug screening. While amphetamine use within 3 days of specimen collection can be

**Table 14.9** Agents implicated in stimulant-dependent sleep disorder

Amphetamine

Methamphetamine

Methylphenidate

Cocaine

Methylenedioxymethamphetamine (MDMA, ecstasy)

Phentermine

Phenylpropanolamine

Propylhexedrine

Theophylline

Ephedrine

Thyroid hormones

Caffeine

Fenfluramine

Pemoline

Diethylpropion

detected, currently available laboratory testing is less sensitive for methylphenidate. The patient did not hide using the prescribed methylphenidate, an agent that was not identified on the drug screen. Taking a careful history from the patient, and if possible obtaining collateral history from family or medical records, remains the most critical part of the sleep evaluation.

The DSM-IV stimulant-dependent sleep disorder describes a reduction of sleep owing to use of, or abstinence from, a long list of agents (Table 14.9). These drugs reduce total and REM sleep time. During binges of stimulant use, a user may not sleep for days, followed by marked hypersomnolence. Stimulant abusers may also abuse sedatives in order to moderate the intensity of their intoxicated state, or obtain sleep. Withdrawal from stimulants can cause excessive daytime sleepiness with coexisting depressed mood and increased appetite. During this phase, polysomnography shows an increase in total and REM sleep time which can result in SOREMPs on an MSLT. Treatment depends on the stimulant abused. Users of potent medications such as amphetamines and cocaine typically need detoxification and rehabilitation. Caffeine users should taper their usage over 1 week to reduce the likelihood of rebound headache.

## ATTENTION DEFICIT HYPERACTIVITY DISORDER

Children with attention deficit hyperactivity disorder (ADHD) exhibit distractibility, inattention and an inability to sit still. The DSM-IV requires the disorder to start before age 7. Affected children typically struggle in several settings, including school, home and social settings. ADHD appears to be more common in boys than girls, but the estimated prevalence rate ranges markedly from 2–18% in published studies[28]. ADHD and sleep are interwined for at least three reasons: first, hyperactive children often have a difficult time slowing down and preparing for sleep as bedtime approaches; second, the psychostimulants that are widely used to treat ADHD can cause insomnia; and third, children who are sleep-deprived, because of either an untreated primary sleep disorder or insufficient sleep, differ from adults in that they sometimes present with hyperactivity instead of excessive daytime sleepiness. Surprisingly, the DSM-IV does not specifically identify or discuss any sleep complaints as part of its diagnostic criteria for the condition.

In addition, recent studies have reported restless legs syndrome and obstructive sleep apnea in children with ADHD, implying that clinicians evaluating a child with presumed ADHD should carefully search for sleep disorders[29]. Whether restless legs syndrome and obstructive sleep apnea cause hyperactivity, thus mimicking ADHD, or truly coexist at high rates with ADHD remains unclear at this time. Patients may benefit from treatment specifically directed to these sleep disorders, when identified. Improving sleep because of targeted treatment may reduce sleep deprivation and improve daytime behavior.

Psychostimulants are widely used to treat ADHD, but clinicians should thoughtfully consider the half-life of the selected agent to avoid causing stimulant-related insomnia. Nevertheless, some children benefit from psychostimulants that remain effective into the evening, to facilitate completion of homework as well as slowing down in preparation for bed. As more pharmacological alternatives to psychostimulants are developed, for example the antidepressant atomoxetine, these agents may be useful for reducing hyperactivity close to bedtime without increasing the risk of insomnia. Behavioral measures that help the child to concentrate and relax are also particularly important close to bedtime.

## REFERENCES

1. First M, ed. *Diagnostic and Statistical Manual of Mental Disorders.* Washington, DC: American Psychiatric Association, 1994:886

2. Buysse D, Reynolds C, Kupfer D, *et al.* Clinical diagnoses in 216 insomnia patients using the International Classification of Sleep Disorders (ICSD), DSM-IV and ICD-10 categories: a report from the APA/NIMH DSM-IV Field Trial. *Sleep* 1994;17:630–7

3. Mellinger G, Balter M, Uhlenhuth E. Insomnia and its treatment. *Arch Gen Psychiatry* 1985;42:225–32

4. Ford D, Cooper-Patrick L. Sleep disturbances and mood disorders: an epidemiologic perspective. *Depression Anxiety* 2001; 14:3–6

5. Rodin J, McAvay G, Timko C. A longitudinal study of depressed mood and sleep disturbances in elderly adults. *J Gerontol Psychol Sci* 1988;43:45–53

6. Giles E, Kupfer D, Rush A. Controlled comparison of electrophysiological sleep in families of probands with unipolar depression. *Am J Psychiatry* 1998;155:192–9

7. Buysse D, Tu X, Cherry C, *et al.* Pretreatment REM sleep and subjective sleep quality distinguish depressed psychotherapy remitters and nonremitters. *Biol Psychiatry* 1999;45:205–13

8. Dolenc L, Besset A, Billiard M. Hypersomnia in association with dysthymia in comparison with idiopathic hypersomnia and normal controls. *Pfluger's Arch Eur J Physiol* 1996;431:R303–4

9. Lewy A. *Seasonal Mood Disorders.* Philadelphia, PA: WB Saunders, 1993

10. Ohayon M, Roth T. Place of chronic insomnia in the course of depressive and anxiety disorders. *J Psychiatr Res* 2003; 37:9–15

11. Kessler R, McGonagle K, Zhao S, *et al.* Lifetime and 12 month prevalence of DSM-III-R psychiatric disorders among persons 15–54 in the United States: results from the national comorbidity study. *Arch Psychiatry* 1994;51:8–19

12. Ohayon M. Prevalence of DSM-IV diagnostic criteria of insomnia: distinguishing insomnia related to mental disorders from sleep disorders. *J Psychiatr Res* 1997; 31:333–46

13. Weissman M, Bland R, Canino G, *et al.* The cross-national epidemiology of panic disorder. *Arch Gen Psychiatry* 1997;54:305–9

14. Schredl M, Kronenberg G, Nonnell P, Heuser I. Dream recall, nightmare frequency, and nocturnal panic attacks in patients with panic disorder. *J Nerv Ment Disord* 2001;189:559–62

15. Stein M, Millar T, Larsen D, Kryger M. Irregular breathing during sleep in patients with panic disorder. *Am J Psychiatry* 1995; 152:1168–73

16. Hauri P, Friedman M, Ravaris C. Sleep in patients with spontaneous panic attacks. *Sleep* 1989;12:323–37

17. Engdahl B, Eberly R, Hurwitz T, Mahowald M, Blake J. Sleep in a community sample of elderly war veterans with and without post-traumatic stress disorder. *Biol Psychiatry* 2000;47:520–5

18. Raskind M, Peskind E, Kanter E, *et al.* Reduction of nightmares and other PTSD symptoms in combat veterans by prazosin: a placebo-controlled study. *Am J Psychiatry* 2003;160:371–3

19. Maixner S, Tandon R, Eiser A, Taylor S, De Quardo J, Shipley J. Effects of antipsychotic treatment on polysomnographic measures in schizophrenia: a replication and extension. *Am J Psychiatry* 1998;155:1600–2

20. Nace EP. Alcoholism: epidemiology, diagnosis, and biological aspects. *Alcohol* 1986;3:83–7

21. Bonora M, St John W, Bledsoe T. Differential elevation by protriptyline and depression by diazepam of upper airway respiratory activity. *Am Rev Respir Dis* 1985;131:41–5

22. Brower K, Aldrich M, Robinson E, Zucker R, Greden JF. Insomnia, self-medication, and relapse to alcoholism. *Am J Psychiatry* 2001;158:399–404

23. Brower K, Hall J. Effects of age and alcoholism on sleep: a controlled study. *J Stud Alcohol* 2001;62:335–43

24. Montagna P, Lugaresi E. Agrypnia excitata: a generalized overactivity syndrome and a useful concept in the neurophysiology of sleep. *Clin Neurophysiol* 2002;113:552–60

25. Liappas I, Malitas P, Dimopoulos N, *et al.* Zolpidem dependence case series: possible neurobiological mechanisms and clinical management. *J Psychopharmacol* 2003; 17:131–5

26. Poyares D, Guilleminault C, Ohayon MM, Tufik S. Can valerian improve the sleep of insomniacs after benzodiazepine withdrawal? *Prog Neuropsychopharmacol Biol Psychiatry* 2002; 26:539–45

27. Brady K, Lydiard R, Malcolm R, Ballenger J. Cocaine-induced psychosis. *J Clin Psychiatry* 1991;52:509–12

28. Rowland A, Lesesne C, Abramowitz A. The epidemiology of attention-deficit/hyperactivity disorder (ADHD): a public health view. *Ment Retard Dev Dis Res Rev* 2002; 8:162–70

29. Chervin R, Dillon J, Bassetti C, Ganoczy D, Pituch K. Symptoms of sleep disorders, inattention, and hyperactivity in children. *Sleep* 1997;20:1185–93

# Section IV
# The patient with excessive movement in sleep

# Chapter 15

# Restless legs syndrome and periodic limb movements of sleep

*Remember: if you can cease all restless activity,*
*your integral nature will appear.*

**Lao Tzu, *The Hua Hu Ching***

In 1945, Dr Karl-Axel Ekbom of Sweden published a monograph on a 'hitherto overlooked disease in the legs' which he called 'restless legs'[1]. For many years considered a rare curiosity, restless legs syndrome (RLS) is today recognized as one of the commonest neurological disorders with a prevalence rate of at least one in 25. With the introduction of polygraphic monitoring of sleep, it became evident that many patients studied in sleep laboratories jerked their legs rhythmically throughout parts of the night. These movements, originally called nocturnal myoclonus, are now known as periodic limb movements of sleep (PLMS). While PLMS can occur in association with RLS, they more often occur independently. The two conditions are frequently confused, and undue significance is often ascribed to the presence of PLMS on a polysomnogram.

## RESTLESS LEGS SYNDROME

### Clinical characteristics

The clinical picture of the disorder is characteristic, and in its full form is easily recognizable. Ekbom described the classic features in 1945: 'The paresthesias are generally described as a creeping, irritating, innervating sensation . . . as though ants were crawling in their skin . . . . The paresthesias . . . set in when the legs have been kept still for a while . . . and the patients are forced to keep moving the legs, which generally gives them some relief'[1]. The International Restless Legs Syndrome Study Group (IRLSSG) has delineated the four cardinal characteristics needed for diagnosis of RLS[2] (Table 15.1).

The essential feature is an irresistible need to move the limbs. This is most commonly experienced in the lower extremities, especially in the calves, but sometimes in the thighs or feet. It may also be present to a

**Table 15.1** International Restless Legs Syndrome Study Group criteria for restless legs syndrome

| |
|---|
| Need to move the legs, accompanied or caused by unpleasant leg sensations |
| Symptoms present during rest or inactivity |
| Relieved by movements such as stretching or walking |
| Symptoms worse in the evening or at night |

lesser extent in the upper extremities, with one study reporting a frequency of almost 50%[3]. The majority experience discomfort in the affected limbs, but occasional patients describe the urge to move without any sensory symptoms. The discomfort is often difficult to characterize, and is usually not perceived as pain. Frequently used descriptors include creeping, crawling, jittery, tingling, burning, aching, deep-seated, 'like bugs under my skin'. Patients often say that it is indescribable, or use bizarre phrases, such as 'soda bubbling through my veins'.

The need to move and the unpleasant sensations are either exclusively present or worsen in severity while lying down or sitting. They may be particularly troublesome in a theater, on a long car journey or during an airplane flight. The symptoms are relieved, at least temporarily, by moving the affected limbs, and patients learn the benefits of stretching or jiggling the legs, walking or riding a stationary bicycle. Forcing the legs to remain still may be impossible and results in an exacerbation of the discomfort and sometimes an involuntary jerk. Massaging the legs or taking hot baths may also relieve the symptoms.

The time of the occurrence of symptoms is also characteristic of the disorder. They are most troublesome in bed before sleep, or on waking during the night. Most patients with RLS will describe resultant sleep onset or sleep maintenance insomnia, clearly due to the limb discomfort. In some patients the symptoms are worst before sleep, while in others they may be most severe a few hours after sleep onset. Symptoms while sitting are most prominent in the evening and least prominent in the morning. A circadian rhythmicity of RLS is responsible for this phenomenon, rather than merely a greater tendency towards patients being at rest later in the day[4].

## Diagnostic pitfalls

Because the diagnosis depends on the patient's history, care should be taken to elicit as accurate a description of the symptoms as possible. Diagnostic difficulties may arise if only some of the four IRLSSG criteria are fulfilled or if atypical features are present.

### Symptoms are described as painful

This is quite compatible with RLS, although most often the discomfort is reported to be painless. A careful history should be taken to rule out neurogenic or vascular claudication, nocturnal leg cramps, pain due to lumbosacral radiculopathy, arthritis or fibromyalgia and the positive symptomatology of peripheral neuropathy (not to be confused

**Table 15.2** Differential diagnosis of restless legs syndrome

| |
|---|
| Nocturnal leg cramps |
| Neurogenic claudication |
| Vascular claudication |
| Acute or chronic lumbosacral radiculopathy |
| Arthritis |
| Fibromyalgia |
| Positive symptomatology of peripheral neuropathy |
| Painful feet and moving toes syndrome |
| Akathisia |

with RLS as a complication of peripheral neuropathy) (Table 15.2). None of these conditions fulfill all four of the IRLSSG criteria for RLS. Patients usually describe a nocturnal leg cramp as a tight hardening of a muscle, usually of sudden onset, relieved by massage of the affected part or by standing firmly on the foot. The burning and tingling experienced in the feet and lower legs of patients with peripheral neuropathy may be severe at rest at night but are usually also present on walking, and are not associated with a desire to move. Painful feet and moving toes syndrome is a rare disorder, often following prior leg trauma, with pain in the feet and athetotic movements of the toes.

### Symptoms are maximal in arms or trunk

Occasional RLS patients describe symptoms maximally or exclusively in the arms and even the low back or abdomen. Again, a careful history can separate RLS from other more common causes of discomfort in these areas. Some patients have both restless legs and an unrelated cause of discomfort elsewhere, such as mechanical back pain or carpal tunnel syndrome.

### Symptoms are asymmetric or unilateral

Many RLS patients describe symptoms that at times are more severe in one leg than in the other. Most often the limbs alternate in terms of severity, but in some patients one limb is consistently more affected than the other. In rare cases, the symptoms are exclusively unilateral. In such cases, other diagnoses should be carefully considered, but if all criteria are fulfilled, the patient should be assumed to have RLS. Clinical experience suggests that unilateral RLS may be associated with underlying local pathology in the affected leg, such as trochanteric bursitis or prior surgery.

### Symptoms do not appear to be relieved by movement

A pitfall for the inexperienced clinician is the patient who denies that walking helps the symptoms. However, often the patient means that after stopping walking, the symptoms recur at the same intensity as before, and careful questioning can reveal that the discomfort is temporarily improved while moving. In some patients with long-standing RLS, movement no longer appears to help even temporarily, but a history of this helping in the past can usually be obtained. Akathisia can mimic RLS, and may be associated with voluntary movements, such as pacing the floor or rocking the body. It most often occurs with the use of dopamine antagonist drugs, but may also be found in Parkinson's disease. Differences between the two conditions[5] are summarized in Table 15.3.

### Case 15.1

A 55-year-old road-repair laborer presented with 2 years' leg pain. The pain was present throughout the thighs and calves of both legs but could not be more precisely localized. It came on while resting after heavy physical work on his job. It was worst in the late afternoons and evenings and often interfered with sleep at night. It was not associated with a compelling desire to move the legs and walking did not help. Investigations for vascular disease and lumbosacral radiculopathies were negative. He did not

**Table 15.3**  Akathisia versus restless legs syndrome (RLS)

|  | Akathisia | RLS |
|---|---|---|
| Desire to move associated with | inner restlessness | limb dysesthesias |
| Night-time exacerbation | minority | majority |
| Worst lying down | minority | majority |
| Sleep disturbance | mild | severe |

respond to levodopa therapy. The patient experienced moderate relief with the use of gabapentin.

The patient fulfilled some, but not all, of the criteria for RLS, including leg discomfort, onset at rest and symptoms worse later in the day. However, there was no compelling restlessness, and moving the legs did not help even temporarily. After other causes were excluded, a trial of a dopaminergic agent was tried unsuccessfully. A diagnosis of a chronic pain syndrome of uncertain cause was made. Gabapentin sometimes provides reasonable relief in such complex patients.

### Epidemiology

Several epidemiological studies in Europe and North America suggest that the prevalence of RLS is as high as 10%, with increasing prevalence with age[6–8]. Most but not all studies suggest a higher prevalence in women, and the disorder appears to be less common in Asian and African-American populations. RLS is often misdiagnosed, with patients reporting a mean of 2 years' delay after seeking medical help before the correct diagnosis is reached. The severity of symptoms tends to worsen with age, with about two-thirds of patients reporting pro-

gression of symptoms with time. RLS may fluctuate in severity, with at least 15% of patients describing remissions lasting a month or more[9].

RLS can start at any age, but about 25% of patients recall symptoms before the age of 20 years[9], sometimes ascribed in childhood to 'growing pains'. Studies have found a relationship between RLS/PLMS and attention deficit hyperactivity disorder in children[10,11] (see Chapter 14). It is unclear whether one of the conditions is primary or whether both are due to the same underlying biochemical or genetic defect.

### Etiology and pathogenesis

RLS can be familial, idiopathic or symptomatic of an underlying disorder[12]. About 50% of patients with RLS have a family history of the condition[13], and clinical experience suggests that the pattern of inheritance is autosomal dominant. However, a family with the first described linkage to a specific chromosome (12q), appeared to have a pseudodominant, autosomal recessive inheritance pattern[14]. Patients with RLS commencing before the age of 45 years are more likely to have first-degree relatives with the disorder than those of later onset[15].

Numerous conditions have been associated with RLS but only a few have been well

**Table 15.4** Etiology of restless legs syndrome

Familial

Idiopathic

Symptomatic
    iron deficiency
    chronic renal failure
    peripheral neuropathy
    pregnancy
    possibly Parkinson's disease

**Table 15.5** Evidence for the relationship of low iron stores and restless legs syndrome (RLS)

Clinical series of patients with iron deficiency and RLS[22]

Correlation of low serum ferritin and severity of RLS[17,18]

Low CSF ferritin in RLS patients[19]

MRI studies showing reduced stores of iron in substantia nigra[20]

Autopsy studies showing low iron in substantia nigra[21]

Improvement in RLS with treatment of iron deficiency[16]

CSF, cerebrospinal fluid; MRI, magnetic resonance imaging

established (Table 15.4). These are iron deficiency (Table 15.5), chronic renal failure, peripheral neuropathy and pregnancy. Ekbom recognized a relationship to iron deficiency, and a trial of intravenous iron therapy was reported as early as 1953[16]. The severity of RLS correlates inversely with serum ferritin concentration less than 45–50 $\mu$/l[17,18], and a study has shown low cerebrospinal fluid (CSF) ferritin concentration in RLS patients with normal serum ferritin concentrations compared with controls[19]. A magnetic resonance imaging (MRI) study has shown reduced brain iron in the substantia nigra in RLS patients, compared with controls, with the reduction proportional to RLS severity[20]. Autopsy studies have also shown reduced iron in substantia nigra[21]. Iron is a necessary cofactor for tyrosine hydroxylase, the rate-limiting step in the synthesis of dopamine, and may be involved in the functioning of the dopamine receptor. Menorrhagia and loss of blood from the alimentary tract are common causes of iron deficiency. A less recognized cause is frequent blood donation, which can precipitate or exacerbate RLS[22].

At least 20% of chronic hemodialysis patients have RLS[23,24], and this essentially resolves after successful kidney transplantation[25]. Low hematocrit and serum ferritin concentration do not appear to predict the occurrence of RLS in chronic renal-failure patients[24]. Evidence for peripheral neuropathy can be detected in one-quarter to one-third of RLS patients by electromyogram (EMG), quantitative thermal testing or biopsies of the sural nerve or cutaneous small-diameter nerve fibers[26,27]. However, the majority of RLS patients do not have clinically detectable peripheral neuropathy, and most peripheral neuropathy patients do not experience restless legs. RLS is common in pregnancy, especially the third trimester, and often resolves after delivery. There is suggestive evidence that RLS may be more common than expected in patients with Parkinson's disease. Less well-established associations of RLS include lumbosacral radiculopathies, rheumatoid arthritis and the use of certain medications, including antidepressants, dopamine antagonists and calcium channel blockers.

The pathogenesis of RLS is uncertain. Various lines of evidence suggest that a disturbance of inhibitory subcortical pathways, such as the reticulospinal tract, may allow expression of a normally suppressed neural generator at spinal cord level. This process may be modulated by abnormal peripheral sensory input from, for instance, a peripheral neuropathy. Functional MRI imaging suggests involvement of the cerebellum and contralateral thalamus[28]. The consistent efficacy of dopaminergic medications in treating RLS strongly implicates the dopamine system, but the anatomical site of dopamine deficiency has not been established. Contradictory results have been obtained with 18-fluorodopa positron emission tomography (PET) scans, with two studies finding reduced dopaminergic activity in the basal ganglia in RLS, but one finding no differences from controls[29–31]. Dopamine deficiency in Parkinson's disease is secondary to a progressive neurodegenerative process in substantia nigra, while that in idiopathic RLS is most likely a non-progressive, primary biochemical deficiency of undetermined mechanism.

### Case 15.2

A 49-year-old woman presented with a 10-year history of a crawling discomfort in her calves, occurring every day on sitting down in the evening and trying to sleep at night. This was associated with an overwhelming desire to move the legs and temporary relief by walking. RLS was not known to occur in her family, and she did not have a history of any gastrointestinal symptoms or menorrhagia. She had donated blood between four and six times a year for the preceding 12 years, and on occasion had been rejected for donation because of a borderline low hemoglobin concentration. Her hemoglobin concentration was slightly low at 12.2 g/dl and her serum ferritin concentration was 8 µg/l (normal ≥ 20 µg/l). She was advised to stop donating blood and was treated with oral ferrous sulfate three times a day in association with vitamin C. After 5 months' treatment, her hemoglobin concentration had risen to 14.5 g/dl and her serum ferritin concentration to 39 µg/l. Eleven months after presentation, minimal RLS was occurring at most once every 2 months.

This case illustrates successful management of RLS related to iron deficiency due to frequent blood donation.

### Management

#### Investigations

Once a careful history establishes a diagnosis of RLS, a limited search for a secondary cause of RLS should be undertaken (Table 15.6). The presence or absence of RLS in the family should be established. Symptoms of peripheral neuropathy, such as numbness, or dysesthesias in the feet, should be elicited. The patient should be asked about a history of anemia, gastrointestinal blood loss, menorrhagia or frequent blood donation. The temporal relationship between onset of RLS and use of medications associated with RLS should be investigated. Dopamine-blocking medications, such as metoclopramide pre-

**Table 15.6** Clinical assessment of restless legs syndrome (RLS)

*History*
Family history of RLS
History of anemia
Observed gastrointestinal blood loss
Conditions predisposing to gastrointestinal blood loss
Menorrhagia
Frequent blood donation
Symptoms of peripheral neuropathy
Use of medications that have been associated with RLS (dopamine blockers, antidepressants, calcium blockers)

*Examination*
Loss of sensation in the feet
Absent ankle reflexes

*Laboratory tests*
Hematocrit
Serum ferritin concentration
Creatinine
Plasma glucose concentration (if neuropathy suspected)

**Table 15.7** Definite indications for measuring serum ferritin concentration in restless legs syndrome (RLS)

Recent onset of RLS
Unexplained worsening of RLS
RLS unresponsive to first-line medications
History of anemia, blood loss, predisposing factors to blood loss or frequent blood donation

scribed for nausea, antidepressants and calcium channel blockers, have all been anecdotally associated with increased severity of RLS. A brief neurological examination of the legs should be performed to determine whether a peripheral neuropathy is present. Electromyography is not indicated if there are no pointers on history or examination to suggest neurological disease. Hematocrit, serum ferritin and creatinine concentration should be measured, especially if the symptoms are of short duration, have recently worsened or are unresponsive to first-line medications (Table 15.7). If a peripheral neuropathy is suspected, tests for a cause should be performed, especially the concentration of plasma glucose.

*Non-pharmacological management*

If serum ferritin concentration is below the lower limit of normal (15–20 µg/l, depending on the testing laboratory), a cause should be sought and iron supplementation supplied. If serum ferritin concentration is between 20 and 50 µg/l, iron supplementation can be considered, especially in patients who appear to be resistant to drug therapy. A common regimen is the use of 325 mg ferrous sulfate administered three times a day between meals. Iron is poorly absorbed from the alimentary tract, especially when taken with food, and 200 mg vitamin C should be added to each dose to aid absorption. However, this dose of iron may produce unacceptable gastrointestinal side-effects, especially in elderly patients, and a lower or less frequent dose, sometimes with food, may be needed. After 2–3 months' treatment, the serum ferritin concentration should be checked; if it has risen to > 45–50 µg/l, iron therapy can be stopped but ferritin concentration should be rechecked 2 months later.

Indefinite use of iron can lead to iatrogenic iron overload states.

There is no evidence that supplementation with any vitamins in the absence of proven vitamin deficiency improves RLS. Many patients report worsening of RLS following unusually severe physical exertion and improvement with a regular exercise program, but these impressions have not been tested scientifically. It has been suggested that cessation of caffeine use or smoking may be beneficial, but these measures are of doubtful benefit based on clinical experience. If medications are believed to be responsible for RLS, substitution of other agents can be attempted. However, antidepressants can usually be continued and RLS managed with conventional drug therapy.

*Pharmacological management*

RLS responds to several classes of medications, allowing the clinician a fairly wide choice of options[32] (Table 15.8). Some of these drugs have been extensively tested in blinded controlled trials, while the efficacy of others is based on open-label studies and clinical experience. In the USA, no medications have been specifically approved by the Food and Drug Administration for the management of RLS, so all drugs are used 'off-label'.

*Dopaminergic agents* Levodopa is used in combination with dopa decarboxylase inhibitors to prevent peripheral catabolism, thus reducing side-effects such as nausea, and allowing the drug to penetrate the central nervous system. Carbidopa is the dopa decarboxylase inhibitor available in the USA, while carbidopa or benserazide are available elsewhere in the world.

**Table 15.8** Drug therapy for restless legs syndrome (RLS)

*Dopaminergic agents*
Levodopa
Dopamine agonists
    ergot agonists (bromocriptine, pergolide, cabergoline)
    non-ergot agonists (pramipexole, ropinirole)
Others (amantadine)

*Opioids*
Low-potency opioids (codeine, propoxyphene, tramadol)
High-potency opioids (oxycodone, hydrocodone, methadone)

*Benzodiazepines and related compounds*
Short-acting agents (zaleplon, zolpidem, triazolam)
Intermediate-acting agents (temazepam)
Long-acting agents (clonazepam)

*Anticonvulsants and others*
Anticonvulsants (carbamazepine, gabapentin)
Adrenergic antagonists (clonidine)

Carbidopa/levodopa has been shown in multiple controlled studies to improve the symptoms of RLS and reduce the frequency of PLMS[33]. If symptoms are especially troublesome before sleep onset, the usual dose is carbidopa/levodopa 25 mg/100 mg before bed. If the predominant problem is waking with RLS later in the night, then a tablet of controlled-release carbidopa/levodopa 25 mg/100 mg is preferable. In some patients a combination of the short-acting and controlled-release forms may be needed[34]. Even the controlled-release form has a relatively short duration of action, and some patients may require an additional dose of medication during the night.

Levodopa should preferentially be administered on an empty stomach to enhance absorption. Minor side-effects such as nausea and insomnia are sometimes seen, but long-term studies have shown that dyskinesias do not generally develop.

Complications specific to RLS have limited the use of levodopa (Table 15.9). The main complication after administration of a predormital dose is the development of worsening symptoms of RLS in the afternoon or evening, despite adequate control at night. This phenomenon, known as restless legs augmentation, may occur in 70% of patients, sometimes within months of commencing therapy. Most often RLS develops progressively earlier in the day, but sometimes augmentation takes the form of increases in severity of pre-existing RLS, or a spread of RLS to involve other parts of the body, such as the arms. The development of restless legs augmentation has been shown to correlate with two factors: first, pretreatment RLS commencing earlier than 6 p.m., and second, the administration of a total daily levodopa dose of 200 mg or more[35]. Once augmentation has occurred, levodopa should be discontinued and a different agent such as a dopamine agonist used. If high doses have been prescribed, the drug should be weaned over 5–7 days rather than abruptly stopped. Reducing the dose and adding a different drug is ineffective in managing augmentation, and administering additional doses of levodopa earlier in the day usually results in further exacerbation of the phenomenon.

Another complication is that of rebound. This is the development of RLS after the effect of a dose of levodopa wears off, especially in the early hours of the morning. It

**Table 15.9** Complications of levodopa in restless legs syndrome (RLS)

*Augmentation* The development or worsening of RLS earlier in the day than the time medication is taken (includes augmentation in time, intensity and anatomical distribution)

*Rebound* The development or worsening of RLS after the effect of a dose has worn off, most commonly in the early morning hours

*Tolerance* The need for increasing doses of the medication to provide relief of the same RLS symptoms

occurs in about 19–35% of patients[35–37] and is also an indication for changing to a different drug. Augmentation and rebound are often confused with the development of tolerance to the medication. This appears to be less common, but natural fluctuations in the severity of RLS make it difficult to determine a true frequency. Because of its short duration of action and the high frequency of augmentation and rebound, levodopa is less commonly used than in the past. It should probably be restricted to patients with intermittent RLS confined to a short period during the day, such as for an hour after going to bed.

**Case 15.3**

A 39-year-old woman with a history of RLS in her mother presented with typical RLS symptoms nightly after going to bed at 10:30 p.m., preventing sleep onset for up to 2 h. A few times a week similar symptoms occurred while she was sitting in a chair watching TV after 8 p.m. She was treated with carbidopa/levodopa

25 mg/100 mg, 30 min before bed, and obtained almost immediate relief. However, 2 months later she reported that her evening symptoms had worsened, so an additional dose of 25 mg/100 mg carbidopa/levodopa was prescribed at 7 p.m. This again provided relief for a few months, but she then reported RLS for the first time while she sat at her desk after 3 p.m. Increasingly frequent doses of the drug were prescribed as the symptoms became more severe and commenced progressively earlier in the day. Eventually she was taking carbidopa/levodopa eight times a day at 2-h intervals (total levodopa dose of 800 mg), and reported immediate RLS if she delayed a dose for even 20 min. In addition, the symptoms had spread from her legs to her arms and even her neck. She became aware that her arms and legs would at times jerk spontaneously. She was weaned off carbidopa/levodopa over 5 days and pramipexole was substituted in a single dose at 8 p.m., commencing at 0.125 mg and increasing over 7 days to 0.5 mg. During the overlap period, she experienced a transient worsening of RLS for 2 days, but by 7 days all augmentation had completely resolved and pramipexole was becoming effective in controlling RLS before sleep.

This case illustrates extremely severe RLS augmentation, precipitated by increasing doses of levodopa. Invariably even profound augmentation disappears with discontinuation of levodopa, but patients should be warned about the possibility of a few days' exacerbation of symptoms at the time of transition to an agonist. If the total daily levodopa dose is 200 mg or less, it can be discontinued immediately, but higher doses should be weaned over a few days.

The newer, non-ergot dopamine agonists are slowly replacing the ergots in the management of RLS. Pramipexole, a non-ergot agonist, binds predominantly to the D-2 and D-3 subtypes of the D2 dopamine receptor subfamily, and has a half-life of 8–12 h. Clinical experience and small controlled trials[33,38] have demonstrated its effectiveness in treating RLS, and it has largely replaced levodopa as a first-line agent for the management of moderate or severe symptoms. Side-effects are uncommon and rarely serious. They may include initial nausea, insomnia, lightheadedness, nasal stuffiness and leg edema. Daytime sleepiness, especially while driving, reported when this drug is used to treat Parkinson's disease, does not seem to be a common problem in RLS, perhaps because the medication is used in lower doses and predominantly in the evening. In a series of 60 patients, only three complained of sleepiness, and none of 'sleep attacks' while driving[39]. Augmentation occurs in 33% of patients usually within the first two and a half years of use, but is less frequent than with levodopa. Also, unlike with levodopa, augmentation is usually treatable with an additional dose earlier in the day without resultant progression. Treatment should commence with 0.125 mg 2 h before the onset of severe symptoms, with this being increased by 0.125 mg every 48–72 h until relief is obtained. Doses required are considerably lower than those needed for the treatment of Parkinson's disease. In a study of 49 patients followed for a mean of 27 months, the median initial dose was 0.38 mg; this had increased by the end of the study to a median dose of 0.63 mg[39]. Most patients require less than 0.75 mg daily, but some may require up to 2 mg. Some patients with RLS occurring during the day may need two doses, such as one in the afternoon and one in the late evening.

Ropinirole, another D-2 and D-3 receptor agonist similar to pramipexole, has also been shown in recent controlled trials[40,41] to be effective in the treatment of RLS, with a similar benign side-effect profile. Dosage should commence at 0.5 mg 2 h before symptoms start, and should be increased by 0.25 mg nightly as needed up to an initial target of 2 mg. Higher equivalent doses are required compared with pramipexole, and many patients may need 3–4 mg daily for effective control of symptoms.

Bromocriptine was the first dopamine agonist to be used in RLS, but is rarely used today. Pergolide, a potent long-acting ergot agonist, has been shown to be effective in controlled trials[33], but because of a much higher frequency of similar side-effects to those with pramipexole and ropinirole, it has largely been replaced by the newer drugs. Treatment should commence with 0.05 mg 2 h before major symptoms start, and this can be increased by 0.05 mg every two nights, until relief is obtained, side-effects develop or a dose of 0.6–0.8 mg is reached. The average effective dose is about 0.15–0.20 mg[42]. Cabergoline is an ultra-long-acting agonist with a half-life of more than 60 h. Open-label studies suggest its effectiveness in combating RLS[43], and its long half-life might theoretically result in less augmentation. Rare reports of fibrotic reactions to the ergot agonists have appeared, including pleuropericardial, retroperitoneal and cardiac valvular fibrosis[44].

Amantadine, a dopaminergic agent of uncertain mechanism, has also been tried for RLS[45].

*Opioids*

These agents have been shown to be effective in controlled trials[33], but side-effects, such as constipation and nausea, and concern regarding potential addiction, somewhat limit their use. Low-potency agents such as codeine (commencing at 30 mg) and propoxyphene (commencing at 65–130 mg) are useful in mild cases, especially when symptoms are often intermittent. Higher-potency agents such as oxycodone (commencing at 5 mg), hydrocodone (commencing at 5 mg) or methadone (commencing at 5–10 mg) have a definite role to play in patients with resistant symptoms when other therapies have failed. The possibility of the drugs worsening obstructive sleep apnea should be considered[46].

*Benzodiazepines*

Clonazepam, a long-acting benzodazepine, was one of the first drugs used for RLS. Experience suggests that the benzodiazepines may be effective, although the few controlled trials have yielded contradictory results[33]. Most studies of periodic limb movements of sleep have shown that benzodiazepines reduce arousals rather than eliminate the movements themselves, and their effectiveness in RLS may also be due to their hypnotic properties. Concerns about their use include their potential to cause daytime sedation, falls at night in the elderly and impotence, especially with longer-acting agents such as clonazepam. They may theoretically exacerbate coexisting obstructive sleep apnea syndrome, and long-term use can result in a degree of physical dependence. Clonazepam should be rarely used today for RLS, but intermediate-acting drugs such as temazepam (7.5–30 mg), or short-acting drugs such as triazolam (0.125–0.25 mg), are sometimes useful in patients with mild or intermittent symptoms, or those who also suffer from psychophysiological insomnia. They may be beneficial in combination with a dopamine agonist in more severely affected patients.

### Anticonvulsants and others

Carbamazepine was found to be superior to placebo in relieving RLS in a controlled study[33], but subsequent clinical experience does not suggest a high degree of efficacy. Gabapentin may in some cases be effective, especially with the painful variant of RLS, confirmed by a controlled trial[47]. The mean daily dose needed was 1300–1800 mg, which can often give rise to daytime sleepiness. However, some patients with mild RLS may obtain relief at lower doses, and the drug may be useful in combination with an agonist in patients with resistant symptoms. Clonidine provided relief from RLS symptoms in controlled studies at doses of 0.15–0.5 mg, but frequent side-effects were noted, including dry mouth, decreased cognition and lightheadedness[48]. Treatment should be initiated at 0.1 mg daily.

Practical management of RLS can be challenging and needs to be adapted to the individual patient. There is no single correct algorithm, but the following approach is suggested, based on personal experience (Table 15.10).

### Mild RLS

Mild RLS can be defined as RLS that is intermittent or only mildly disruptive to sleep initiation or maintenance. Non-pharmacological techniques can be tried. If the symptoms are intermittent, consider carbidopa/levodopa, a benzodiazepine, gabapentin or a low-potency opioid. The development of augmentation with levodopa should be carefully monitored. If RLS is continuous, consider the use of gabapentin.

### Moderate or severe RLS

This is RLS that is present most days and is moderately or severely disruptive to sleep onset or maintenance. Generally treatment is commenced with a non-ergot dopamine agonist such as pramipexole or ropinirole.

### Resistant RLS

This is RLS that does not respond adequately to a dopamine agonist, or when uncontrollable daytime augmentation or tolerance has developed with an agonist. Strategies at this stage include changing to another dopamine agonist, adding a second medication such as a benzodiazepine or gabapentin or changing to a high-potency opioid.

---

**Case 15.4**

A 56-year-old woman with severe RLS was referred for agitated behavior after surgery. She had long-standing RLS and had developed over time augmentation with levodopa, pergolide, pramipexole and ropinirole. Eventually reasonable control of her highly resistant RLS was obtained

---

with a combination of 3 mg ropinirole daily and 10 mg oxycodone before bed. She underwent a surgical procedure and was maintained on parenteral narcotics for 3 days postoperatively. On the night of the fourth day she developed an intense exacerbation of RLS and fell out of bed while trying to obtain relief from her discomfort. Intravenous lorazepam was administered without benefit and two nurses were needed to hold her still. A number of factors contributed to her RLS exacerbation. First, parenteral opioids were abruptly stopped and oral oxycodone not restarted. Second, she had received parenteral dopamine-blocking medication in the form of metoclopramide to treat opioid-related nausea, and third, she had experienced blood loss at the time of surgery with her hemoglobin concentration falling to 7.8 g/l. Parenteral narcotics were recommenced, metoclopramide therapy stopped and a blood transfusion administered. Within hours RLS had resolved. She was discharged on her previous regimen and her symptoms remained under fair control.

This case illustrates some of the problems that can occur in the management of very resistant RLS. In particular, surgeons should be aware that RLS medications should be continued postoperatively, that abrupt discontinuation of parenteral opioids can worsen RLS, that drugs which can exacerbate RLS should be avoided and that acute iron deficiency from blood loss may need correction.

## PERIODIC LIMB MOVEMENTS OF SLEEP

### Description

The characteristic movement of PLMS is extension of the great toe with dorsiflexion of the ankle and flexion of the knee and hip. The movements last from 0.5 to 5.0 s and occur in clusters once every 20–40 s for minutes to hours. Although usually both legs move simultaneously, often one leg predominates for long periods. PLMS persist through all stages of non-rapid eye movement (NREM) sleep, but usually become less frequent or are not present during rapid eye movement (REM) sleep. The movements are often more frequent in the first half of the night. Empirical criteria are used for the purposes of scoring sleep studies (Table 15.11). The number of movements per hour of sleep is counted (periodic limb movement

**Table 15.10** Restless legs syndrome (RLS) management algorithm

Establish diagnosis of RLS

Assess for treatable secondary causes

Decide if RLS is mild, moderate to severe or resistant, and use appropriate agents

*Mild RLS* non-pharmacological strategies; if RLS intermittent, consider levodopa, low-potency opioids, or benzodiazepines; if RLS continuous, consider gabapentin

*Moderate or severe RLS* use a non-ergot dopamine agonist, such as pramipexole or ropinirole

*Resistant RLS* change to a different dopamine agonist, add a second agent such as gabapentin or a benzodiazepine, or use a high-potency opioid

**Table 15.11** Polysomnogram criteria for periodic limb movements of sleep[49,50]

| |
| --- |
| Electromyogram (EMG) activity in one or both anterior tibial muscles recorded with surface EMG electrodes |
| Amplitude > 25% of a calibration signal produced by voluntary dorsiflexion of the great toe |
| Movement duration of 0.5–5.0 s |
| Intermovement interval of 4–90 s |
| At least four consecutive movements |
| Simultaneous movements in both limbs counted as a single movement |

**Table 15.12** Differential diagnosis of periodic limb movements of sleep

| |
| --- |
| Sleep starts |
| Apnea-induced arousals |
| REM sleep behavior disorder |
| Rhythmic movement disorder |
| Nocturnal seizures |
| Myoclonus and other hyperkinetic movement disorders |
| Misperception by a bed partner of normal changes of position during sleep |

REM, rapid eye movement

index), as well as the percentage associated with arousals (Figure 15.1). A frequency of greater than five per hour is traditionally considered abnormal, but this cut-off is too low in a population older than 50 years. A number of other movements during sleep can be confused with PLMS, and sometimes a polysomnogram is required to make the correct diagnosis (Table 15.12). In particular, arousals at the termination of obstructive apneas or hypopneas may incorporate jerks of the limbs or body indistinguishable from PLMS on a polysomnogram unless their consistent relationship to sleep-disordered breathing is noted.

## Clinical associations

The clinical significance of PLMS is controversial. In a study of 100 asymptomatic subjects, 5% of those between 30 and 49 years old had PLMS, compared with 29% of those older than 49 years. No patient younger than 30 years had PLMS. (PLMS were defined as at least 30 periodic movements over the course of the night, approximately

the same as the more conventional figure of at least five per hour[51].) A study of 427 volunteers aged 65 years or older revealed five or more PLMS per hour in 45%. Limb movements at the termination of disordered breathing events were counted as PLMS, but only 10% of the subjects had apnea indexes of 5/h or more[52]. At least 80% of patients with restless legs syndrome will have PLMS[53], but the majority of patients with PLMS on a clinical polysomnogram do not give a history of restless legs (Figure 15.2). Twenty-two elderly insomniacs had a mean PLMS index of 34.5/h, but there was no correlation between the PLMS index and number of arousals, total sleep time or other polysomnogram parameters[54]. PLMS were found in 13% of a large study of 409 consecutive patients studied in a clinical sleep laboratory. These were equally distributed between patients complaining of insomnia, excessive daytime sleepiness and other symptoms, and between those eventually diagnosed with narcolepsy and sleep apnea and other disorders[55]. No correlation was found between mean sleep latencies on a

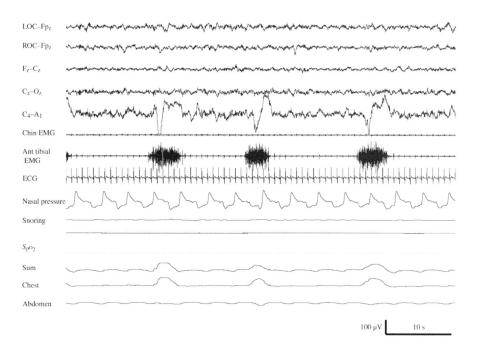

LOC–Fp$_z$
ROC–Fp$_z$
F$_z$–C$_z$
C$_z$–O$_z$
C$_4$–A$_1$
Chin EMG
Ant tibial EMG
ECG
Nasal pressure
Snoring
S$_p$O$_2$
Sum
Chest
Abdomen

100 μV    10 s

**Figure 15.1**  Periodic limb movements of sleep. This 60-s polysomnogram (PSG) fragment shows three periodic limb movements of sleep resulting in sufficient body movement to cause movement artifacts in the C4–A1 and plethysmography channels. Arousal did not occur. Channel labels as in Figure 4.1

multiple sleep latency test (MSLT) and the PLMS index in 67 patients with a variety of sleep disorders[56]. A more homogeneous group of 34 patients with PLMS complaining of excessive daytime sleepiness but no symptoms of RLS, sleep apnea or narcolepsy underwent a MSLT. There was no correlation between the PLMS index and either the mean MSLT latency or polysomnogram sleep efficiency, and the eventual diagnosis was that of idiopathic hypersomnia[57]. Various studies have shown a high prevalence of PLMS in samples of patients with narcolepsy, obstructive sleep apnea syndrome, and REM sleep behavior disorder, as well as in Parkinson's disease[58]. Thus, PLMS are common in the elderly and in patients with a wide range of different sleep symptoms and disorders. The movements themselves may be largely epiphenomena of often little clinical significance.

## PLMS and arousals

The relationship between PLMS and the electroencephalogram (EEG) is complex. Some movements appear to be closely followed by an EEG arousal (usually a K-complex and subsequent short run of alpha rhythm), some appear to be preceded by an

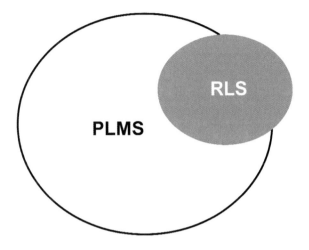

**Figure 15.2** Relationship between restless leg syndrome (RLS) and periodic limb movements of sleep (PLMS). This Venn diagram indicates schematically that about 80% of RLS patients will have PLMS on a polysomnogram polysomnogram, but the majority of people with PLMS on a polysomnogram will not have RLS

arousal and some have no clear relationship to arousals. A consistent increase in heart rate and delta power on the EEG is seen at, or just prior to, the onset of a periodic limb movement, even when the conventionally analyzed EEG does not show any features of arousal[59]. One study has shown that bursts of K–alpha may persist, even if the PLMS are successfully treated[60]. A functional MRI study suggested that PLMS were associated with activation of subcortical structures, including the midbrain and pons[28]. Thus, PLMS do not appear to be primary motor phenomena resulting in sleep fragmentation, but rather manifestations of a cyclical disruption of an underlying oscillatory neural network[59]. It is uncertain whether auto-

nomic changes associated with PLMS result in any clinical consequences for patients.

## Classification of periodic limb movements of sleep

Table 15.13 outlines a clinical classification of PLMS. PLMS associated with RLS is placed in a category separate from other sleep and neurological disorders because of the high frequency of PLMS in RLS, the presence of periodic limb movements of wakefulness in RLS and rare cases of RLS developing earlier in the day after treatment of PLMS with dopaminergic agents. In the absence of RLS, care should be exercised in ascribing a patient's symptoms to PLMS. In

**Table 15.13** Classification of periodic limb movements of sleep (PLMS). Modified from reference 61

Asymptomatic PLMS in normal subjects, especially the elderly

PLMS associated with restless legs syndrome

PLMS associated with other sleep or neurological disorders (including sleep apnea, narcolepsy, idiopathic hypersomnia, REM sleep behavior disorder, Parkinson's disease)

Periodic limb movement disorder (see text for criteria)

REM, rapid eye movement

order to diagnose periodic limb movement disorder, patients must exhibit symptoms conceivably caused by PLMS, such as insomnia, hypersomnia or, most typically, a clear perception of leg movements causing disruption of the sleep of the patient or bed partner. No other sleep disorders should be present that could cause the symptoms. A polysomnogram should show a higher frequency of PLMS than expected in normal subjects of the same age, and a reasonable percentage of the PLMS should be associated with EEG arousals. Dopaminergic agents should result in resolution of the primary symptoms and this should be sustained to avoid placebo effect. If so defined, rare cases of periodic limb movement disorder do exist, but are few and far between.

## Case 15.5

A 45-year-old man was referred for periodic limb movement disorder, unresponsive to medications. He had originally presented with a 5-year history of exces-sive daytime sleepiness commencing at age 33 years. He did not appear to be sleep-deprived and did not complain of cataplexy. There was no history of RLS. A polysomnogram had shown no evidence of disordered breathing, but 27 periodic limb movements per hour of which 20% were associated with EEG arousals. A diagnosis of periodic limb movement disorder was made, and treatment commenced with controlled release carbidopa/levodopa before bed. There was no improvement in his sleepiness and pergolide, clonazepam and dextropropoxyphene were used successively in increasing doses, again without benefit. All medications were discontinued and a repeat polysomnogram followed by an MSLT was performed. The PLMS index was 19/h with 15% causing arousals. The mean sleep latency on the MSLT was 4.3 min with no sleep-onset REM periods. A diagnosis of idiopathic hypersomnia was reached. Treatment was commenced with modafinil, with marked improvement in daytime sleepiness.

This case illustrates the incorrect diagnosis of periodic limb movement disorder in a patient without RLS, based on polysomnogram findings. The correct diagnosis was idiopathic hypersomnia, and the PLMS were asymptomatic epiphenomena.

## Presence of PLMS as a diagnostic test for restless legs syndrome

Can the presence of PLMS be used as a diagnostic test for RLS? PLMS (> 5/h) will be recorded on a single-night polysomnogram in 80% of patients with a clinical diagnosis of

RLS, and in 88% after two studies[53]. Thus, the presence of PLMS on a polysomnogram is moderately sensitive but non-specific as a predictor of RLS, and is rarely appropriate as a diagnostic test for the disorder. However, when the primary complaint is that of disruptive leg movements during sleep without RLS, a polysomnogram may be helpful.

Two other diagnostic tests for RLS have been described. These are based on the fact that periodic limb movements can continue during wakefulness in patients with RLS if the legs are held still. In the fixed immobilization test, the patient lies on a bed during wakefulness with the legs immobilized in a stretcher for 30–60 min, while involuntary leg movements are monitored via anterior tibial surface EMG. This can result in severe discomfort, so in the suggested immobilization test (SIT), no stretcher is used and instead the patient is asked to remain still voluntarily. The scoring criteria are slightly different from PLMS, with periodic limb movements lasting 0.5–10.0 s being counted. More than 40 leg movements per hour in the SIT are suggestive of RLS, with 81% sensitivity and 81% specificity[62]. The SIT is rarely used clinically, both because of its only moderate sensitivity and specificity, and because it should optimally be performed in the evening when most sleep laboratories are at their busiest.

## Management of PLMS

When it is felt necessary to treat PLMS, medications that are successful in treating RLS are generally effective. In particular, dopamine agonists, controlled-release carbidopa/levodopa or benzodiazepines are often used.

## REFERENCES

1. Ekbom KA. *Restless Legs*. Stockholm: Ivar Hoeggstroms, 1945

2. Allen RP, Picchietti D, Hening WA, Trenkwalder C, Walters AS, Montplaisir J. Restless legs syndrome: diagnostic criteria, special considerations, and epidemiology. A report from the restless legs syndrome diagnosis and epidemiology workshop at the National Institutes of Health. *Sleep Med* 2003;4:101–19

3. Michaud M, Chabli A, Lavigne G, Montplaisir J. Arm restlessness in patients with restless legs syndrome. *Mov Disord* 2000;15:289–93

4. Trenkwalder C, Hening WA, Walters AS, Campbell SS, Rahman K, Chokroverty S. Circadian rhythm of periodic limb movements and sensory symptoms of restless legs syndrome. *Mov Disord* 1999;14:102–10

5. Walters AS, Hening W, Rubinstein M, Chokroverty S. A clinical and polysomnographic comparison of neuroleptic-induced akathisia and the idiopathic restless legs syndrome. *Sleep* 1991;14:339–45

6. Phillips B, Young T, Finn L, Asher K, Hening WA, Purvis C. Epidemiology of restless legs symptoms in adults. *Arch Intern Med* 2000;160:2137–41

7. Lavigne GJ, Montplaisir JY. Restless legs syndrome and sleep bruxism: prevalence and association among Canadians. *Sleep* 1994;17:739–43

8. Rothdach AJ, Trenkwalder C, Haberstock J, Keil U, Berger K. Prevalence and risk factors of RLS in an elderly population: the MEMO study. Memory and Morbidity in Augsburg Elderly. *Neurology* 2000; 54:1064–8

9. Walters AS, Hickey K, Maltzman J, *et al.* A questionnaire study of 138 patients with restless legs syndrome: the 'Night-Walkers' survey. *Neurology* 1996;46:92–5

10. Picchietti DL, Underwood DJ, Farris WA, *et al.* Further studies on periodic limb movement disorder and restless legs syndrome in children with attention-deficit hyperactivity disorder. *Mov Disord* 1999;14:1000–7

11. Picchietti D, Underwood DJ, Farris WA, *et al.* Further studies on periodic limb movement disorder and restless legs syndrome in children with attention-deficit hyperactivity disorder. *Mov Disord* 2002;14:1000–7

12. Ondo W, Jankovic J. Restless legs syndrome: clinicoetiologic correlates. *Neurology* 1996; 47:1435–41

13. Winkelmann J, Wetter TC, Collado-Seidel V, *et al.* Clinical characteristics and frequency of the hereditary restless legs syndrome in a population of 300 patients. *Sleep* 2000; 23:597–602

14. Desautels A, Turecki G, Montplaisir J, Sequeira A, Verner A, Rouleau GA. Identification of a major susceptibility locus for restless legs syndrome on chromosome 12q. *Am J Hum Genet* 2001;69:1266–70

15. Allen R, Earley C. Defining the phenotype of the restless legs syndrome (RLS) using age-of-symptom-onset. *Sleep Med* 2000; 1:11–19

16. Norlander NB. Therapy in restless legs. *Acta Med Scand* 1953;145:453–7

17. O'Keeffe ST, Gavin K, Lavan JN. Iron status and restless legs syndrome in the elderly. *Age Ageing* 1994;23:200–3

18. Sun ER, Chen CA, Ho G, Earley CJ, Allen RP. Iron and the restless legs syndrome. *Sleep* 1998;21:371–7

19. Earley CJ, Connor JR, Beard JL, Malecki EA, Allen RP. Abnormalities in CSF concentrations of ferritin and transferrin in restless legs syndrome. *Neurology* 2000;54: 1698–700

20. Allen RP, Barker PB, Wehrl F, Song HK, Earley CJ. MRI measurement of brain iron in patients with restless legs syndrome. *Neurology* 2001;56:263–5

21. Connor JR, Boyer PJ, Menzies SL, *et al.* Neuropathological examination suggests impaired brain iron acquisition in restless legs syndrome. *Neurology* 2003;61:304–9

22. Silber M, Richardson JW. Multiple blood donations associated with iron deficiency in patients with restless legs syndrome. *Mayo Clin Proc* 2003;78:52–4

23. Winkelman JW, Chertow GM, Lazarus JM. Restless legs syndrome in end-stage renal disease. *Am J Kidney Dis* 1996;28:372–8

24. Collado-Seidel V, Kohnen R, Samtleben W, Hillebrand GF, Oertel WH, Trenkwalder C. Clinical and biochemical findings in uremic patients with and without restless legs syndrome. *Am J Kidney Dis* 1998;31:324–8

25. Winkelmann J, Stautner A, Samtleben W, Trenkwalder C. Long-term course of restless legs syndrome in dialysis patients after kidney transplantation. *Mov Disord* 2002; 17:1072–6

26. Iannaccone S, Zucconi M, Marchettini P, *et al.* Evidence of peripheral axonal neuropathy in primary restless legs syndrome. *Mov Disord* 1995;10:2–9

27. Polydefkis M, Allen RP, Hauer P, Earley CJ, Griffin JW, McArthur JC. Subclinical sensory neuropathy in late-onset restless legs syndrome. *Neurology* 2000; 55:1115–21

28. Bucher SF, Seelos KC, Oertel WH, Reiser M, Trenkwalder C. Cerebral generators

involved in the pathogenesis of the restless legs syndrome. *Ann Neurol* 1997;41:639-45

29. Trenkwalder C, Walters AS, Hening WA, *et al.* Positron emission tomographic studies in restless legs syndrome. *Mov Disord* 1999;14:141–5

30. Turjanski N, Lees AJ, Brooks DJ. Striatal dopaminergic function in restless legs syndrome: 18F-dopa and 11C-raclopride PET studies. *Neurology* 1999;52:932–7

31. Ruottinen HM, Partinen M, Hublin C, *et al.* An FDOPA PET study in patients with periodic limb movement disorder and restless legs syndrome. *Neurology* 2000;54:502–4

32. Chesson AL Jr, Wise M, Davila D, *et al.* Practice parameters for the treatment of restless legs syndrome and periodic limb movement disorder. An American Academy of Sleep Medicine Report. Standards of Practice Committee of the American Academy of Sleep Medicine. *Sleep* 1999; 22:961–8

33. Hening W, Allen R, Earley C, Kushida C, Picchietti D, Silber M. The treatment of restless legs syndrome and periodic limb movement disorder. An American Academy of Sleep Medicine Review. *Sleep* 1999; 22:970–99

34. Collado-Seidel V, Kazenwadel J, Wetter TC, *et al.* A controlled study of additional *sr*-L-dopa in L-dopa-responsive restless legs syndrome with late-night symptoms. *Neurology* 1999;52:285–90

35. Allen RP, Earley CJ. Augmentation of the restless legs syndrome with carbidopa/levodopa. *Sleep* 1996;19:205–13

36. Becker PM, Jamieson AO, Brown WD. Dopaminergic agents in restless legs syndrome and periodic limb movements of sleep: response and complications of extended treatment in 49 cases. *Sleep* 1993;16:713–16

37. Guilleminault C, Cetel M, Philip P. Dopaminergic treatment of restless legs and rebound phenomenon. *Neurology* 1993; 43:445

38. Montplaisir J, Nicolas A, Denesle R, Gomez-Mancilla B. Restless legs syndrome improved by pramipexole: a double-blind randomized trial. *Neurology* 1999;52: 938–43

39. Silber M, Girish M, Izurieta R. Pramipexole in the management of restless legs syndrome: an extended study. *Sleep* 2003; 26:819–21

40. Walters AS, Ondo W, Sethi K, Dreykluft T, Grunstein R. Ropinerole versus placebo in the treatment of restless legs syndrome (RLS): a 12 week multicenter double-blind placebo controlled study conducted in 6 countries [Abstract]. *Sleep* 2003;26:A344

41. Trenkwalder C, Garcia-Borreguero D, Montagna P, *et al.* Ropinirole in in the treatment of restless legs syndrome: results from the TREAT RLS 1 study, a 12-week randomized, placebo-controlled study in 10 European countries. *Journal Neurosurg Psychiatry* 2004;75:92–7

42. Silber MH, Shepard JW Jr, Wisbey JA. Pergolide in the management of restless legs syndrome: an extended study. *Sleep* 1997;20:878–82

43. Zucconi M, Oldani A, Castronovo C, Ferrini-Strambi L. Cabergolire is an effective single-drug treatment for restless legs syndrome: clinical and actigraphic evaluation. *Sleep* 2003;26:815–18

44. Pritchett A, Morrison JF, Edwards WD, Schaff HV, Connolly HM, Espinosa EE. Valvular heart disease in patients taking pergolide. *Mayo Clin Proc* 2002;77:1280–6

45. Evidente VG, Adler CH, Caviness JN, Hentz JG, Gwinn-Hardy K. Amantadine is beneficial in restless legs syndrome. *Mov Disord* 2000;15:324–7

46. Walters AS, Winkelmann J, Trenkwalder C, *et al.* Long-term follow-up on restless legs syndrome patients treated with opioids. *Mov Disord* 2001;16:1105–9

47. Garcia-Borreguero D, Larrosa E, De la Llave Y, Verger K, Masramon X, Hernandez G. Treatment of restless legs syndrome with gabapentin. A double-blind, cross-over study. *Neurology* 2002;59:1573–9

48. Wagner ML, Walters AS, Coleman RG, Hening WA, Grasing K, Chokroverty S. Randomized, double-blind, placebo-controlled study of clonidine in restless legs syndrome. *Sleep* 1996;19:52–8

49. Coleman RM. Periodic movements in sleep (nocturnal myoclonus) and restless legs syndrome. In Guilleminault C, ed. *Sleeping and Waking Disorders: Indications and Techniques.* Menlo Park: Addison-Wesley, 1982:265–95

50. Recording and scoring leg movements. The Atlas Task Force. *Sleep* 1993;16:748–59

51. Bixler EO. Nocturnal myoclonus and nocturnal myoclonic activity in a normal population. *Res Commun Chem Path Pharmacol* 1982;36:129–40

52. Ancoli-Israel S, Kripke DF, Klauber MR, Mason WJ, Fell R, Kaplan O. Periodic limb movements in sleep in community-dwelling elderly. *Sleep* 1991;14:496–500

53. Montplaisir J, Boucher S, Poirier G, Lavigne G, Lapierre O, Lesperance P. Clinical, polysomnographic, and genetic characteristics of restless legs syndrome: a study of 133 patients diagnosed with new standard criteria. *Mov Disord* 1997;12:61–5

54. Youngstedt SW, Kripke DF, Klauber MR, Sepulveda RS, Mason WJ. Periodic leg movements during sleep and sleep disturbances in elders. *J Gerontol* 1998;53A:M391–4

55. Coleman RM, Pollack CP, Weitzman ED. Periodic movements in sleep (nocturnal myoclonus): relation to sleep disorders. *Ann Neurol* 1980;8:416–21

56. Mendelson W. Are periodic limb movements associated with clinical sleep disturbances? *Sleep* 1996;19:219–23

57. Nicolas A, Lesperance P, Montplaisir J. Is excessive daytime sleepiness with periodic leg movements during sleep a specific diagnostic category? *Eur Neurol* 1998;40:22–6

58. Montplaisir J, Michaud M, Denesle R, Gosselin A. Periodic leg movements are not more prevalent in insomnia or hypersomnia but are specifically associated with sleep disorders involving a dopaminergic mechanism. *Sleep Med* 2000;1:163–7

59. Sforza E, Juony C, Ibanez V. Time-dependent variation in cerebral and autonomic activity during periodic leg movements in sleep: implications for arousal mechanisms. *Clin Neurophysiol* 2002;113:883–91

60. Montplaisir J, Boucher S, Gosselin A, Poirier G, Lavigne G. Persistence of repetitive EEG arousals (K–alpha complexes) in RLS patients treated with L-dopa. *Sleep* 1996;19:196–9

61. Silber MH. Controversies in sleep medicine: periodic limb movements. *Sleep Med* 2001;2:367–9

62. Montplaisir J, Boucher S, Nicolas A, *et al.* Immobilization tests and periodic leg movements in sleep for the diagnosis of restless leg syndrome. *Mov Disord* 1998;13:324–9

# Chapter 16

# The parasomnias

*From ghoulies and ghosties,*
*And three leggity beasties,*
*And things that go bump in the night,*
*Good Lord, deliver us.*

**Old Scottish prayer**

Parasomnias are undesirable, intermittent motor or sensory phenomena occurring during sleep. They range from simple visual imagery at sleep onset to complex and co-ordinated motor activity, such as running and punching. Some parasomnias can be terrifying to the patient or an observer, and in the past were ascribed to supernatural forces. Although, technically, periodic limb movements (Chapter 15) and nocturnal seizures (Chapter 18) could be considered parasomnias under this definition, they are usually considered to be separate conditions. Parasomnias can be classified according to the state of sleep from which they arise: non-rapid eye movement (NREM) parasomnias, rapid eye movement (REM) parasomnias and parasomnias that are not state dependent (Table 16.1).

## DIAGNOSTIC CONSIDERATIONS

Common parasomnias can be diagnosed by history from the patient and an observer, but in more complex situations, a modified polysomnogram (PSG) known as an electroencephalogram (EEG) video-polysomnogram is required. For parasomnia PSGs (Table 16.2), additional EEG and electromyogram (EMG) derivations are

**Table 16.1** Classification of parasomnias

*Parasomnias of NREM sleep*

Disorders of arousal
    classic disorders
        sleepwalking
        sleep terrors
        confusional arousals
    variant disorders
        sleep-related eating disorder
        complex nocturnal visual hallucinations
        nocturnal panic attacks

Wake–sleep transition disorders
    sleep starts (hypnic jerks)
    sensory starts (including exploding head syndrome)

*Parasomnias of REM sleep*

Nightmares

Sleep paralysis

REM sleep behavior disorder

Sleep-related painful erections

Catathrenia (nocturnal expiratory groaning)

*Non-state dependent parasomnias*

Rhythmic movement disorder
(body rocking, head banging)

Bruxism

Nocturnal enuresis

NREM, non-rapid eye movement; REM, rapid eye movement

**Table 16.2** Requirements for the polysomnographic study of parasomnias

---

Appropriate cardiorespiratory monitoring

Sufficient extra EEG derivations to record ictal and interictal activity (preferably 16)

Additional EMG derivations on the upper extremities

Ability to display signals at varying time windows including a 10-s screen to define EEG activity accurately

Time-synchronized video and audio recordings

Interpreters able to score sleep accurately

Interpreters able to interpret abnormalities of sleep-disordered breathing

Interpreters able to interpret ictal and interictal EEG abnormalities

---

EEG, electroencephalogram; EMG, electromyogram

required. In most cases, 16 extra EEG derivations should be used to rule out epileptic events. In addition to submental and tibialis anterior EMG, at least one muscle in each upper extremity, such as extensor digitorum communis, should be monitored. Full respiratory monitoring is needed, as arousals at the termination of apneas can be associated with dramatic motor activity, and an obstructive sleep apnea can actually precipitate sleepwalking or sleep terrors. The recording system should have the capacity to display signals at varying time windows, ranging from a 10-s screen for ictal and interictal activity to a 120-s screen for respiratory events with slow periodicity. Time-synchronized video and audio recording (ideally with a digital video system) is essential, as

the electrophysiological findings are often non-specific and the diagnosis dependent on actually seeing and hearing the event. These studies require special expertise, as the interpreter needs to be skilled in sleep staging and cardiorespiratory monitoring, as well as in ictal and interictal EEG.

## NON-RAPID EYE MOVEMENT PARASOMNIAS

### Disorders of arousal

*Clinical features*

These disorders are characterized by abnormal behavior occurring with sudden partial arousals from deep NREM sleep, most often stage 4[1]. On the basis of clinical features, the behaviors are usually classified as sleepwalking, sleep terrors or confusional arousals. However, many events overlap, making classification difficult, and patients often experience more than one type of event. Sleepwalking consists of complex, co-ordinated motor behaviors, most commonly walking, but sometimes sitting and standing. Sleepwalkers usually wander around the bedroom, but may move to other rooms or even leave the building. Sleep terrors are characterized by a piercing scream or cry accompanied by autonomic and motor manifestations of intense fear, including tachycardia, tachypnea and diaphoresis. Patients may sit up or throw themselves off the bed. Confusional arousals consist of brief episodes of confusion and disorientation, with neither the complex motility of sleepwalking nor the intense fear of sleep terrors. Patients will often raise the head from the pillow and briefly look around before returning to sleep.

Most events arise in the first third of the night, when slow-wave sleep is maximal, and commonly occur within the first hour of sleep onset. Patients do not react normally to external stimuli, and appear confused, unresponsive and sometimes combative if efforts are made to awaken them. They generally do not remember the events, or describe preceding dreams[2]. However, some patients will describe fragmentary imagery, often involving a situation of danger, and very occasionally will recall a more vivid, complex dream.

### Epidemiology

Sleepwalking occurs in at least 6% of children up to the age of 12 years[3], and single episodes may be sufficiently common to be considered a variant of normal development. As many as 2% of adults sleepwalk[4], and about 20% of childhood sleepwalkers continue somnambulism during adulthood[3]. The frequency of sleep terrors is less established, but they are thought to occur in at least 1% of children.

### Etiology and pathogenesis

Even a normal adult has considerable difficulty making a rapid transition between slow-wave sleep and full alertness if suddenly woken, for example, by a ringing telephone. This is not surprising when one considers the widespread differences between the physiology of deep NREM sleep and that of wakefulness. In patients with disorders of arousal, an abnormality appears to exist in the arousal mechanism, resulting in the patient becoming 'entrapped' in an abnormal state of consciousness between deep NREM sleep and full wakefulness. The causative abnormalities at pathophysiological or neurochemical levels have not been delineated. Possible hypotheses include a diminished responsiveness of the reticular activating system or an increased facilitation of the neural networks maintaining slow-wave sleep. A single positron emission computed tomography (SPECT) study of one patient during an episode of sleepwalking showed increased blood flow in the anterior cerebellum and posterior cingulate cortex compared with slow-wave sleep, and decreased blood flow in the frontoparietal cortices compared with wakefulness[5]. These findings confirm that sleepwalking is a dissociated state, sharing some features of both states.

Certain maturational, genetic and psychological factors predispose to the occurrence of arousal disorders (Table 16.3). Disorders of arousal are commonest during the first decade, and may be due to immature cerebral development of sleep and waking mechanisms. A family history of somnambulism or sleep terrors in first-degree relatives is a predisposing factor, but the mode of genetic transmission has not been delineated. Psychopathology is rare in children, but psychiatric disease may be present in adults, especially if the parasomnia starts only in adulthood.

Episodes may arise spontaneously, but are often precipitated by factors that increase either the depth or the duration of slow-wave sleep, prevent full awakenings or result in sleep fragmentation. Prior sleep deprivation or unusual sleep–wake schedules may deepen slow-wave sleep. The use of alcohol or central nervous system (CNS)-depressant medications, especially combination

**Table 16.3** Predisposing and precipitating factors in arousal parasomnias

*Predisposing factors*

Genetic factors

Maturational factors

*Precipitating factors*

Deepening slow–wave sleep

    prior sleep deprivation

    unusual sleep–wake cycles

Preventing complete awakening

    CNS-depressant drugs, including alcohol, major tranquilizers, lithium and short-acting hypnotics, often in combination

Increasing arousals

    environmental stimuli

    medical disorders, including febrile illnesses, OSA, and gastroesophageal reflux

    psychiatric disorders, including short-term anxiety and stress

CNS, central nervous system; OSA, obstructive sleep apnea

psychotropic agents, may prevent awakenings to full alertness. Arousals may be precipitated by environmental stimuli, especially noise, mental stress and medical disorders including fever, obstructive sleep apnea and gastroesophageal reflux.

*Violence during arousal parasomnias*

The vast majority of sleepwalkers do not engage in injurious behavior, but violence during sleep may be more common than suspected. In a sample of 4972 subjects from the UK, 2.1% reported violent or injurious behavior to themselves or their bed partner[6]. This was commoner in males and in younger subjects (aged 15–44 years). Homicide while sleepwalking has been reported since at least the 18th century[7], and sexual offenses while sleepwalking have also been described, including indecent exposure and assaults[8,9].

Violence during sleepwalking appears to take place under two circumstances. First, most cases occur abruptly, immediately on arousal. Some patients leap out of bed and through a window, with either no memory of a dream or a brief recollection of reacting to a dangerous situation. Sometimes the arousal is precipitated by the actions of a bed partner; patients have been described who have assaulted or killed the person who has unexpectedly woken them. Second, violence has been described later in a more prolonged episode of sleepwalking, apparently when the victim is attempting to restrain the patient. Extremely complex motor activity has been described during violent parasomnias, including driving. The best-documented case is that of a man who drove 23 km to the house of his parents-in-law and stabbed and beat his mother-in-law to death, possibly while she was confronting him[10]. A number of criteria must be fulfilled before a legal defense of sleepwalking can be seriously considered (Table 16.4). Additional helpful factors include the event occurring within the first 3 h of falling asleep, the presence of prior sleep deprivation and alcohol or drug use.

### Case 16.1

A 33-year-old woman traveled to Europe on vacation. She obtained, at most, 2 h sleep on the flight, and did not nap dur-

**Table 16.4** Criteria for a sleepwalking defense. Adapted with permission from references 7 and 11

A history of sleepwalking behavior is present before the event

Polysomnogram studies confirm a tendency to abnormal arousals from slow-wave sleep

The event was apparently motiveless and senseless

At least partial amnesia was present for the event

The assailant reacted to the event with perplexity and horror, and no attempt was made to conceal the crime

**Table 16.5** Indications for video-electroencephalogram polysomnography in suspected disorders of arousal

*Consequences of the behavior*

Behavior resulting in injuries to the patient or others

Behavior resulting in damage to objects

Behavior seriously disturbing the sleep of others

*Unclear diagnosis*

Seizures considered

Obstructive sleep apnea considered

REM sleep behavior disorder considered

Other parasomnias considered

REM, rapid eye movement

ing the subsequent day. She had two glasses of wine with dinner, and went to sleep in a hotel at 10 p.m. One hour later she woke to find she had thrown herself across the room, smashing the thick glass of the bedroom window and severely lacerating her face. She remembered a brief image of a terrible danger from which she needed to flee, but had no other dream recall. She had sleepwalked only once before in her life while she was at college. There was no family history of sleepwalking.

This event was almost certainly an arousal parasomnia, which occurred at a time of night when slow-wave sleep could have been expected. There was a background history of a prior event of sleepwalking. Precipitating factors were severe sleep deprivation, increasing the intensity and duration of slow-wave sleep, and alcohol, which may have prevented a full awakening. Because the event was isolated and clearly associated with recovery sleep from sleep deprivation, a PSG was not performed and treatment not prescribed. However, the patient was urged to avoid sleep deprivation and to consider the temporary use of an intermediate-acting benzodiazepine medication on the night following future trips across time zones.

*Diagnosis*

In most children, the diagnosis can be made by a careful history from parents and the child, and a similar approach is possible in some adults. PSG is indicated if the events have been injurious to the patient or others, have resulted in damage to inanimate objects or seriously disturb the sleep of others in the household, including bed partners, parents or siblings. PSG should also be considered if the diagnosis is unclear, especially if epilepsy or REM sleep behavior disorder are being considered (Table 16.5).

The interpreter should review the entire PSG record, even if the technologist does not note any events, as minor confusional arousals can easily be missed. The additional EEG derivations should be read, especially around the time of recorded events. All arousals from slow-wave sleep should be reviewed on the videotape. The PSG does not always show minor events, and a negative single-night study does not rule out the diagnosis of an arousal parasomnia. Some laboratories use the technique of arousing the patient during slow-wave sleep by means of a loud noise, in the hope of precipitating an event.

At the start of an event, the PSG shows sudden arousals from slow-wave sleep, sometimes accompanied by bursts of hypersynchronous delta waves. A study of 252 arousals from slow-wave sleep in patients with sleepwalking or sleep terrors showed a single high-amplitude delta wave in the scoring channel in the 10 s before arousal in only 47%, while two or more such delta waves occurred in only 15.5% of arousals[12]. Multichannel high-amplitude delta occurred in only 2% of arousals. Thus, hypersynchronous delta waves should not be considered essential for the diagnosis, and represent a non-specific arousal pattern seen in some instances. The EEG after arousal may show varied patterns, including rhythmic delta activity (6%), irregular mixed frequency activities, predominantly delta and theta (38%), alpha rhythm (36%) or muscle artifact (20%). It should be strongly emphasized that alpha rhythm recorded during a parasomnia does not imply that the patient is fully awake and aware, and does not prove that the event is of psychogenic origin. The

PSG appearance of sleepwalking, sleep terrors and confusional arousals is identical, and a video recording is needed to categorize them further. In addition, other causes of arousals, such as pain from carpal tunnel syndrome, may result in very similar PSG appearances (Figure 16.1).

Compared with normal age-matched controls, the background PSG of patients with disorders of arousal shows a higher percentage of slow-wave sleep, more frequent arousals from slow-wave sleep and a more even distribution of slow-wave sleep throughout the night[14]. Power spectral analysis has shown a lower amount of slow-wave activity in the first sleep cycle compared with controls, perhaps due to increased fragmentation by arousals[15,16]. However, the amount of delta activity increases just before a confusional arousal. These findings shed interesting light on the pathogenesis of the disorder, but are not specific enough to be of diagnostic help.

The differential diagnosis includes nightmares, REM sleep behavior disorder, nocturnal seizures, dissociative disorders, nocturnal panic attacks, obstructive sleep apnea syndrome and periodic limb movements of sleep. In difficult cases, the video-EEG PSG helps to resolve the diagnosis.

*Management*

Management of arousal disorders, especially in children, involves primarily reassurance. Parents should understand that the phenomena are common, and do not usually indicate the presence of neurological or psychiatric disease. Any possible precipitating factors should be identified and corrected. The bed environment should be made safe, including securing of bedroom windows, use of stair

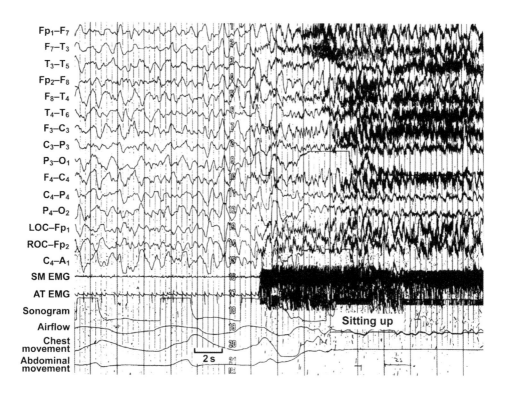

**Figure 16.1** Arousal parasomnia. This 30-s polysomnogram (PSG) fragment has an extended electroencephalogram (EEG) montage. It was recorded from a 9-year-old boy with stridor (see sonogram channel) as a result of vocal cord paralysis following surgery for a posterior fossa medulloblastoma. He presented with episodes of sleep terror, some precipitated by stridor. Note the sudden arousal from slow-wave sleep preceded by a series of hypersynchronous delta waves. Although muscle artifact partially obscures the recording after the arousal, some slow EEG activity can be seen to continue. Epileptiform activity is absent. LOC, left outer canthus; ROC, right outer canthus; SM, submental; AT, anterior tibial; EMG, electromyogram. Reproduced with permission from reference 13

gates and additional locks on external doors, as indicated by the particular child's sleepwalking pattern. No attempt should be made to wake the patient, who may be gently redirected back to bed. In the case of sleep terrors, the child should be held and consoled, but the parents should not be distressed if confusion and apparent fear continue despite their reassurances. Parents should be informed that the patient is usually amnesic for the occurrences and that the disorder does not generally result in daytime sleepiness.

Forms of behavioral therapy have been studied, and are often preferred by patients and parents to the use of drugs. Scheduled anticipatory awakenings is a technique of transiently waking the patient about 15 min before the expected time of the parasomnia. After 1–4 weeks' treatment, events become fewer or cease in the majority of children[17,18]. Hypnosis has also been used with success, especially in adults. After 1–6 initial sessions, the patient is taught self-hypnosis, and continues to apply the technique. In a series of 27 patients, 77% were much or very much improved after 9–24 months' follow-up[19].

Drug therapy should be used selectively, for behavior either potentially injurious to the patient or others, or intensely disruptive to the sleep of the rest of the household. Otherwise in children it should usually be restricted to situations when it is highly desirable to suppress the behavior, such as during sleepovers or at summer camps. In young adults, treatment may be needed to avoid social embarrassment at college or in new sexual relationships. Both benzodiazepines and antidepressants have been used, but no controlled trials have been performed. Diazepam, clonazepam, flurazepam, alprazolam, imipramine and paroxetine have been reported to be effective in short series or single cases. The largest study reported was of 58 patients treated with an average of 1.16 mg clonazepam for a mean of 3.3 years[20]. Drugs should be administered a sufficient time before sleep onset to allow for full absorption, as arousal events can occur within the first hour of sleep. Short-acting hypnotics should be used with caution, as they may occasionally precipitate events, perhaps by preventing full awakenings.

## Variants of arousal parasomnias

### Sleep-related eating disorder

Sleep-related eating disorder (SRED) consists of episodes of eating during the night with partial or complete amnesia. It is commoner in women. The patients will walk to the kitchen, prepare food, usually high in calories and sometimes consisting of idiosyncratic concoctions, and then eat it, often sloppily. PSG studies show that the events arise from NREM and most often slow-wave sleep, with the eating behavior always occurring during alpha rhythm. Food should be placed at the bedside when performing PSG on suspected SRED patients. SRED is often associated with other sleep disorders, including other sleepwalking (60%), restless legs syndrome and period limb movements of sleep (13%) and obstructive sleep apnea (11%). Affective disorders (37%), anxiety disorders (18%) and prior substance abuse (24%) are common[21]. SRED in association with use of the short-acting hypnotic, zolpidem, has been described[22]. Management can be challenging. Associated sleep disorders should be identified and treated. Short-acting hypnotics should be discontinued. Behavioral techniques, such as locking the kitchen door or chaining shut the refrigerator can be tried, but are usually unsuccessful. Psychotherapy is generally unhelpful. Treatment with intermediate or long-acting benzodiazepines, such as clonazepam or temazepam, is sometimes successful. There have been reports of success with combinations of codeine and levodopa, but these patients may have had associated periodic limb movements of sleep[21].

**Table 16.6** The spectrum of sleep and eating

Sleep-related eating disorder (SRED)

Night (nocturnal) eating syndrome (NES)

Daytime anorexia/bulimia nervosa with night eating

Kleine–Levin syndrome

---

SRED should be differentiated from other conditions linking sleep and eating (Table 16.6). Night (nocturnal) eating syndrome (NES) is characterized by recurrent awakenings with an inability to return to sleep without eating, but no amnesia for the behavior. In infants this may be a form of sleep-onset association disorder, while in adults it is linked to obesity. Morning anorexia is common, with more than 50% of daily energy intake being consumed during the night[23]. Melatonin and leptin levels have been reported to be low during the night, perhaps accounting for increased appetite and poor sleep consolidation. Anorexia and bulimia nervosa must be excluded before a diagnosis of either SRED or NES can be made. Kleine–Levin syndrome may be associated with hyperphagia during waking periods (see Chapter 7).

### Case 16.2

A 52-year-old woman had experienced severe sleep-onset insomnia due to restless legs syndrome (RLS) for more than 10 years. About 3 years before presentation, she was prescribed 5 mg zolpidem before bed and this allowed her to initiate sleep within 15 min. Soon after starting zolpidem treatment, she began eating nightly in her sleep. She had no recollection of the events but would wake in the morning to find a knife covered with cheese in the kitchen, a cookie box in her bed or food remnants scattered on the floor. She did not have a past history of sleepwalking. A PSG was performed with food left at her bedside. She awoke 90 min after sleep onset from stage 4 NREM sleep. She sat up, ate some cookies while the EEG demonstrated alpha rhythm and returned to sleep. She did not recall the event in the morning. The PSG also showed 26 periodic limb movements per hour, of which 30% caused arousals. Zolpidem was discontinued and temazepam (15 mg) substituted. Prami-pexole was prescribed, which controlled RLS at a dose of 0.5 mg taken 2 h before bed. Sleep-eating ceased, and had not recurred on follow-up 9 months later.

This case illustrates the precipitation of sleep-eating by the use of a short-acting hypnotic in the setting of RLS and periodic limb movements of sleep (PLMS). Substituting a longer-acting benzodiazepine and treating the underlying sleep disorder resulted in complete alleviation of the eating behavior.

*Nocturnal visual hallucinations*

A rare parasomnia is the occurrence of complex visual hallucinations on waking during the night. These usually consist of vivid, detailed, relatively immobile images of people or animals without auditory accompaniments. Hallucinations can last minutes to an hour, and disappear promptly if the lights are switched on. At least initially, patients have reduced insight into their unreality, but full recall of the events. The hallucinations may be intensely frightening, and some patients spring out of bed to grab the images. In one of our patients hallucinations arose in alpha rhythm from stages 2 and 3 NREM sleep[24], and from stage 3 sleep in another reported patient[2]. This is a heterogeneous disorder with varied etiologies, including dementia with Lewy bodies (see Chapter 17), anxiety disorders and the use of beta-blockers. However, in other patients it appears to be an idiopathic parasomnia, sometimes associated with other parasomnias, including sleepwalking, sleep-talking, REM sleep behavior disorder and sleep paralysis. The hallucinations are similar to those described during wakefulness in patients with blindness (Charles–Bonnet hallucinations) and from thalamic or midbrain pathology (peduncular hallucinations). A common mechanism may be reduced afferent input into the visual association areas at night[25].

## Case 16.3

An 80-year-old woman presented with a 5-year history of waking in the middle of the night, about three times a week, with vivid complex visual hallucinations, not arising from dreams. She would see images of witches hovering over her bed, dead hands, birds and butterflies. She realized that the hallucinations were not real, and learned that they would vanish if she turned on the light. Hallucination did not occur during the day and there were no symptoms to suggest a psychosis. Her mental state examination was normal with no evidence for dementia. She had severe macular degeneration, with bilaterally reduced visual acuity. She was not taking beta-blockers. She had learned to adapt her sleep to these occurrences and declined a trial of medication.

This case illustrates typical complex nocturnal visual hallucinations. In an older patient, one needs to consider dementia with Lewy bodies, but the patient had normal cognitive function. The most likely explanation was that these were so-called release hallucinations, also named Charles–Bonnet hallucinations, caused by blindness from macular degeneration.

### Nocturnal panic disorder

Nocturnal panic attacks can arise in association with daytime panic disorder, or in isolation (see Chapter 14). Patients awake suddenly from NREM sleep, often at the transition between stages 2 and 3 sleep[26], complaining of dyspnea, palpitations, paresthesias, diaphoresis and feelings of profound fear. They do not usually recall dream imagery. Obstructive sleep apnea syndrome, nocturnal stridor, paroxysmal nocturnal dyspnea from cardiac failure and REM sleep nightmares should also be considered in the differential diagnosis. Management is similar to that of daytime panic disorder.

## Wake–sleep transition disorders

### Sleep starts (hypnic jerks)

These are sudden brief contractions of multiple muscles of the legs, arms or trunk at

**Table 16.7** Differential diagnosis of nightmares

|  | Nightmares | Sleep terrors | REM sleep behavior disorder |
|---|---|---|---|
| Stage of sleep | REM sleep | slow-wave sleep | REM sleep |
| Dreams | vivid, frightening | none, or simple image | vivid, usually defending self against attack |
| Vocalization | minimal | marked screaming | speech, shouts or yells |
| Movements | minimal | sit up, stand, jump or run | punch, kick, jump out of bed |
| Responsiveness on arousal | fully alert | unresponsive | alert |
| Recall of events | full recall | little recall | recall of dream if awoken during episode |
| Commonest time of night | last third | first third | last third |

REM, rapid eye movement

sleep onset, and may be asymmetric. They may be associated with a brief impression of falling. They are a normal phenomenon and may occur in as many as 60% of subjects of all ages. They should not be confused with bed partners' descriptions of periodic limb movements of sleep. Very occasionally, they may occur many times in succession, and be sufficiently intense that they result in sleep-onset insomnia. Management usually involves reassurance, but in troublesome cases, a rapid-onset, short-acting benzodiazepine may be helpful.

### Sensory starts

A related phenomenon at sleep onset is the occurrence of brief sensory experiences, which may be visual (flashes of light) or auditory (loud bangs). 'Exploding head syn-drome' is the perception of a sudden painless explosion in the head, sometimes accompanied by a loud noise, usually occurring at sleep–wake transition[27]. It probably represents a variant of sensory starts.

## PARASOMNIAS OF RAPID EYE MOVEMENT SLEEP

### Nightmares

Nightmares are frightening dreams that awaken the sleeper from REM sleep. They are common in childhood, and the lifetime prevalence of occasional nightmares is probably close to 100%. Frequent nightmares occur in about 4% of the adult population[28], with a higher frequency in patients with psychopathology or substance abuse. Post-traumatic stress disorder (PTSD) should especially be considered, particularly if there is a recurring theme to the dreams. Clusters of nightmares may occur during periods of stress or as a result of certain medications, including levodopa, beta-blockers and withdrawal of REM-suppressant drugs.

Nightmares can usually be easily differentiated from sleep terrors (Table 16.7). After arousal from a nightmare, a complex vivid dream can be recalled, while either no dream or only a short frightening image is remembered after a sleep terror. Arousal from a nightmare, in contrast to a sleep terror, is not usually associated with motility, vocalization, intense autonomic discharges or confusion. Nightmares arise from REM sleep, while arousal disorders arise predominantly from slow-wave sleep. Therefore, most nightmares occur in the last third of the night, while most arousal disorders occur in the first third. Nightmares can be differentiated from REM sleep behavior disorder by the absence of dream enactment behavior, however vivid the recall of movement in the dream.

If necessary, management involves psychotherapy, including behavioral techniques and hypnosis. A commonly used technique involves asking the patient to rewrite their dreams with a happy ending, and to rehearse these before sleep[29].

## Sleep paralysis

Sleep paralysis consists of episodes of paralysis of skeletal muscle without loss of consciousness, occurring either at sleep onset or upon awakening during the night or in the morning. Most commonly, all skeletal muscles with the exception of respiratory and extraocular muscles are involved. The expe-

rience is usually frightening, and is associated with hypnagogic visual or auditory hallucinations in about 20% of patients[30]. Episodes may last for several minutes, and can sometimes be aborted by someone touching the patient. The largest epidemiological study suggests a lifetime prevalence of 6%[30], but other studies report a higher frequency in young adults. Very occasional reports of familial sleep paralysis have appeared. About 60% of patients with narcolepsy and cataplexy have repeated sleep paralysis, but the attacks usually commence only after the onset of sleepiness (see Chapter 7). Although this parasomnia occurs at sleep–wake transition, it is classified with the REM-related parasomnias as it is thought to be due to intrusion of REM skeletal muscle atonia into wakefulness. Drug therapy is not usually needed, but tricyclic antidepressants such as protriptyline are often effective.

## REM sleep behavior disorder

REM sleep behavior disorder (RBD) is characterized by loss of normal REM sleep skeletal muscle atonia, and the resultant occurrence of complex motor activity associated with dream mentation[31]. Close to 90% of patients with RBD are male. It is predominantly a disorder of middle to older age, with the mean age of onset being reported in different series as 53 and 61 years[32,33]. However, RBD has been reported in younger patients, including children.

### Case 16.4

A 62-year-old man presented to a sleep clinic at the urging of his wife, who reported that he moved excessively in his sleep. He had punched and kicked her and frequently screamed aloud. On one occasion he knocked the lamp off the nightstand, bruising his fingers. As best as she could understand his shouting, he appeared to be warding off attacks. These events had been occurring for the preceding 2 years and had increased in frequency, now occurring almost nightly. He and his wife had noticed some difficulties with short-term memory over the preceding year, but they believed this was 'due to age'.

Neurological examination revealed full orientation, mild problems with attention, normal learning and difficulty copying a complex figure. He could recall only two out of four words, 5 min after learning them. He had no tremor. Tone at rest was normal, but when he shook his head, cogwheel-type rigidity built up in the right wrist. Rapid alternating movement rates were normal. His face appeared somewhat immobile, but his speech was normal. Gait and tests of postural stability were normal. A PSG showed increased phasic motor activity during REM sleep, and one episode of screaming and punching his arms in the air was recorded. No epileptiform activity was seen. After neuropsychometric testing and an magnetic resonance imaging (MRI) scan of the brain, a diagnosis of REM sleep behavior disorder in the setting of early dementia with Lewy bodies was reached. Therapy with 0.5 mg clonazepam controlled most of the events without causing worsening of his cognitive functioning.

This case illustrates typical RBD in an older man. RBD was the initial manifestation of a neurodegenerative disorder, which was diagnosed as dementia with Lewy bodies.

### Clinical features

Bed partners describe intermittent episodes of motor activity during the night, usually commencing at least 90 min after sleep onset and most frequently in the second half of the night. The patient will vocalize and often talk, laugh, yell, shout or scream. Movements include flailing of the arms, punching, kicking and jumping or falling out of bed. Sleepwalking or nocturnal wandering may occur in 10% of patients, but many of these have an overlap parasomnia disorder with both RBD and a slow-wave sleep arousal disorder[34]. About a third of patients report injuries to themselves during sleep, either while falling out of bed or by striking furniture or walls (Table 16.8)[32]. Injuries include lacerations or ecchymoses to the head, face or limbs, and fractured bones have been reported. One of our patients lacerated his hands, grabbing venetian blinds, and one kicked a hole in the bedroom wall. One patient fired an unloaded gun, while another attempted to set fire to his bed. A few patients have experienced subdural hematomas from falling out of bed. Two-thirds of sleeping partners report being assaulted; about 15% report injuries caused by punching, slapping, kicking, pulling of hair and attempted strangulation. The wife of one of our patients required dental work, while others were injured by a falling vase or picture. In contrast to sleepwalking, however, homicide has not been reported in association with RBD. Patients have constructed barriers to separate themselves from their wives, and others have tied them-

**Table 16.8**  Clinical features of 93 patients with rapid eye movement (REM) sleep behavior disorder (RBD). Reproduced with permission from reference 32

| | |
|---|---|
| Gender (93 patients) | 81 (87%) male; 12 (13%) female |
| Mean age of onset (years) (56 patients) | 60.9 (range 36–84) |
| Mean age at diagnosis (years) (93 patients) | 64.4 (range 37–85) |
| Injuries to self | 30/93 (32%) |
| Assaults on sleeping partner | 53/83 (64%) |
| Injuries to sleeping partner | 13/83 (16%) |
| Dreams associated with RBD activity | 62/67 (93%) |
| Dream content described | 37/67 (55%) |
|     defense against attack by people | 57% |
|     defense against attack by animals | 30% |
|     adventure dreams | 9% |
|     sports dreams | 2% |
|     aggression by the dreamer | 2% |

selves to the bed. Many spouses choose to sleep in a separate room. If aroused, the patient describes vivid and often violent, action-filled dreams, with his behavior frequently correlating with dream mentation. The patient usually dreams he is attempting to protect himself against attack by humans or animals. Adventure and sports dreams are sometimes reported, but the patient very rarely dreams that he is the primary aggressor. If allowed to remain asleep, the patient rarely remembers the events or dreams in the morning.

*Diagnosis and differential diagnosis*

Although the diagnosis can be suspected clinically, it is wise to confirm it by PSG. Reasons include the importance of excluding nocturnal seizures and other parasomnias, and the risk of worsening the severity of undetected sleep apnea with the use of benzodiazepines. PSG recordings should be per-

**Table 16.9**  Diagnostic criteria for rapid eye movement (REM) sleep behavior disorder[33]

| |
|---|
| PSG abnormality consisting of elevated tonic or excessive phasic muscle tone in submental or limb leads during REM sleep |
| *Either* a history of injurious or disruptive sleep behaviors *or* observation of abnormal REM sleep behaviors during the PSG |
| Absence of EEG epileptiform activity during REM sleep |

PSG, polysomnogram; EEG, electroencephalogram

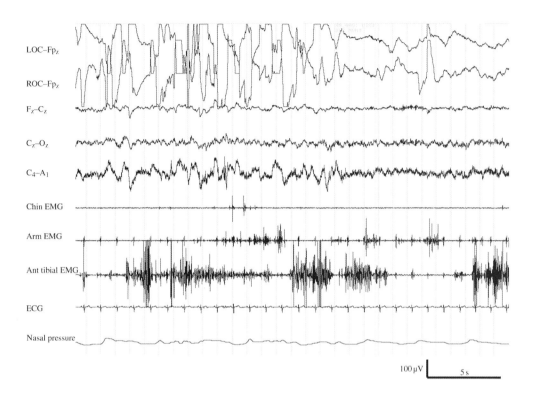

**Figure 16.2** Rapid eye movement (REM) sleep behavior disorder. This 30-s polysomnogram (PSG) fragment shows abnormally increased phasic twitching in the anterior tibial and arm electromyogram (EMG) derivations during REM sleep. Such REM sleep without atonia is the neurophysiological substrate for REM sleep behavior disorder. Channel labels as in Figure 4.1

formed with multiple EMG derivations, with recordings from at least a single muscle of each arm in addition to the usual anterior tibial and submental electrodes. If seizures are suspected in the differential diagnosis, additional EEG derivations should be used. The typical PSG findings are increased phasic twitching in REM sleep, which may be seen in limb or submental EMG leads as well as in the form of EMG artifact in the EEG derivations (Figure 16.2). Occasionally, sustained tonic muscle tone in REM sleep is present, and sometimes in patients with neurodegenerative disorders, ambiguous sleep is present with intermixing of the neurophysiological findings of REM and NREM sleep. Video and audio recordings will show gross motor activity in about half the patients studied for a single night, but the presence of abnormal EMG tone in REM sleep together with reports of abnormal nocturnal behavior from observers at home are sufficient to establish the diagnosis (Table 16.9). REM sleep without atonia is some-

**Table 16.10** Differential diagnosis of rapid eye movement (REM) sleep behavior disorder

Arousal at termination of obstructive apneas

Nocturnal seizures

Sleep terrors and sleepwalking

Nightmares

Rhythmic movement disorder

Periodic limb movements of sleep

Psychogenic dissociative states

Post-traumatic stress disorder

Malingering

**Table 16.11** Evidence that rapid eye movement (REM) sleep behavior disorder (RBD) is associated with alpha-synucleinopathies

High frequency of alpha-synucleinopathies in case series of RBD patients

High frequency of RBD in case series of patients with Parkinson's disease

High frequency of RBD in case series of patients with multiple system atrophy

Clinical and psychometric findings in patients with dementia and RBD similar to those of dementia with Lewy bodies and dissimilar to Alzheimer's disease

Autopsies of patients with RBD show alpha-synucleinopathies

PET and SPECT scans of idiopathic RBD patients show decreased striatal dopaminergic activity

PET, positron emission tomography; SPECT, single positron emission computed tomorgraphy

times seen in PSG recordings of patients without any history of dream enactment behavior or observation of such behavior in the laboratory. This finding is of uncertain significance, but in some patients it may represent an asymptomatic prodrome of RBD. MRI scans frequently show non-specific areas of increased water content, but these have not been shown to be more common in an RBD population compared with age-matched controls[32,35].

The differential diagnosis of RBD (Table 16.10) includes sudden arousals at the termination of obstructive apneas, which may involve considerable motor activity of the trunk and limbs. Seizures are rare in REM sleep, but have been occasionally reported in association with dreaming. Sleepwalking, sleep terrors, periodic limb movements of sleep, nightmares, PTSD (see Chapter 14) and rhythmic movement disorder may sometimes mimic RBD, as may psychogenic dissociative disorders.

*Etiology*

A high percentage of patients with RBD have underlying neurological disease. Case series and a review of the world literature suggest that the percentage is as high as 50–60%[36], but these figures may be inflated, as they are derived from academic centers with a higher probability of seeing patients with serious neurological disorders. A number of lines of evidence suggest that the majority of such patients will have a neurodegenerative disorder in the class known as the alpha-synucleinopathies (Table 16.11). Alpha-synuclein is a protein constituent of intracellular inclusion bodies found in Parkinson's disease

**Table 16.12** Characteristics of alpha-synucle-inopathies*

*Parkinson's disease*
Parkinsonism (rigidity, bradykinesia, rest tremor, loss of postural control)
Usually asymmetric
Idiopathic
Responsive to levodopa
Lewy body inclusions

*Dementia with Lewy bodies*
Dementia with deficits of attention and visuo-spatial ability
Fluctuating cognition
Visual hallucinations
Delusions
Depression
Parkinsonism

*Multiple system atrophy*
Combinations of:
    parkinsonism[†]
    dysautonomia[†]
    cerebellar dysfunction
    upper motor neuron dysfunction

*Neurodegenerative illnesses with inclusion bodies containing alpha-synuclein; [†]parkinsonism and dysautonomia often referred to as Shy–Drager syndrome

(PD), dementia with Lewy bodies (DLB) and multiple system atrophy (MSA) (Table 16.12 and Chapter 17). In contrast, tauopathies, not usually associated with RBD, are characterized by the presence of phosphorylated tau protein inclusion bodies, and include progressive supranuclear palsy (PSP), frontotemporal dementias and corticobasal degeneration (CBD). In one series of 53 RBD patients with neurological disease, 25 (47%) had PD (with or without dementia), seven (13%) had dementia without parkinsonism and 14 (26%) had MSA[32]. The frequency of RBD in patients with PD is 15–33%[37,38], and 58% of PD patients may have the polysomnographic finding of REM sleep without atonia. In MSA, the frequency of REM motor dyscontrol is even higher: 69–90% of MSA patients have RBD, and 90–95% have REM sleep without atonia[39,40]. RBD in MSA occurs equally in men and women, while the male predominance persists in other neurodegenerative disorders[32].

RBD in the presence of dementia suggests the presence of DLB rather than pure Alzheimer's disease (AD). A study has shown a high frequency of fluctuations, depression, delusions, visual hallucinations and parkinsonism, all features of DLB[41]. Psychometric tests of patients with dementia and RBD have been compared with controls with autopsy-proven AD[42]. The RBD group showed significantly worse performance in measures of perceptual organization, attention and visual memory, and better performance on measures of verbal memory, again similar to the pattern seen in DLB. Seven of 14 RBD patients with dementia who were followed for up to 6 years developed signs of parkinsonism[43].

Eighteen autopsies of patients with RBD have been reported[43–48]. All demonstrated the presence of alpha-synucleinopathies, and none pure AD or tauopathies. DLB was present in 13 cases (six with concomitant AD changes), PD in one, diffuse Lewy bodies but no neurological or cognitive abnormalities before death in one and MSA in three. No autopsy cases of RBD with pure AD or tauopathies have been reported. It is not known why the alpha-synucleinopathies should be associated with RBD; it is possible that the anatomical site of the pathology may be important. In particular, Lewy bodies are found in the pedunculopontine nucleus in the pontine tegmentum, an area of the brainstem involved in the control of REM atonia.

Isolated cases of other diseases associated with RBD have been reported, including brainstem vascular disorders, astrocytoma and multiple sclerosis. It can be seen in patients with narcolepsy, but the frequency has not been determined. RBD has been reported in a few clinically diagnosed cases of suspected PSP and CBD, without pathological confirmation[32,49,50]. Acute episodes of RBD may follow abrupt discontinuation of alcohol, amphetamines, barbiturates and cocaine. RBD may be associated with the use of selective serotonin reuptake inhibitors, venlafaxine and perhaps tricyclic anti-depressants. The presence of REM sleep without atonia in PTSD is controversial.

What pathology underlies idiopathic RBD? There is reason to suspect that alpha-synuclein pathology may also be present in many RBD cases without neurological abnormalities. In a retrospective study, RBD was recalled as the first neurological symptom in 52% of patients with RBD and PD, 60% of cases of dementia and RBD and 36% of cases of RBD and MSA[32]. The median time from onset of RBD to onset of other symptoms of the neurological disorder was 3–4 years. In a prospective study of 29 RBD patients with normal neurological examinations, 65% had developed parkinsonism or dementia after a mean of about 13 years from RBD onset[51]. A single case has been reported of an 84-year-old man with a 20-year history of RBD and a normal neurological examination, but autopsy findings of diffuse Lewy bodies, including in the locus ceruleus and pedunculopontine nuclei[45]. Position emission tomography (PET) and SPECT scan studies of patients with idiopathic RBD showed decreased striatal dopamine innervation compared with controls, with the degree of abnormality being less than in symptomatic PD[52,53]. The most likely explanation is that some of the patients had presymptomatic PD, but a primary involvement of the basal ganglia in the pathogenesis of RBD is a possible alternative explanation.

*Management*

Not all patients with RBD require drug treatment, and the first step in management involves improving the safety of the sleep environment. Furniture should be moved away from the bedside, a mattress placed on the floor next to the bed and weapons kept out of the bedroom. Bed partners of patients with RBD may need to move into a separate bed. The standard medical treatment of RBD is the use of clonazepam in doses of 0.25–2.0 mg before sleep. Close to 90% of patients have complete or partial relief of symptoms with the medication[32,33]. Side-effects, such as daytime sedation, cognitive impairment, gait unsteadiness during the night and impotence, limit its use, especially in older patients. Clonazepam reduces phasic twitching in RBD, but does not restore REM atonia[54]. It should be used with considerable caution in patients with dementia, gait difficulties, untreated obstructive sleep

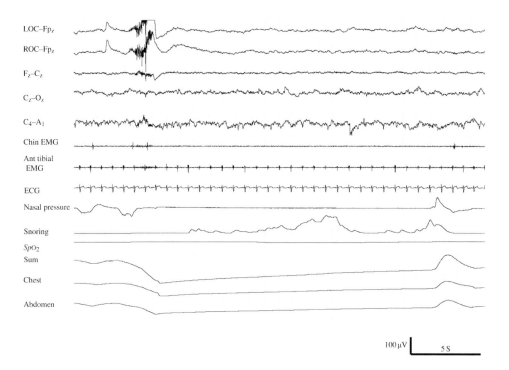

**Figure 16.3** Catathrenia (nocturnal expiratory groaning). This 30-s polysomnogram (PSG) fragment shows catathrenia (prolonged expiratory groaning) in rapid eye movement (REM) sleep. Expiration is indicated by upward deflections on the airflow and impedance plethysmography channels. Note the 20-s prolonged expiration with slowly rising signals on the airflow and plethysmography channels, commencing at the end of an inspiratory breath. The sonogram channel demonstrates accompanying vocalization during the expiration, which on an audio recording would sound like a prolonged moan. Channel labels as in Figure 4.1

apnea syndrome or nocturnal stridor (as may be seen in MSA, see Chapter 17). Other benzodiazepines have been used in small numbers of patients, but their efficacy is less well established. Agents such as clozapine and quetiapine have been used, especially in patients who also have dementia-related nocturnal confusion. A number of open trials of melatonin in doses of 3–12 mg before bed have been reported with apparent success[55–57].

## Sleep-related painful erections

These are characterized by penile pain causing arousals during erections associated with REM sleep. This very rare condition is not usually associated with apparent penile pathology, although Peyronie's disease may occasionally be present. If no local pathology can be detected, REM-suppressant agents such as tricyclic antidepressants can be used.

## Catathrenia (nocturnal expiratory groaning)

This rare idiopathic condition is characterized by high-pitched, monotonous, irregular groans, which occur during prolonged expirations[58,59]. They follow deep inspirations and last a median of 10 s, although some may continue for almost a minute (Figure 16.3). They occur in repeated clusters, each lasting several minutes to an hour. They arise mainly in REM sleep, but are not associated with abnormal muscle tone or any other sleep-disordered breathing. They commence in the first to the third decade, and severely disturb the sleep of the bed partner. The sound is felt to be due to partial glottic closure of uncertain origin. Treatment with benzodiazepines, antidepressants and nasal continuous positive airway pressure (nCPAP) has been unsuccessful.

## NON-STATE-DEPENDENT PARASOMNIAS

### Rhythmic movement disorder

This category of parasomnia includes conditions previously known as head banging, body rocking and jactatio capitis nocturna. It comprises a group of stereotyped, repetitive movements of large muscles, usually of the head, neck and trunk, but sometimes the legs. It may occur in any stage of sleep, including REM sleep, but most often occurs prior to the onset of sleep and persists into light sleep. In some patients it seems to be semivoluntary, and is utilized as a sleep-inducing aid, while in others it occurs entirely during sleep. While it is common in infants and usually resolves by about 4 years of age, it may sometimes persist through childhood and into adulthood. It is especially common in mentally handicapped children, and occasionally skull injuries can occur in this group. The cause is unknown. On PSG it appears as high-amplitude rhythmic movement artifact at 0.5–2 Hz, usually visible in all EEG derivations as well as in respiratory and other channels. It should not be confused with spike and wave activity. Treatment usually involves reassurance, and padding around the crib, but protective headgear may sometimes be necessary. Benzodiazepines and tricyclic antidepressants have been tried with variable success.

### Bruxism

Intermittent clenching or grinding of the teeth during sleep is common, with a reported prevalence of 8%[60]. It may occur at any age and during any stage of sleep. Consequences can include damage to the teeth and gums, facial pain and disturbance of the bed partner. The etiology is unknown, although anxiety may play a role in some patients. It occasionally occurs at termination of obstructive apneas, leading to the hypothesis that it may be a non-specific arousal phenomenon. It is easily recognized on a PSG as approximately 1 Hz rhythmic activity recorded from the electro-oculogram (EOG) and $A_1$ or $A_2$ EEG electrodes, and consisting of movement artifact with superimposed EMG activity (Figure 16.4). Therapy most often involves the use of a dental occlusal appliance.

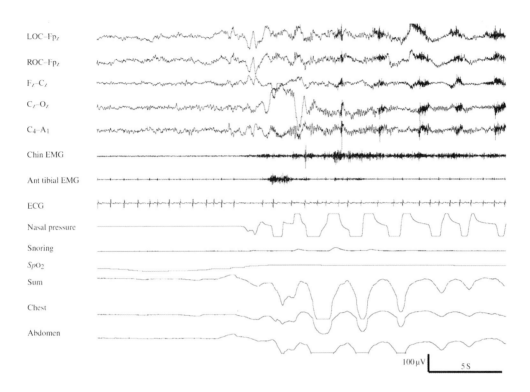

LOC–Fp_1

ROC–Fp_1

F_1–C_1

C_1–O_1

C_4–A_1

Chin EMG

Ant tibial EMG

ECG

Nasal pressure

Snoring

SpO_2

Sum

Chest

Abdomen

100 µV   5 S

**Figure 16.4** Bruxism. This 30-s polysomnogram (PSG) fragment shows an arousal following termination of an obstructive apnea. Five bursts of electromyogram (EMG) activity can be seen in the electroencephalogram (EEG) and electro-oculogram (EOG) derivations following the arousal. This activity is typical of bruxism, which may be associated with arousals from apneas. Channel labels as in Figure 4.1.

## Nocturnal enuresis

Recurrent involuntary micturition during sleep is normal during early childhood, and is only considered a possible disorder after the age of 5 years. However, up to 8% of boys and 4% of girls are still enuretic at age 12 years[61]. Enuresis can occur during NREM or REM sleep. Genetic factors appear to play a role in persistent enuresis, and enuretic children have a small functional bladder capacity. Organic urinary conditions should be ruled out, especially in rare cases of secondary enuresis (enuresis reoccurring after a period of continence). Behavioral techniques are usually effective, especially in motivated families. These include the use of a urine alarm, scheduled awakenings with the child guided to the bathroom before enuresis occurs and retention control training. Imipramine has been used, but provides only temporary relief with the potential for side-effects. Desmopressin acetate, a vasopressin analog, given intranasally before bed may reduce urine volume, but also works only as long as the drug is administered.

## REFERENCES

1. Broughton RJ. Sleep disorders: disorders of arousal? Enuresis, somnambulism, and nightmares occur in confusional states of arousal, not in 'dreaming sleep'. *Science* 1968;159:1070–8

2. Kavey NB, Whyte J. Somnambulism associated with hallucinations. *Psychosomatics* 1993;34:86–90

3. Hublin C, Kaprio J, Partinen M, Heikkila K, Koskenvuo M. Prevalence and genetics of sleepwalking: a population-based twin study. *Neurology* 1997;48:177–81

4. Ohayon MM, Guilleminault C, Priest RG. Night terrors, sleepwalking, and confusional arousals in the general population: their frequency and relationship to other sleep and mental disorders. *J Clin Psychiatry* 1999;60:268–76

5. Bassetti C, Vella S, Donati F, Wielepp P, Weder B. SPECT during sleepwalking [Letter]. *Lancet* 2000;356:484–5

6. Ohayon MM, Caulet M, Priest RG. Violent behavior during sleep. *J Clin Psychiatry* 1997;58:369–76

7. Bonkalo A. Impulsive acts and confusional states during incomplete arousal from sleep: criminological and forensic implications. *Psychiatr Q* 1974;48:400–9

8. Fenwick P. Sleep and sexual offending. *Med Sci Law* 1996;36:122–34

9. Rosenfeld DS, Elhajjar AJ. Sleepsex: a variant of sleepwalking. *Arch Sex Behav* 1998; 27:269–78

10. Broughton R, Billings R, Cartwright R, *et al.* Homicidal somnambulism: a case report. *Sleep* 1994;17:253–64

11. Mahowald MW, Bundlie SR, Hurwitz TD, Schenck CH. Sleep violence – forensic science implications: polygraphic and video documentation. *J Forens Sci* 1990;35:413–32

12. Schenck CH, Pareja JA, Patterson AL, Mahowald MW. Analysis of polysomnographic events surrounding 252 slow-wave sleep arousals in thirty-eight adults with injurious sleepwalking and sleep terrors. *J Clin Neurophysiol* 1998;15:159–66

13. Daube JR, Cascino GD, Dotson RM, Silber MH, Westmoreland BF. Clinical neurophysiology. *Continuum* 1998;4:149–72

14. Espa F, Ondze B, Deglise P, Billiard M, Besset A. Sleep architecture, slow wave activity, and sleep spindles in adult patients with sleepwalking and sleep terrors. *Clin Neurophysiol* 2000;111:929–39

15. Gaudreau H, Joncas S, Zadra A, Montplaisir J. Dynamics of slow-wave activity during the NREM sleep of sleepwalkers and control subjects. *Sleep* 2000;23:755–60

16. Guilleminault C, Poyares D, Abat F, Palombini L. Sleep and wakefulness in somnambulism – a spectral analysis study. *J Psychosom Res* 2001;51:411–16

17. Frank NC, Spirito A, Stark L, Owens-Stively J. The use of scheduled awakenings to eliminate childhood sleepwalking. *J Pediatr Psychol* 1997;22:345–53

18. Lask B. Novel and non-toxic treatment for night terrors. *Br Med J* 1988;297:592

19. Hurwitz TD, Mahowald MW, Schenck CH, Schluter JL, Bundlie SR. A retrospective

outcome study and review of hypnosis as treatment of adults with sleepwalking and sleep terror. *J Nerv Ment Dis* 1991; 179:228–33

20. Schenck CH, Mahowald MW. Long-term, nightly benzodiazepine treatment of injurious parasomnias and other disorders of disrupted nocturnal sleep in 170 adults. *Am J Med* 1996;100:333–7

21. Schenck CH, Hurwitz TD, O'Connor KA, Mahowald MW. Additional categories of sleep-related eating disorders and the current status of treatment. *Sleep* 1993; 16:457–66

22. Morgenthaler TI, Silber MH. Amnestic sleep related eating disorder associated with zolpidem. *Sleep Med* 2002;3:323–8

23. Birketvedt GS, Florholmen J, Sundsfjord J, *et al.* Behavioral and neuroendocrine characteristics of the night-eating syndrome. *J Am Med Assoc* 1999;282:657–63

24. Silber MH, Hansen MR, Girish M. Complex nocturnal visual hallucinations. *Sleep* 2002; 25:A484

25. Manford M, Andermann F. Complex visual hallucinations. Clinical and neurobiological insights. *Brain Res* 1998;121:1819–40

26. Hauri PJ, Friedman M, Ravaris CL. Sleep in patients with spontaneous panic attacks. *Sleep* 1989;12:323–37

27. Pierce JMS. Clinical features of the exploding head syndrome. *J Neurol Neurosurg Psychiatry* 1989;52:907–10

28. Janson C, Gislason T, De Backer W, *et al.* Prevalence of sleep disturbances among young adults in three European countries. *Sleep* 1995;18:589–97

29. Krakow B, Johnston L, Melendrez D, *et al.* An open-label trial of evidence-based cognitive behavioral therapy for nightmares and insomnia in crime victims with PTSD. *Am J Psychiatry* 2001;158:2043–7

30. Ohayon MM, Zulley J, Guilleminault C, Smirne S. Prevalence and pathologic associations of sleep paralysis in the general population. *Neurology* 1999;52:1194–2000

31. Schenck CH, Mahowald MW. REM sleep behavior disorder: clinical, developmental, and neuroscience perspectives 16 years after its formal identification in SLEEP. *Sleep* 2002;25:120–38

32. Olson EJ, Boeve BF, Silber MH. Rapid eye movement sleep behavior disorder: demographic, clinical and laboratory findings in 93 cases. *Brain* 2000;123:331–9

33. Schenck CH, Hurwitz TD, Mahowald MW. REM sleep behaviour disorder: an update on a series of 96 patients and a review of the world literature. *J Sleep Res* 1993;2:224–31

34. Schenck CH, Boyd JL, Mahowald MW. A parasomnia overlap disorder involving sleepwalking, sleep terrors, and REM sleep behavior disorder in 33 polysomnographically confirmed cases. *Sleep* 1997;20:972–81

35. Culebras A, Moore JT. Magnetic resonance findings in REM sleep behavior disorder. *Neurology* 1989;39:1519–23

36. Schenck CH, Mahowald MW. REM sleep parasomnias. *Neurol Clin* 1996;14:697–720

37. Comella CL, Nardine TM, Diederich NJ, Stebbins GT. Sleep-related violence, injury, and REM sleep behavior disorder in Parkinson's disease. *Neurology* 1998;51: 526–9

38. Gagnon J, Bedard M, Fantini M, *et al.* REM sleep behavior disorder and REM sleep without atonia in Parkinson's disease. *Neurology* 2002;59:585–9

39. Plazzi G, Corsini R, Provini F, *et al.* REM sleep behavior disorders in multiple system atrophy. *Neurology* 1997;48:1094–7

40. Tachibana N, Kimura K, Kitajima K, Shinde A, Kimura J, Shibasaki H. REM sleep motor dysfunction in multiple system atrophy: with special emphasis on sleep talk as its early clinical manifestation. *J Neurol Neurosurg Psychiatry* 1997;63:678–81

41. Boeve BF, Silber MH, Ferman TJ, *et al.* REM sleep behavior disorder and degenerative dementia: an association likely reflecting Lewy body disease. *Neurology* 1998;51:363–70

42. Ferman TJ, Boeve BF, Smith GE, *et al.* REM sleep behavior disorder and dementia: cognitive differences when compared with AD. *Neurology* 1999;52:951–7

43. Ferman TJ, Boeve BF, Smith GE, *et al.* Dementia with Lewy bodies may present as dementia and REM sleep behavior disorder without Parkinsonism or hallucinations. *J Int Neuropsychol Soc* 2002;8:907–14

44. Boeve B, Silber MH, Parisi JE, *et al.* Synucleinopathy pathology and REM sleep behavior disorder plus dementia or parkinsonism. *Neurology* 2003;61:40–5

45. Uchiyama M, Isse K, Tanaka K, *et al.* Incidental Lewy body disease in a patient with REM sleep behavior disorder. *Neurology* 1995;45:709–12

46. Schenck CH, Mahowald MW, Anderson ML, Silber MH, Boeve BF, Parisi JE. Lewy body variant of Alzheimer's disease (AD) identified by postmortem ubiquitin staining in a previously reported case of AD associated with REM sleep behavior disorder [Letter]. *Biol Psychiatry* 1997;42:527–8

47. Arnulf I, Bonnet AM, Damier P, *et al.* Hallucinations, REM sleep, and Parkinson's disease: a medical hypothesis. *Neurology* 2000;55:281–8

48. Turner RS, D'Amato CJ, Chervin RD, Blaivas M. The pathology of REM sleep behavior disorder with comorbid Lewy body dementia. *Neurology* 2000;55:1730–2

49. Pareja JA, Caminero AB, Masa JF, Dobato JL. A first case of progressive supranuclear palsy and pre-clinical REM sleep behavior disorder presenting as inhibition of speech during wakefulness and somniloquy with phasic muscle twitching during REM sleep. *Neurologia* 1996;11:304–6

50. Kimura K, Tachibana N, Aso T, Kimura J, Shibasaki H. Subclinical REM sleep behavior disorder in a patient with corticobasal degeneration. *Sleep* 1997;20:891–4

51. Schenck CH, Bundlie SR, Mahowald MW. REM behavior disorder (RBD): delayed emergence of Parkinsonism and/or dementia in 65% of older men initially diagnosed with idiopathic RBD, and an analysis of the minimum and maximum tonic and/or phasic electromyographic abnormalities found during REM sleep [Abstract]. *Sleep* 2003;26:A316

52. Albin RL, Koeppe RA, Chervin RD, Consens FB, Wernette K, Frey KA. Decreased striatal dopaminergic innervation in REM sleep behavior disorder. *Neurology* 2000;55:1410–12

53. Eisensehr I, Linke R, Noachtar S, Scwarz J, Gildehaus FJ, Tatsch K. Reduced striatal dopamine transporters in idiopathic rapid eye movement sleep behaviour disorder – comparison with Parkinson's disease and controls. *Brain Res* 2000;123:1155–60

54. Lapierre O, Montplaisir J. Polysomnographic features of REM sleep behavior disorder: development of a scoring method. *Neurology* 1992;42:1371–4

55. Boeve BF, Silber MH, Ferman TJ. Melatonin for treatment of REM sleep behavior disorder in neurologic disorders: results in 14 patients. *Sleep Med* 2003;4:281–4

56. Kunz D, Bes F. Melatonin as a therapy in REM sleep behavior disorder patients: an open-labeled pilot study on the possible influence of melatonin on REM-sleep regulation. *Mov Dis* 1999;14:507–11

57. Takeuchi N, Uchimura N, Hashizume Y, *et al*. Melatonin therapy for REM sleep behavior disorder. *Psychiatr Clin Neurosci* 2001; 55:267–9

58. Vertrugno R, Provini F, Plazzi G, *et al*. Catathrenia (nocturnal groaning): a new type of parasomnia. *Neurology* 2001;56: 681–3

59. Pevernagie DA, Boon PA, Mariman AN, Verhaeghen DB, Pauwels RA. Vocalization during episodes of prolonged expiration: a parasomnia related to REM sleep. *Sleep Med* 2001;2:19–30

60. Lavigne GJ, Montplaisir JY. Restless legs syndrome and sleep bruxism: prevalence and association among Canadians. *Sleep* 1994;17:739–43

61. Friman PC. Nocturnal enuresis in the child. In Ferber R, Kryger M, eds. *Principles and Practice of Sleep Medicine in the Child*. Philadelphia: WB Saunders, 1995

# Chapter 17

# Sleep in patients with parkinsonism and dementia

*When you are old and gray and full of sleep,*
*And nodding by the fire,…*

**W.B. Yeats, *When you are Old***

It has become increasingly clear that sleep disturbances are integral components of many of the common degenerative disorders of the nervous system that affect the elderly. As the distribution of the population shifts upwards in age, understanding and management of these sleep disorders will become more important. This chapter considers sleep issues in disorders causing parkinsonism and dementia.

Parkinsonism is a clinical syndrome with diverse causes characterized by at least two of the following four physical signs: rest tremor, rigidity, bradykinesia and loss of postural reflexes. The commonest cause of parkinsonism is Parkinson's disease (PD), but less common causes of parkinsonism such as multiple system atrophy and progressive supranuclear palsy are also associated with abnormalities of sleep. About 60–80% of patients with dementia have Alzheimer's disease (AD). Dementia with Lewy bodies (DLB) is now considered the second most common irreversible cause of dementia, accounting for approximately 15–25% of cases.

## PARKINSON'S DISEASE

Parkinson's disease is a neurodegenerative disorder with specific pathology (Lewy inclusion bodies), initial asymmetry of clinical features and responsiveness to levodopa therapy. The motor manifestations of PD are caused by degeneration of dopaminergic neurons of the substantia nigra that project to the striatum. PD is managed by the administration of levodopa (converted to dopamine in the neurons of the substantia nigra) or dopamine agonists, which act postsynaptically by binding to dopamine receptors on cells of the striatum.

Sleep disorders are common in PD, being reported in 76–86% of patients in clinic-based series and 60% of community patients[1–3]. They may be due to the symptoms of PD, primary sleep disorders (some related and some unrelated to PD), medication effects, depression or circadian dysrhythmias, usually associated with dementia. The following account is a symptom-based approach to the sleep problems most com-

**Table 17.1** Sleep problems in Parkinson's disease

Insomnia

Hypersomnia

Excessive motor activity at night

Hallucinations and behavioral problems at night

**Table 17.2** Mechanisms of insomnia in Parkinson's disease

Symptoms of Parkinson's disease

    bradykinesia

    tremor

    nocturia

    early-morning dystonia

Primary sleep disorders

    restless legs syndrome

Effects of medication

    dopaminergic agents

Depression

Circadian dysrhythmias

monly experienced in patients with PD (Table 17.1). A careful sleep history from the patient and sleeping partner or care-giver often helps to dissect out which of the many factors are the most important.

## Insomnia

### Symptoms of Parkinson's disease

The symptoms of PD themselves (Table 17.2) can result in insomnia if they are subopti-mally treated. A normal adult sleeper changes position two or three times an hour[4]. Bradykinesia during the night can result in difficulty with turning over in bed, resulting in awakenings and complaints of pain and stiffness. Parkinsonian tremor can persist during the night, resulting in diffi-culty in maintaining sleep continuity. It most often occurs during periods of wakefulness, during epochs of sleep preceding wakeful-ness or during epochs in which there is a transition from deeper to lighter stages of sleep[5]. Nocturia is more commonly reported in PD patients than in age-matched con-trols[1]. While this may be partly the result of awakenings from other causes, detrusor hyperreflexia is commonly found on urody-namic studies in PD. Uncomfortable early-morning dystonia may also wake a PD patient from sleep. If parkinsonian symp-toms are suspected as the cause for insom-nia, increased doses of PD medications are required before sleep, including controlled-release forms of levodopa, and long-acting dopamine agonists.

### Primary sleep disorders: restless legs syndrome

Restless legs syndrome (RLS) may be more common in PD than in age-matched con-trols[6], although this has not been assessed adequately with current criteria. However, RLS occurs sufficiently frequently in older persons for this condition to be considered carefully in the differential diagnosis of PD patients with insomnia. Associated periodic limb movements may also be present, some-times causing sleep fragmentation[7]. The management of uncontrolled RLS in PD can be challenging, as most patients are already taking levodopa, often in doses likely to cause daytime augmentation (see Chapter

15). In this situation, a change from levodopa to a dopamine agonist such as pramipexole or ropinirole is often desirable, but this may result in less satisfactory control of motor symptoms. Alternatively, addition of an opioid, gabapentin or a benzodiazepine may provide relief.

### Effect of medication

Levodopa and the dopamine agonists are alerting agents, and in some patients may cause sleep-onset or sleep-maintenance insomnia. Affected patients will describe being wide-awake or feeling 'wired'. It is often possible to obtain a clear history of the insomnia starting immediately after initiation of the drug or an increase in the dose. It is sometimes possible to reduce evening doses of dopaminergic agents without causing an increase in the motor symptoms at night, but otherwise the addition of a benzodiazepine such as temazepam or a sedating antidepressant such as trazodone may prevent the drug-induced insomnia.

### Depression

Depression is more common in PD than in controls, and may occur more frequently than in other chronic neurological disorders[2]. It should be actively considered in any PD patient complaining of insomnia. It may be challenging to diagnose in PD, as some of the neurovegetative symptoms of depression may be ascribed to the bradykinesia of the underlying disorder. The presence of anxiety should also be considered. If depression is suspected, a trial of antidepressant therapy should be undertaken. No specific groups of antidepressants have been shown to be superior in the management of depression in PD, and tricyclic antidepressants, selective serotonin reuptake inhibitors, trazodone and other agents have been successfully used.

### Circadian dysrhythmias

Disturbances of circadian sleep–wake rhythms with inappropriate wakefulness during the night and sleep during the day may occur in PD, especially if an associated dementia is present. Management is discussed below in the section on 'Hallucinations and behavioral problems at night'.

## Hypersomnia

### Symptoms of Parkinson's disease

Disrupted sleep from inadequately controlled motor symptoms at night may cause secondary daytime sleepiness (Table 17.3). However, this does not seem to be the major

**Table 17.3** Mechanisms of hypersomnia in Parkinson's disease (PD)

| |
|---|
| Symptoms of Parkinson's disease |
|     sleep disturbance from bradykinesia, tremor or nocturia |
|     an intrinsic disorder of hypersomnia in PD |
| Primary sleep disorders |
|     obstructive sleep apnea syndrome |
|     periodic limb movements of sleep |
| Effects of medication |
|     dopaminergic agents |
| Depression |
| Circadian dysrhythmias |

cause in most sleepy PD patients, and it appears likely that, in some, sleepiness may be a primary symptom of the disease itself. A community-based study of PD showed that 27% of patients complained of daytime sleepiness. Compared with those without sleepiness, somnolence did not appear to be related to nocturnal sleeping complaints or to the use of dopamine agonists. The sleepy patients had more severe parkinsonism, lower cognitive functioning and more hallucinations[8]. A study of 27 treated PD patients revealed[9] mean multiple sleep latency test (MSLT) latencies of less than 5 min in 19% of patients, with shorter latencies correlating with higher sleep efficiency and longer nocturnal total sleep time. Patients with short MSLT latencies were more likely to have longer disease duration, hallucinations and sleep-onset rapid eye movement (REM) periods (SOREMPs). In a study of ten treated PD patients with vivid hallucinations compared with ten PD patients without hallucinations[10], the hallucinating patients were more likely to have shorter sleep latencies and SOREMPs on MSLT. Cerebrospinal fluid (CSF) hypocretin-1 was found to be absent in nine of 19 patients with advanced PD, and low compared with age-matched controls in the other ten[11]. In contrast, levels were normal in three sleepy PD patients with early disease[12]. These and other reports have led to the hypothesis that PD may be associated with an intrinsic, narcolepsy-like disorder of sleepiness, commoner in patients with more advanced disease.

### Primary sleep disorders

As respiratory function tests demonstrate upper airway obstruction during wakefulness in PD[13], one could predict that obstructive sleep apnea syndrome (OSAS) might be a common problem. However, few data are available on the prevalence of sleep-disordered breathing in PD, and in one study, OSAS did not appear to be more common in PD than in controls[14]. Nevertheless, OSAS is sufficiently common in older patients that a careful history of snoring, snort arousals and observed apneas should be taken in any sleepy PD patient. If present, management of OSAS is similar to that in a patient without PD (see Chapter 8). Periodic limb movements of sleep in PD are discussed below under 'Excessive motor activity at night'.

### Effects of medication

An influential report appeared in 1999 describing eight PD patients treated with pramipexole or ropinirole who experienced sudden, overwhelming episodes of sleepiness while driving[15]. The episodes ceased after the medication was discontinued or the dose reduced. This led to considerable concern that non-ergot dopamine agonists could cause 'sleep attacks'. However, other case reports of sleepiness induced by bromocriptine, pergolide and levodopa indicate that any dopaminergic agent may sometimes induce hypersomnolence[16,17]. In a study of 236 PD patients, episodes of sudden, irresistible sleepiness correlated on multivariate analysis with the use of ropinirole and bromocriptine[18]. A retrospective chart review of patients receiving pramipexole during a clinical trial showed no significant difference in the frequency of hypersomnia in patients taking the drug compared with placebo. However, in the open-label phase of the study, 38% of 37 patients complained of moderate or severe sleepiness[19]. In contrast, no 'sleep attacks' were identified in a study of 55 PD patients, and sleepiness measured by the Epworth sleepiness scale was not associated with any medication, and specifically not with pramipexole[20]. A multicenter study of 638 PD patients revealed no correlation between sleepiness and any specific dopaminergic medication, while falling asleep at the wheel without warning occurred in only 0.7% of drivers[21]. A polysomnogram recorded in a PD patient with sudden episodes of sleep, but not taking non-ergot dopaminergic agents, revealed a rapid transition from wakefulness to stage 2 non-rapid eye movement (NREM) sleep[22]. A study of a large cohort of PD patients showed that sleepiness correlated with levodopa dose, the use of agonists and disease severity[23]. However, together these three factors accounted for only 9% of the sleepiness, suggesting the presence of other as yet undetermined factors.

The concept of 'sleep attacks' is controversial; most patients with any cause of sleepiness will experience a prodrome of drowsiness before falling asleep, although some may fall asleep abruptly without warning. There is little evidence to suggest that the sleepiness induced by dopaminergic agents in a minority of patients is different from that caused by other problems such as obstructive sleep apnea syndrome, narcolepsy or sleep deprivation. Dopamine generally produces arousal, and the mechanism of paradoxical drowsiness is uncertain. In order to determine the exact prevalence of drug-induced sleepiness in PD, large studies excluding other causes of hypersomnolence will be needed.

Other causes of sleepiness, such as OSAS, should be considered before determining that it is due to medication or the disease itself. Dopaminergic agents should be used at the lowest effective dose, patients should be warned about this potential side-effect before commencing treatment and questions about sleepiness should be routinely asked at return visits. Should sleepiness develop, the dose should be reduced, other causes sought and driving restricted until the problem is elucidated[17]. Stimulant therapy with modafinil or methylphenidate should be considered if hypersomnolence persists or dopaminergic therapy is essential for the well-being of the patient[24]. A placebo-controlled trial of sleepy PD patients showed significant decreases in the Epworth sleepiness scale with modafinil treatment, but no change in the maintenance of wakefulness test[25].

## Depression

Some patients with depression complain of fatigue and sleepiness, and this diagnosis should always be considered in hypersomnolent PD patients.

## Circadian dysrhythmias

As discussed above under 'Insomnia', PD patients with reversal of sleep–wake rhythms may present with wakefulness at night and excessive sleep during the day.

### Case 17.1

A 62-year-old woman presented with an asymmetric rest tremor of her hands, slowness in walking and reduced intensity of her speech. A diagnosis of Parkinson's disease was made and she was treated with one tablet of carbidopa/levodopa

25/100 mg three times a day. After a year her symptoms worsened, and the dose of medication was slowly increased to two and a half tablets three times a day (total daily levodopa dose of 750 mg). She then noticed a period of intense somnolence occurring about 30 min after each dose, lasting 60–90 min. This was severe enough that she had to lie down and sleep. She had no symptoms to suggest sleep-disordered breathing or restless legs, and slept relatively undisturbed for 8 h each night. Cognitive function was normal and she had not experienced hallucinations. Reduction in the dose of carbidopa/levodopa resulted in resolution of the sleepiness but unacceptable control of her motor symptoms. Her medication was changed to pramipexole with better control of parkinsonism and no recurrence of hypersomnolence.

This case illustrates how occasionally any dopaminergic medication, including levodopa, can paradoxically cause sleepiness. The diagnosis in this patient was easy because of the onset of hypersomnia after the increase in dose, the clear temporal relationship to the time of administration of the drug and resolution of the symptom on reducing the dose. In many patients, especially with more advanced disease, multiple mechanisms may contribute, and sleep studies may be needed to help untangle the factors responsible.

## Excessive motor activity at night

*Symptoms of Parkinson's disease and effects of medications*

A careful history from a bed partner and the patient can usually establish whether the abnormal movements observed during the night are due to tremor or drug-induced dyskinesias (Table 17.4). If tremor is responsible, then an increased dose of controlled-release levodopa or a dopamine agonist before sleep is required. In contrast, if the symptoms are due to peak-dose dyskinesias, then a reduction of levodopa dose is needed. Sometimes the presleep dose needs to be given as two smaller doses, one before bed and the other on waking during the night. Alternatively, a dopamine agonist before bed can be substituted for levodopa.

*REM sleep behavior disorder*

As early as 1971, a case of 'violent dreams' in PD was reported[26], and in 1975 it was recog-

**Table 17.4** Mechanisms of excessive motor activity at night in Parkinson's disease

| |
| --- |
| Symptoms of Parkinson's disease |
|     tremor |
| Primary sleep disorders |
|     REM sleep behavior disorder |
|     periodic limb movements of sleep |
| Effects of medication |
|     levodopa-induced dyskinesias |

REM, rapid eye movement

nized that the electromyogram (EMG) continued to show muscle activity during REM sleep in PD patients[27]. As discussed in Chapter 16, REM sleep behavior disorder (RBD) occurs in 15–33% of PD patients[28,29], and PD is identified in 13–27% of RBD patients[30,31]. Dream enactment behavior commenced before any other symptoms of PD in 52% of 25 patients with both PD and RBD[30], and 38% of 29 patients with RBD of apparently uncertain cause had developed parkinsonism 6 years later[32].

The diagnosis and management of RBD is discussed in Chapter 16. While a polysomnogram (PSG) is generally required for diagnosis, RBD can sometimes be presumed to be present in the setting of PD when a classic history is obtained. Clonazepam should be used with caution in the presence of gait instability, and alternatives such as improving the safety of the bed environment or recommending other medications should be considered.

*Periodic limb movements of sleep*

Periodic limb movements of sleep (PLMS) have been shown to be more frequent in PD patients compared with controls[7]. While PLMS can fragment sleep, they are common in asymptomatic older subjects, and care should be taken not to overemphasize their clinical significance, especially if the majority are not accompanied by arousals (see Chapter 15). Indications for treatment include associated troublesome restless legs syndrome or disturbance of the sleep of a bed partner. Management includes the use of dopamine agonists, gabapentin or a benzodiazepine.

**Table 17.5** Mechanisms of hallucinations and behavioral problems at night

| |
| --- |
| Primary sleep disorders |
|     REM sleep behavior disorder |
| Effect of medications |
|     dopaminergic agents |
| Circadian dysrhythmia |
|     confusion with dementia |

REM, rapid eye movement

## Hallucinations and behavioral problems at night

Levodopa can cause a spectrum of increasingly severe abnormalities of perception and behavior as PD advances. Vivid dreams and nightmares are common; in one study, 24% of PD patients on medication complained of unpleasant or frightening dreams, compared with less than 2% of controls[1]. Patients on levodopa can also experience waking hallucinations, that are usually visual and can be well formed and vivid. At least initially, their sense of reality is preserved, and they perceive the experiences to be hallucinatory. Later, however, levodopa can cause confusional states, often manifest during the night. Dopaminergic agonists can have similar effects (Table 17.5).

Approximately one-third of PD patients develop, with time, a dementing illness characterized pathologically by diffuse Lewy bodies, sometimes with associated Alzheimer changes. Confusional behavior can occur, which is often perceived by care-givers to be worse at night, as it interferes with their sleep. This has given rise to the term 'sun-

Table 17.6 Distinguishing rapid eye movement (REM) sleep behavior disorder (RBD) from nocturnal confusion and wandering in Parkinson's disease patients

| Insomnia | RBD | Nocturnal confusion and wandering |
|---|---|---|
| Duration | less than 30 min | more than 30 min |
| Site | usually in bed | usually out of bed |
| Type of behavior | flailing, kicking, shouting | wandering, talking |
| Perception to observer | asleep and dreaming | awake but confused |
| Polysomnogram | typical behavior during REM sleep without atonia | typical behavior during wakefulness, often with slow EEG rhythms |

EEG, electroencephalogram

downing', but objective observations have shown that confusion in dementia can occur at any time. It is important to distinguish this nocturnal confusional behavior from REM sleep behavior disorder, as the management is different (Table 17.6). This can most often be achieved by a careful history from a care-giver, and polysomnography is rarely needed. Most RBD behavior occurs in bed, while confusion is often manifested by wandering behavior. In RBD, observers will describe the patient as asleep, but acting out dreams, while 'sundowning' patients appear to be awake but confused. RBD episodes usually last minutes, while confused wanderings often continue for hours. If a PSG is performed, RBD behavior is seen to occur during REM sleep without atonia, while 'sundowning' occurs during wakefulness, often with abnormally slow background electroencephalogram (EEG) rhythms, after waking from NREM sleep. As a high percentage of PD patients have REM sleep without atonia, even without a history of abnormal motor activity, the actual behavior described by care-givers must be observed during the sleep study before a definite conclusion can be reached regarding its nature.

The management of abnormal behavior at night in a patient with PD can be challenging. Once RBD has been excluded, either by history or a PSG, consideration should be given to reducing the dose of dopaminergic agents. Occasionally, these drugs may have to be at least temporarily discontinued altogether, often during a hospital admission, in case overwhelming rigidity and akinesia develop. If this is ineffective, then confusion should be treated directly, initially by behavioral methods. Conventional neuroleptics may worsen PD, and should be avoided if at all possible. Quetiapine, with minimal extrapyramidal effects, is usually the first agent used, commencing at a dose of 25 mg before sleep (see below under 'Alzheimer's disease' for more details).

## MULTIPLE SYSTEM ATROPHY

Multiple system atrophy (MSA) is a neurodegenerative disease characterized by combinations of progressive parkinsonism, dys-autonomia, cerebellar dysfunction and pyramidal signs. When the predominant features are dysautonomia and parkinsonism, it is sometimes referred to as Shy–Drager syndrome. Degenerative cell loss and gliosis is present in the substantia nigra, various pontomedullary nuclei and cerebellar Purkinje cells, with characteristic glial or neuronal inclusions, but no Lewy bodies. The mean duration of disease from onset to death is 8–10 years[33]. Respiratory and motor sleep disorders (Table 17.7) are extremely common in all forms of MSA, with 70% of patients complaining of sleep disturbances[34].

### Sleep-disordered breathing

A range of centrally mediated disturbances in respiration are seen in MSA. These include vocal cord dysfunction, obstructive and central sleep apnea syndrome, respiratory dysrhythmias and central neurogenic hypoventilation. Abnormal patterns of respiration reported include periodic breathing in the erect position, Cheyne–Stokes, apneustic, cluster and irregular breathing. The $CO_2$ response curve may be flattened[35]. Central neurogenic alveolar hypoventilation causing hypercapnic respiratory failure during sleep and later during wakefulness may occur, and can result in death. Degeneration of the neuronal circuitry in the pons and medulla controlling respiration is the presumed pathophysiological mechanism responsible for these disorders.

One of the most important respiratory sleep disorders in MSA is nocturnal stridor. It was noted to be present in 13% of 203 pathologically proven cases of MSA[36], but the actual prevalence may be higher. It may present at any stage of the disease, and can occasionally be the presenting feature. A sleeping partner will describe a strained, high-pitched, harsh inspiratory sound, different from any previously noted snoring. In some patients, stridor may also be present during wakefulness. Laryngoscopy awake shows a spectrum of findings, ranging from normal vocal cord movement through restriction of cord abduction and paradoxical cord movement to complete paramedian cord fixation with critically reduced airway diameter. Occasionally only one cord is involved initially, with later progression to both[37].

The pathogenesis of stridor in MSA is controversial, with both peripheral and central factors having been implicated. Abduction of the cords results from contraction of the posterior cricoarytenoid (PCA) muscles innervated by branches of the recurrent laryngeal nerves arising from the nucleus ambiguus in the medulla. Pathological studies of the PCA muscles in MSA with stridor, have yielded contradictory results, with neurogenic atrophy present in some but not all

**Table 17.7** Sleep problems in multiple system atrophy

| |
| --- |
| *Sleep-disordered breathing* |
| Nocturnal stridor |
| Sleep apnea syndromes |
| Respiratory dysrhythmias |
| Central neurogenic hypoventilation |
| *Motor dysfunction* |
| REM sleep behavior disorder |
| Periodic limb movements of sleep |

REM, rapid eye movement

**Table 17.8** Proposed respiratory management of patients with multiple system atrophy (MSA) Modified from reference 48

Question all patients with MSA and their bed partners about stridor, snoring, apneas, nocturnal or daytime dyspnea and daytime sleepiness

If stridor or sleep apnea are suspected, perform a PSG. If daytime or nocturnal dyspnea is present, perform overnight oximetry (if a PSG is not planned) and measure arterial blood gases

If stridor is heard on PSG or if an observer reports daytime stridor, perform laryngoscopy. Consider tracheostomy, especially if the vocal cords are abnormal or daytime stridor is present. If the patient declines tracheostomy, use nCPAP, monitoring compliance and the elimination of stridor

If sleep apnea is detected, treat appropriately, usually with n-CPAP

If arterial blood gas analysis and overnight oximetry reveal respiratory failure with nocturnal hypoxemia due to central hypoventilation, consider nocturnal ventilation, either via a nasal mask (see Chapter 9) or a tracheostomy

For patients without evidence of respiratory problems, monitor for stridor and dyspnea

PSG, polysomnogram; nCPAP, nasal continuous positive airway pressure

specimens[38–40]. Similarly, reduced axons in the recurrent laryngeal nerve[38–40] and loss of neurons in nucleus ambiguus[38,41,42] have been reported in some cases, while there have been no abnormalities in others. In contrast, surface[43] and wire electrode[44,45] recordings of the laryngeal muscles during stridor have shown paradoxical EMG activity in the adductor thyroarytenoid and cricothyroid muscles with inspiration, a phase when they should be relaxed. These studies suggest that abnormal central control of the complex system controlling the laryngeal musculature during breathing may be responsible for the phenomenon.

Because some MSA patients with stridor die in their sleep[46–48], tracheostomy has been the standard recommended treatment. In one study[41], five of eight patients with vocal cord paralysis who did not undergo tracheostomy died suddenly, a mean of 1.1 years after diagnosis, while nine of 11 patients who underwent tracheostomy were alive, a maximum of 5 years later. In a study of 30 patients, those with stridor had a significantly shorter survival from the time of the sleep evaluation[48]. Nine of 11 with stridor died, a median of 1.8 years after the sleep evaluation, compared with 16 without stridor.

A recommendation to perform tracheostomy is tempered by the experience that many MSA patients, themselves unaware of stridor, are difficult to convince of the need for the procedure, and fear it will result in decreasing quality of life. Nasal continuous positive airway pressure (CPAP) has been used with variable results; in three patients stridor was eliminated without recurrence after 6 months[49], but in another study all five patients died[48]. A single study has been reported of unilateral injection of botulinum toxin into the thyroarytenoid muscle, and improvement of the stridor and reduction in tonic EMG activity in the muscle was noted 1 month later in three of four patients[45]. It is recommended that a PSG be performed if stridor or OSAS are suspected in MSA (Table 17.8). If stridor is present, tracheostomy should be strongly considered, especially if the vocal cords move abnormally on laryngoscopy or daytime stridor is heard. If the patient declines tracheostomy, nasal CPAP should be used at a pressure that eliminates stridor, but care should be taken to ensure as near perfect compliance as possible, and that stridor does not recur.

## Motor dysfunction

REM sleep without atonia occurs in 90–95% of MSA patients, and REM sleep behavior disorder in 69–90%[50,51]. RBD can occur in both male and female RBD patients in contrast to PD patients with RBD who are predominantly male[30,51]. As in PD, RBD symptoms may be the initial manifestation of MSA (see Chapter 16). The presence of RBD can be used to establish a diagnosis of MSA in patients presenting with autonomic failure[52]. Motor dyscontrol in NREM sleep in the form of periodic limb movements is also common in this disorder[48].

### Case 17.2

The wife of a 60-year-old man woke one night to hear him breathing with a loud, crowing, inspiratory sound. The sound continued to be audible at night over the next week, and also developed during wakefulness in the evening, associated with a feeling of dyspnea. On questioning, his wife also described dream enactment behavior for the preceding 10 years, with her husband screaming, kicking and punching. He had also developed progressive gait unsteadiness, urinary incontinence and impotence over 1–2 years. Examination revealed gait ataxia without evidence for parkinsonism. A thermoreg-

ulatory sweat test showed marked reduction of sweating over most of the body. A PSG demonstrated severe inspiratory stridor and increased muscle tone in REM sleep. Indirect laryngoscopy revealed reduced abduction of the vocal cords during inspiration.

A diagnosis of multiple system atrophy was made. The patient consented to tracheostomy, which was plugged during the day. Over the next 2 years, dyspnea developed on effort. Arterial blood gases demonstrated mild hypercapnic respiratory failure. Overnight oximetry showed hypoxemia during probable REM sleep. The patient used 1 l/min oxygen at night via his tracheostomy, and breathed through an open tracheostomy tube with oxygen supplementation when walking. Hypercapnia did not worsen with oxygen therapy. Three and a half years later, the patient was still able to walk on a treadmill for 10 min at a time.

This case illustrates how nocturnal stridor can complicate MSA of all types, as the patient had cerebellar and autonomic in-volvement but no parkinsonism. He tolerated tracheostomy well and was alive with a reasonable quality of life 3.5 years later, despite also developing mild centrally mediated respiratory failure. If oxygen is used in such patients, care should be taken to ensure that hypercapnia does not worsen (see Chapter 9).

## PROGRESSIVE SUPRANUCLEAR PALSY

Progressive supranuclear palsy (PSP) is a rare neurodegenerative disorder characterized by a rigid akinetic parkinsonian syndrome with prominent axial rigidity and lack of responsiveness to levodopa, early gait instability with falls, supranuclear (especially downward) vertical gaze palsies, pseudobulbar palsy and a frontal lobe-type dementia. Sleep disturbances are an integral part of PSP. A questionnaire study of 437 patients with a clinical diagnosis of PSP revealed that 50% of patients more than 3 years after diagnosis reported changed sleeping patterns or difficulty in sleeping[53].

Sleep architecture is disrupted, with decreased total sleep time, very low sleep efficiency, increased wake time after sleep onset and increased percentage stage 1 NREM and REM sleep[54,55]. A characteristic feature is the reduction in abundance and amplitude of sleep spindles. PSG-confirmed RBD has been reported in only two cases of clinically diagnosed PSP and no autopsy cases[30,56], suggesting that it is a rare phenomenon. In contrast to MSA, the EMG tone in REM is normal in PSP[54,57]. Sleep-disordered breathing is also uncommon. The pathophysiology of the sleep disturbances is presumably linked to the extensive brainstem pathology.

## ALZHEIMER'S DISEASE

Alzheimer's disease, the commonest cause of dementia, usually manifests initially with problems of short-term memory, and then progresses slowly to generalized failure of intellectual and social functioning over a period of years. Sleep disturbances in AD may manifest as nocturnal insomnia, daytime sleepiness, confused, agitated and wandering behavior at night or combinations of these problems. The cognitive impairment characteristic of the dementia may often result in the patient having reduced insight

**Table 17.9** Mechanisms of sleep disturbances in Alzheimer's disease

Circadian dysrhythmias

Intercurrent medical conditions

Primary sleep disorders
    obstructive sleep apnea
    restless legs syndrome

Medications

Depression

into the symptoms, and collateral history from a bed partner or care-giver may be essential. Sleep disturbances may worsen cognitive difficulties and further reduce the quality of the patient's life. They also cause considerable care-giver burden, and are a major factor leading to nursing home placement[58]. Multiple mechanisms may be involved (Table 17.9).

### Circadian dysrhythmias

Reversal of day–night rhythms with wakefulness at night and sleep during the day is very common in AD[59,60]. These symptoms are thought to be due primarily to degenerative changes in the biological clock in the suprachiasmatic nuclei of the hypothalamus[59,61,62]. However, environmental factors in nursing homes may also play a role in institutionalized patients, including lack of light exposure, exercise and intellectual stimulation during the day and forced early bedtimes at night.

Empirical treatment with exogenous melatonin and phototherapy has been tried. However, a multicenter placebo-controlled trial of low-dose and high-dose melatonin for sleep disturbances (particularly circadian dysrhythmias) in Alzheimer's disease[63] found no significant differences in nocturnal sleep time, sleep efficiency, wake time after sleep onset or day–night sleep ratio between either treatment group and placebo-treated patients. Melatonin was well tolerated, and it is possible that it may be beneficial in occasional patients. Phototherapy has shown some promise in the management of circadian dysrhythmias in demented individuals, although the optimal timing, duration and intensity of light have not been determined[64–66].

When the predominant problem is insomnia with other causes excluded (see below), then agents such as trazodone may be helpful. Benzodiazepines should be used with caution in dementia, as they may worsen cognitive impairment, cause gait unsteadiness and induce daytime sleepiness. When the predominant problem is nocturnal wandering or agitation, and medical, psychiatric or sleep disorders have been excluded, behavioral management such as distraction and gentle redirection should be attempted. If this fails, the atypical neuroleptic agents can be useful. Quetiapine, which does not have extrapyramidal or hematological side-effects, can be used in a dose of 25 mg before sleep, increasing as needed to 100 mg. Risperidone and olanzapine may also be used, although they have a higher frequency of extrapyramidal problems. Clozapine can induce blood dyscrasias and needs frequent laboratory monitoring. Although the anticholinesterase agents, such as donepezil and rivastigmine, are used predominantly to help cognition, they appear in practice sometimes to reduce behavioral dyscontrol in dementia as well. Anticonvulsants, such as valproic acid or carbamazepine, may also

sometimes stabilize disruptive behavior. When the predominant problem is daytime hypersomnia, and no other cause can be determined, empirical use of stimulants such as modafinil has been tried.

## Intercurrent medical conditions

The development of nocturnal confusion or daytime sleepiness in a patient with dementia should raise the possibility of the presence of an intercurrent medical disorder. These include infections, such as cystitis, aspiration or hypostatic pneumonia or occasionally staphylococcal osteitis and bacteremia. Metabolic disorders, such as hyponatremia, uremia, hepatic failure or disturbances in glucose metabolism should be considered. Occult gastrointestinal blood loss may cause reduced oxygen carrying capacity and cerebral hypoxemia. Constipation and urinary retention may not be recognized by a demented patient, and pain may manifest as agitation. Rarely, a serious injury such as a fractured hip may present with confusion and inability to walk.

### Case 17.3

A 71-year-old woman was noted by her family to have developed mild memory problems over the preceding year, not severe enough to interfere particularly with her life-style. Over 2 days she developed worsening predominantly nocturnal confusion, severe enough to need hospitalization. She was found to be anemic (hemoglobin concentration 9 g/dl), and a bleeding duodenal ulcer was identified as the cause. Following a blood transfusion, her acute confusion cleared entirely. She returned home, but memory continued to worsen slowly, and eventually a diagnosis of AD was made.

This case illustrates how an acute medical problem, especially one involving decreased blood oxygen-carrying capacity, may cause severe nocturnal confusion in a patient with even early dementia. Identification and treatment of the cause is essential.

### Primary sleep disorders

*Obstructive sleep apnea syndrome*

A number of studies have shown cognitive impairment in severe OSAS[67–69]. In contrast, patients with mild or moderate OSAS show considerably fewer cognitive problems[67,70]. These effects may be due to either chronic intermittent hypoxemia or to sleep deprivation and daytime sleepiness[71]. Successful treatment of severe OSAS with nasal CPAP results in reversal of cognitive deficits in most domains[68,72].

Whether OSAS is more frequent in AD than in age-matched controls is uncertain[73,74], but severity of dementia correlates with the apnea–hyponea index[75]. At the least, OSAS and AD are likely to coincide frequently, as the incidence of both conditions increases with age. There are also a few reports of patients diagnosed with delirium or dementia recovering full cognitive functioning after treatment of OSAS[76–78].

*Restless legs syndrome*

The frequency of RLS in AD is not known, but its high prevalence in the elderly results in the two conditions frequently co-occurring. Demented patients may not give a clear history of RLS, and its presence may have to be inferred by insomnia associated with restless movements of the legs in bed and a desire to walk. It should be considered in the differential diagnosis of nocturnal wanderings. Dopaminergic drugs are relatively well tolerated in patients with dementia, especially in a low dose, but clinicians must be aware of their theoretical potential to exacerbate insomnia and nocturnal hallucinations or confusion.

### Effects of medications

Many medications may cause confusion in AD. In particular, anticholinergic drugs should be avoided and dopaminergic agents used with care. Sometimes multiple sedatives have been prescribed in an attempt to stop the nocturnal behavior, but may in fact be a contributing cause. The anticholinesterase agents may cause insomnia if administered at night.

### Depression

Depression, often difficult to diagnose in a patient with dementia, may present with a variety of sleep disturbances. It may be a cause of insomnia or daytime sleepiness. If agitated depression is present, nocturnal confusion and wandering may result. A trial of antidepressant medication, preferably avoiding the tricyclic agents because of their anticholinergic activity, should be considered if the suspicion of depression is high.

## DEMENTIA WITH LEWY BODIES

Dementia with Lewy bodies (DLB) is characterized by a generalized dementia with an emphasis on visuospatial disturbances, hallucinations, delusions, depression and day-to-day fluctuations. Signs of parkinsonism are sometimes, but not always, present. Lewy bodies are found in cortical neurons. The most characteristic sleep feature of DLB is the presence of RBD, which has now been included as a supportive feature for the diagnosis[79]. A number of clinical, psychometric and autopsy studies have demonstrated that the occurrence of RBD in a demented patient predicts the presence of cortical Lewy bodies, with or without associated Alzheimer changes, even if there are no clinical signs of parkinsonism[80–83]. The diagnosis and management of RBD are discussed in Chapter 16. Distinctions between RBD and nocturnal confusion and wandering are described above in this chapter under 'Parkinson's disease'. Clonazepam should be used with caution in demented patients, because of the risk of increasing cognitive impairment.

## REFERENCES

1. Van Hilten JJ, Weggeman M, Van der Velde EA, Kerkhoff GA, Van Dijk JG, Roos RAC. Sleep, excessive daytime sleepiness and fatigue in Parkinson's disease. *J Neural Transm* 1993;5:235–44

2. Tandberg E, Larsen JP, Karlsen K. A community-based study of sleep disorders in patients with Parkinson's disease. *Mov Disord* 1998;13:895–9

3. Factor SA, McAlarney T, Sanchez-Ramos JR, Weiner WJ. Sleep disorders and sleep effect in Parkinson's disease. *Mov Disord* 1990;5:280–5

4. DeKoninck J, Lorrain D, Gagnon P. Sleep positions and position shifts in five age groups: an ontogenic picture. *Sleep* 1992; 15:143–9

5. Fish DR, Sawyers D, Allen PJ, Blackie JD, Lees AJ, Marsden CD. The effect of sleep on the dyskinetic movements of Parkinson's disease, Gilles de la Tourette syndrome, Huntington's disease and torsion dystonia. *Arch Neurol* 1991;48:210–14

6. Menza MA, Rosen RC. Sleep in Parkinson's disease: the role of depression and anxiety. *Psychosomatics* 1995;36:262–6

7. Wetter TC, Collado-Seidel V, Pollmacher T, Yassouridis A, Trenkwalder C. Sleep and periodic leg movement patterns in drug-free patients with Parkinson's disease and multiple system atrophy. *Sleep* 2000;23: 361–7

8. Tandberg E, Larsen JP, Karlsen K. Excessive daytime sleepiness and sleep benefit in Parkinson's disease: a community-based study. *Mov Disord* 1999;14:922–7

9. Rye DB, Bliwise DL, Dihenia B, Gurecki P. Daytime sleepiness in Parkinson's disease. *J Sleep Res* 2000;9:63–9

10. Arnulf I, Bonnet AM, Damier P, et al. Hallucinations, REM sleep, and Parkinson's disease: a medical hypothesis. *Neurology* 2000;55:281–8

11. Drouot X, Moutereau S, Nguyen JP, et al. Low levels of ventricular CSF orexin/hypocretin in advanced PD. *Neurology* 2003;61:540–3

12. Overeem S, Van Hilten JJ, Ripley B, Mignot E, Nishino S, Lammers GJ. Normal hypocretin-1 levels in Parkinson's disease patients with excessive daytime sleepiness. *Neurology* 2002;58:498–9

13. Hovestadt A, Bogaard JM, Meerwaldt JD, Van der Meche FGA. Pulmonary function in Parkinson's disease. *J Neurol Neurosurg Psychiatry* 1989;52:329–33

14. Apps MCP, Sheaff PC, Ingram DA, Kennard C, Empey DW. Respiration and sleep in Parkinson's disease. *J Neurol Neurosurg Psychiatry* 1989;48:1240–5

15. Frucht S, Rogers JD, Greene PE, Gordon MF, Fahn S. Falling asleep at the wheel: motor vehicle mishaps in persons taking pramipexole and ropinirole. *Neurology* 1999;52:1908–10

16. Schapira AH. Sleep attacks (sleep episodes) with pergolide. *Lancet* 2000;355:1332–3

17. Olanow CW, Schapira AH, Roth T. Waking up to sleep episodes in Parkinson's disease. *Mov Disord* 2000;15:212–15

18. Montastruc JL, Brefel-Courbon C, Senard JM, *et al.* Sleep attacks and antiparkinsonian drugs: a pilot prospective pharmaco-epidemiologic study. *Clin Neuropharmacol* 2001;24:181–3

19. Hauser RA, Gauger L, Anderson WM, Zesiewicz TA. Pramipexole-induced somnolence and episodes of daytime sleep. *Mov Disord* 2000;15:658–63

20. Tracik F, Ebersbach G. Sudden daytime sleep onset in Parkinson's disease: polysomnographic recordings. *Mov Disord* 2001;16:500–6

21. Hobson DE, Lang AE, Martin WRW, Razmy A, Rivest J, Fleming J. Excessive daytime sleepiness and sudden-onset sleep in Parkinson disease. A survey by the Canadian Movement Disorders Group. *J Am Med Assoc* 2002;287:455–63

22. Pal S, Bhattacharya KF, Agapito C, Chaudhuri KR. A study of excessive daytime sleepiness and its clincial significance in three groups of Parkinson's disease patients taking pramipexole, cabergoline and levodopa mono and combination therapy. *J Neural Transm* 2001;198:71–7

23. O'Suilleabhain PE, Dewey RBJ. Contributions of dopaminergic drugs and disease severity to daytime sleepiness in Parkinson disease. *Arch Neurol* 2002;59: 986–9

24. Adler CH, Caviness JN, Hentz JG, Lind M, Tiede J. Randomized trial of modafinil for treating subjective daytime sleepiness in patients with Parkinson's disease. *Mov Disord* 2003;18:287–93

25. Hogl B, Saletu M, Brandauer E, *et al.* Modafinil for the treatment of daytime sleepiness in Parkinson's disease: a double-blind, randomized, crossover, placebo-controlled polygraphic trial. *Sleep* 2002;25: 905–9

26. Kales A, Ansel RD, Markham CH, Scharf MB, Tan T. Sleep in Parkinson's disease and normal subjects prior to and following levodopa administration. *Clin Pharmacol Ther* 1971;12:397–406

27. Mouret J. Differences in sleep in patients with Parkinson's disease. *Electroenceph Clin Neurophysiol* 1975;38:653–57

28. Comella CL, Nardine TM, Diederich NJ, Stebbins GT. Sleep-related violence, injury, and REM sleep behavior disorder in Parkinson's disease. *Neurology* 1998; 51:526–9

29. Gagnon J, Bedard M, Fantini M, *et al.* REM sleep behavior disorder and REM sleep without atonia in Parkinson's disease. *Neurology* 2002;59:585–9

30. Olson EJ, Boeve BF, Silber MH. Rapid eye movement sleep behavior disorder: demographic, clinical and laboratory findings in 93 cases. *Brain* 2000;123:331–9

31. Schenck CH, Hurwitz TD, Mahowald MW. REM sleep behaviour disorder: an update on a series of 96 patients and a review of the world literature. *J Sleep Res* 1993;2:224–31

32. Schenck CH, Bundlie SR, Mahowald MW. Delayed emergence of a parkinsonian disorder in 38% of 29 older men initially diagnosed with idiopathic rapid eye movement sleep behaviour disorder. *Neurology* 1996; 46:388–93

33. Bower JH, Maraganore DM, McDonnell SK, Rocca WA. Incidence of progressive supranuclear palsy and multiple system atrophy in Olmsted County, Minnesota, 1976 to 1990. *Neurology* 1997;49:1284–8

34. Ghorayeb I, Yekhlef F, Chrysostome V, Balestre E, Bioulac B, Tison F. Sleep disorders and their determinants in multiple system atrophy. *J Neurol Neurosurg Psychiatry* 2002;72:798–800

35. McNicholas WT, Rutherford R, Grossman R, Moldofsky H, Zamel N, Phillipson EA. Abnormal respiratory pattern generation during sleep in patients with autonomic dysfunction. *Am Rev Respir Dis* 1983; 128: 429–33

36. Wenning GK, Ben Shlomo Y, Magalhaes M, Daniel SE, Quinn NP. Clinical features and natural history of multiple system atrophy. An analysis of 100 cases. *Brain* 1994; 117:835–45

37. Williams A, Hanson D, Calne DB. Vocal cord paralysis in the Shy–Drager syndrome. *J Neurol Neurosurg Psychiatry* 1979;42:151–3

38. Bannister R, Gibson W, Michaels L, Oppenheimer DR. Laryngeal abductor paralysis in multiple system atrophy. A report on three necropsied cases, with observations on the laryngeal muscles and the nuclei ambigui. *Brain* 1981;104:351–68

39. DeReuck J, Van Landegem W. The posterior crico-arytenoid muscle in two cases of Shy–Drager syndrome with laryngeal stridor. Comparison of the histological, histochemical and biometric findings. *J Neurol* 1987;234:187–90

40. Hayashi M, Isozaki E, Oda M, Tanabe H, Kimura J. Loss of large myelinated nerve fibres of the recurrent laryngeal nerve in patients with multiple system atrophy and vocal cord palsy. *J Neurol Neurosurg Psychiatry* 1997;62:234–8

41. Isozaki E, Miyamoto K, Osanai R, Hayashida T, Tanabe H. [Clinical studies of 23 patients with multiple system atrophy presenting with vocal cord paralysis]. *Rinsho Shinkeigaku – Clin Neurol* 1991;31:249–54

42. Lapresle J, Annabi A. Olivopontocerebellar atrophy with velopharyngeal paralysis: a contribution to the somatopy of the nucleus ambiguus. *J Neuropathol Exp Neurol* 1979; 38:401–6

43. Isozaki E, Osanai R, Horiguchi S, Hayashida T, Hirose K, Tanabe H. Laryngeal electromyography with separated surface electrodes in patients with multiple system atrophy presenting with vocal cord paralysis. *J Neurol* 1994;241:551–6

44. Plazzi G, Provini F, Montagna P, *et al.* Video-polygraphic recording of sleep-related stridor [Abstract]. *Sleep Res* 1996;25:439

45. Merlo IM, Occhini A, Pacchetti C, Alfonsi E. Not paralysis, but dystonia causes stridor in multiple system atrophy. *Neurology* 2002; 58:649–52

46. Hughes RGM, Gibbon KP, Lowe J. Vocal cord abductor paralysis as a solitary and fatal manifestation of multiple system atrophy. *J Laryngol Otol* 1998;112:177–8

47. Kavey NB, Whyte J, Blitzer A, Gidro-Frank S. Sleep-related laryngeal obstruction presenting as snoring or sleep apnea. *Laryngoscope* 1989;99:851–4

48. Silber MH, Levine S. Stridor and death in multiple system atrophy. *Mov Disord* 2000; 15:699–704

49. Iranzo A, Santamaria J, Tolosa E. Continuous positive airway pressure eliminates nocturnal stridor in multiple system atrophy. *Lancet* 2000;356:1329–30

50. Tachibani N, Kimura K, Kitajima K, Shinde A, Kimura J, Shibasaki H. REM sleep motor dysfunction in multiple system atrophy: with special emphasis on sleep talk as its early clinical manifestation. *J Neurol Neurosurg Psychiatry* 1997;63:678–81

51. Plazzi G, Corsini R, Provini F. REM sleep behavior disorders in multiple system atrophy. *Neurology* 1997;48:1094–7

52. Plazzi G, Cortelli P, Montagna P. REM sleep behaviour disorder differentiates pure autonomic failure from multiple system atrophy with autonomic failure. *J Neurol Neurosurg Psychiatry* 1998;64:683–5

53. Santacruz P, Uttl B, Litvan I, Grafman J. Progressive supranuclear palsy. A survey of the disease course. *Neurology* 1998;50:1637–47

54. Montplaisir J, Petit D, Decary A, *et al*. Sleep and quantitative EEG in patients with progressive supranuclear palsy. *Neurology* 1997;49:999–1003

55. Aldrich MS, Foster NL, White RF, Bluemlein L, Prokopowicz G. Sleep abnormalities in progressive supranuclear palsy. *Ann Neurol* 1989;25:577–81

56. Pareja JA, Caminero AB, Masa JF, Dobato JL. A first case of progressive supranuclear palsy presenting as inhibition of speech during wakefulness and somniloquy with phasic muscle twitching during REM sleep. *Neurologia* 1996;11:304–6

57. Leygonie F, Thomas J, Degos JD, Bouchareine A, Barbizet J. Troubles de somneil dans la maladie de Steele-Richardson. *Rev Neurol* 1976; 132:125–36

58. Severson MA, Smith GE, Tangalos EG, *et al*. Patterns and predictors of institutionalization in community-based dementia patients. *J Am Geriatr Soc* 1994;42:181–5

59. Vitiello M, Bliwise D, Prinz P. Sleep in Alzheimer's disease and the sundown syndrome. *Neurology* 1992;42(Suppl 6):83–94

60. Ancoli-Israel S, Klauber M, Jones D, *et al*. Variations in circadian rhythms of activity, sleep, and light exposure related to dementia in nursing-home patients. *Sleep* 1997; 20:18–23

61. Stopa E, Volicer L, Kuo-Leblanc V, *et al*. Pathologic evaluation of the human suprachiasmatic nucleus in severe dementia. *J Neuropathol Exp Neurol* 1999;58:29–39

62. Swaab D, Fliers E, Partman T. The suprachiasmatic nucleus of the human brain in relation to sex, age and senile dementia. *Brain Res* 1985;342:37–44

63. Singer C, Tractenberg R, Kaye J, *et al*. A multicenter, placebo-controlled trial of melatonin for sleep disturbance in Alzheimer's disease. *Sleep* 2003;27:893–901

64. Van Someren E, Kessler A, Mirmiran M, Swaab D. Indirect bright light improves circadian rest–activity rhythm disturbances in demented patients. *Biol Psychiatry* 1997; 41:955–63

65. Lyketsos C, Lindell Veiel L, Baker A, Steele C. A randomized, controlled trial of bright light therapy for agitated behaviors in dementia patients residing in long-term care. *Int J Geriatr Psychiatry* 1999;14:520–5

66. Satlin A, Volicer L, Ross V, Herz L, Campbell S. Bright light treatment of behavioral and sleep disturbances in patients with Alzheimer's disease. *Am J Psychiatry* 1992;149:1028–32

67. Bedard MA, Montplaisir J, Richer F, Rouleau I, Malo J. Obstructive sleep apnea

syndrome: pathogenesis of neuropsychological deficits. *J Clin Exp Neuropsychol* 1991; 13:950–64

68. Feuerstein C, Naegele B, Pepin JL, Levy P. Frontal lobe-related cognitive functions in patients with sleep apnea syndrome before and after treatment. *Acta Neurol Belg* 1997; 97:96–107

69. Naegele B, Thouvard V, Pepin JL, *et al.* Deficits of cognitive executive functions in patients with sleep apnea syndrome. *Sleep* 1995;18:43–52

70. Redline S, Strauss ME, Adams N, *et al.* Neuropsychological functioning in mild sleep-disordered breathing. *Sleep* 1997; 20:160–7

71. Roehrs T, Merrion M, Pedrosi B, Stepanski E, Zorick F, Roth T. Neuropsychological function in obstructive sleep apnea syndrome (OSAS) compared to chronic obstructive pulmonary disease (COPD). *Sleep* 1995;18:382–8

72. Bedard MA, Montplaisir J, Malo J, Richer F, Rouleau I. Persistent neuropsychological deficits and vigilance impairment in sleep apnea syndrome after treatment with continuous positive airways pressure (CPAP). *J Clin Exp Neuropsychol* 1993;15:330–41

73. Reynolds CF III, Kupfer DJ, Taska LS, *et al.* Sleep apnea in Alzheimer's dementia: correlation with mental deterioration. *J Clin Psychiatry* 1985;46:257–61

74. Bliwise DL, Yesavage JA, Tinklenberg JR, Dement WC. Sleep apnea in Alzheimer's disease. *Neurobiol Aging* 1989;10:343–6

75. Ancoli-Israel S, Klauber MR, Butters N, Parker L, Kripke DF. Dementia in institutionalized elderly: relation to sleep apnea. *J Am Geriatr Soc* 1991;39:258–63

76. Scheltens P, Visscher F, Van Keimpema ARJ, Lindeboom J, Taphoorn MJB, Wolters EC. Sleep apnea syndrome presenting with cognitive impairment. *Neurology* 1991;41: 155–6

77. Munoz X, Marti S, Sumalla J, Bosch J, Sampol G. Acute delirium as a manifestation of obstructive sleep apnea syndrome. *Am J Respir Crit Care Med* 1998;158:1306–7

78. Lee JW. Recurrent delirium associated with obstructive sleep apnea. *Gen Hosp Psychiatry* 1998;20:120–2

79. McKeith IG, Perry EK, Perry RH. Report of the second dementia with Lewy body international workshop: diagnosis and treatment. Consortium on Dementia with Lewy Bodies. *Neurology* 1999;53:902–5

80. Boeve BF, Silber MH, Ferman TJ, *et al.* REM sleep behavior disorder and degenerative dementia: an association likely reflecting Lewy body disease. *Neurology* 1998; 51:363–70

81. Boeve BF, Silber MH, Ferman TJ, Lucas JA, Parisi JE. Association of REM sleep behavior disorder and neurodegenerative disease may reflect an underlying synucleinopathy. *Mov Disord* 2001;16:622–30

82. Ferman TJ, Boeve BF, Smith GE, *et al.* REM sleep behavior disorder and dementia: cognitive differences when compared with AD. *Neurology* 1999;52:951–7

83. Ferman TJ, Boeve BF, Smith GE, *et al.* Dementia with Lewy bodies may present as dementia and REM sleep behavior disorder without parkinsonism or hallucinations. *J Int Neuropsychol Soc* 2002;8:907–14

# Chapter 18

# Sleep in patients with epilepsy and headaches

*Sleep hath its own world,*
*and a wide realm of wild reality.*

**Lord Byron,** *The Dream*

## SLEEP AND EPILEPSY

Sleep and epilepsy are intimately related. It has been known since antiquity that seizures occur commonly at night, but the explanation had to await an understanding of cerebral neuronal activity during sleep. Certain seizure types arise almost exclusively from sleep, and nocturnal seizures may mimic parasomnias. Epilepsy results in changes of sleep architecture, while antiseizure medications have varied effects on sleep and wakefulness.

## Classification of seizures and epilepsy

### Classification of epileptic seizures

The International League against Epilepsy (ILAE) classification of seizures is universally accepted (Table 18.1). Seizures are divided into partial seizures (also called focal) and generalized seizures. Partial seizures arise from a specific system of neurons in a part of one cerebral hemisphere. They are subdivided into simple partial seizures (no impairment of consciousness) and complex partial seizures (consciousness impaired). Simple

**Table 18.1** International League against Epilepsy classification of seizures

*Partial seizures*

Simple partial seizures
    motor signs
    sensory symptoms
    autonomic symptoms
    psychic symptoms

Complex partial seizures
    with impairment of consciousness only
    with additional automatisms

Partial seizures with secondary generalization

*Generalized seizures*

Absence seizures
Tonic–clonic seizures
Myoclonic seizures
Tonic seizures
Clonic seizures
Atonic seizures

partial seizures are further classified according to their symptomatology (motor, sensory, autonomic or psychic), while complex partial seizures are divided into those with only impairment of consciousness and those with additional motor behavior (automatisms). A simple partial seizure can evolve into a complex partial seizure and either can evolve into a secondary generalized seizure.

Generalized seizures are those in which the first clinical manifestations indicate involvement of both cerebral hemispheres. Motor behavior is bilateral, and consciousness is often impaired at the onset of the seizure. Absence seizures are characterized by transient loss of consciousness with or without minor motor activity and associated with generalized spike and wave discharges on the electroencephalogram (EEG). Generalized tonic–clonic seizures are characterized by sudden loss of consciousness followed by tonic contraction of muscles and then rhythmic clonic jerks and postictal drowsiness. Myoclonic, tonic, clonic and atonic seizures are rarer subtypes of generalized seizures.

*Classification of epilepsies and epileptic syndromes*

It is important to differentiate a classification of seizures from that of epilepsies and epileptic syndromes (Table 18.2). Patients may have more than one type of seizure, yet have a well-defined clinical syndrome with consistent etiology, course and prognosis. The ILAE classification of the epilepsies divides them into localization-related and generalized. Localization-related epilepsies are characterized by seizures with a localized origin, most commonly from a region of one cerebral hemisphere. Generalized epilepsies are epileptic disorders characterized by generalized seizures. Both localization-related

**Table 18.2** International League against Epilepsy classification of epilepsies and epileptic syndromes (selected examples)

*Localization-related*

Symptomatic
    temporal lobe epilepsies (TLE)*
    frontal lobe epilepsies*
    occipital lobe epilepsies
    parietal lobe epilepsies

Idiopathic
    benign childhood epilepsy with centrotemporal spikes*
    childhood epilepsy with occipital paroxysms

*Generalized*

Idiopathic
    benign neonatal convulsions
    absence epilepsies
    juvenile myoclonic epilepsy (JME)*
    epilepsy with generalized tonic–clonic seizures on awakening*

Symptomatic
    West syndrome (infantile spasms)
    Lennox–Gastaut syndrome

*Undetermined origin*

Epilepsy with continuous spike waves during slow-wave sleep*

*Epilepsies with a strong relationship to the sleep–wake cycle

and generalized epilepsies are subdivided into idiopathic epilepsies (no underlying neurological lesion and probable genetic etiology) and symptomatic epilepsies (resulting from a structural disorder of the brain). Most localization-related epilepsies are symptomatic and most generalized epilepsies are idiopathic.

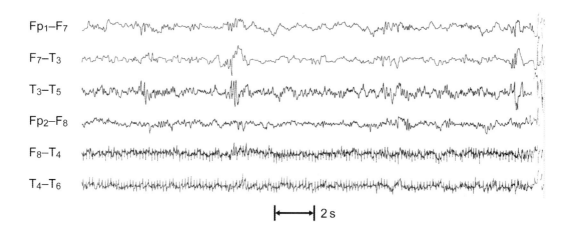

Fp₁–F₇

F₇–T₃

T₃–T₅

Fp₂–F₈

F₈–T₄

T₄–T₆

⊢⟶⊣ 2 s

**Figure 18.1** Interictal epileptiform spikes. This fragment of electroencephalogram (EEG) recording, obtained during a polysomnogram with additional EEG derivations, shows multiple interictal spike and wave discharges arising from the left mid-temporal region. See Figure 4.2 for location of the different electrodes

## Effects of sleep on epilepsy

*Temporal lobe epilepsies*

*Interictal epileptic discharges* Focal spike and sharp-wave discharges on an EEG are electrophysiological markers for partial seizures, but do not produce any clinical effects themselves (Figure 18.1). A number of studies have examined the frequency of these interictal epileptic discharges (IEDs) during different stages of sleep in patients with complex partial seizures arising from the temporal lobes[1–4]. All studies have shown that the most frequent rate of discharge is during stages 3 and 4 non-rapid eye movement (NREM) sleep and the least frequent rate is during rapid eye movement (REM) sleep. IEDs fire at an intermediate rate during stages 1 and 2 NREM sleep, while discharges during wakefulness occur at about

the same frequency as during REM sleep. NREM sleep also activates discharges that were not present in wakefulness. A normal wake EEG may be associated with an IED during NREM sleep while a record showing a unilateral IED during wake may also show a new contralateral spike discharge during NREM sleep. During REM sleep, bilateral IEDs sometimes revert to unilateral discharges, and in one study the side of discharges during REM sleep predicted the side of origin of most of the patient's seizures[4].

The ability of NREM sleep to activate IEDs is the reason that daytime sleep recordings are frequently used in EEG laboratories in the diagnosis of epilepsy. NREM and especially slow-wave sleep appear to predispose to epileptiform discharges because of the intense neuronal synchronicity that occurs between brainstem, thalamus and cortex in this state. The normal phenomena of sleep spindles and high-amplitude delta waves produced by the burst-firing of thalamic and cortical neurons (see Chapter 1) form the substrate that allows pathological rhythmic epileptic discharges to develop.

*Seizures*  As with IEDs, nocturnal partial seizures occur predominantly in NREM sleep and rarely during REM sleep. However, in contrast to IEDs, seizures are more common in stages 1 and 2 rather than in stages 3 and 4 NREM sleep[5]. The reason is not fully understood, but sleep fragmentation may predispose to seizure occurrence, and arousals are more frequent during lighter stages of NREM sleep. Partial seizures generalize more often during sleep than wakefulness, and last longer when occurring in slow-wave sleep compared with stage 2 NREM sleep and wakefulness[6].

*Frontal lobe epilepsies*

Nocturnal seizures are more common in frontal lobe compared with temporal lobe epilepsy[7]. Frontal lobe seizures may vary widely in clinical manifestation depending on their exact site of origin. An important subtype consists of seizures arising predominantly or entirely during sleep[8]. Because many of these seizures arise from deep cortical structures, the events are often not accompanied by abnormalities in the scalp EEG, and thus may resemble non-epileptic parasomnias. The disorder is sometimes familial, and is then known as autosomal dominant nocturnal frontal lobe epilepsy. A number of families have been described, and the gene locus has been mapped to the nico-tinic acetylcholine receptor α4 subunit on chromosome 20[9].

The most characteristic motor behavior in nocturnal frontal lobe seizures consists of bizarre asymmetric dystonic posturing of the limbs and trunk arising out of NREM sleep and lasting less than a minute, usually with preservation of consciousness. The seizures may recur several times a night. When these events were first identified in the 1980s, they were believed to be a form of movement disorder, and were given the name paroxysmal nocturnal dystonia[10]. A number of lines of evidence eventually led to the correct conclusion that the disorder was a form of epilepsy[11]. While most events are not associated with scalp EEG seizure discharges, these can be present in occasional patients with similar motor activity. The EEGs of some patients show interictal frontal spike activity, and some patients have occasional similar daytime events. Most important, the events are stereotyped with the same clinical manifestations across different nights. The majority of affected patients obtain partial or complete relief with the use of carbamazepine.

In the borderland between frontal lobe epilepsy and parasomnias lie a few ill-defined conditions. The term episodic nocturnal wanderings has been used to describe patients with frequent sleepwalking behaviors responsive to anticonvulsants and associated with interictal EEG spike activity[12]. Paroxysmal arousals, often with transient posturing of the limbs, may mimic the NREM parasomnia of confusional arousals[8] (see Chapter 16). 'Epileptic K-complexes' have been described, with possible epileptiform sharp-wave activity superimposed on the arousal complex[13]. It may be extremely difficult to be certain whether such events are epileptic or not, and some patients may have both a seizure disorder and a parasomnia.

## Case 18.1

A 32-year-old man presented with nocturnal episodes. These had commenced at the age of 16 years, and occurred on at least five nights every week. On a specific night the number of episodes varied between one and three. The events were all similar, with the patient developing twisting movements of the trunk, arms and legs, resulting in him gyrating around the bed. He appeared to have recall of the episodes, which lasted about 45 s. He had never had daytime seizures and had not experienced sleepwalking. There were no risk factors for epilepsy, including no family history of similar events.

With video-EEG polysomnography, two events were captured. They arose out of stage 2 NREM sleep and were completely stereotyped, appearing as described above. No ictal changes were seen on the 16-channel EEG, and no interictal spikes were recorded. A magnetic resonance imaging (MRI) scan of the head was normal. A diagnosis of nocturnal frontal lobe epilepsy was made. A combination of carbamazepine and valproic acid therapy resulted in elimination of the seizures.

This case illustrates the features of nocturnal frontal lobe epilepsy. Despite the lack of EEG findings, the diagnosis was established by the typical dystonic motor activity, the stereotyped nature of the attacks and their frequency. The response to therapy confirmed the diagnosis.

### Benign childhood epilepsy with centrotemporal spikes

This common condition is an example of an idiopathic localization-related epileptic syndrome possibly following an autosomal dominant inheritance pattern. It usually commences in the late years of the first decade or early years of the second and is a benign illness, usually remitting before adulthood. The child usually awakens shortly after sleep onset with unilateral paresthesias of the mouth and face followed by clonic jerking of the lower face, drooling of saliva and speech arrest if the dominant hemisphere is involved. Occasionally secondary generalization may occur. The interictal EEG shows a diagnostic pattern of sleep activated synchronous spikes in both the central and temporal regions, often with an unusual distribution across both hemispheres.

### Juvenile myoclonic epilepsy

Juvenile myoclonic epilepsy is a genetically determined form of generalized epilepsy, inherited in an autosomal dominant pattern with a gene locus on the short arm of chromosome 6. Onset is usually in adolescence. Patients develop myoclonic jerks of the upper body, generalized tonic–clonic seizures and absence seizures, all occurring predominantly upon awakening in the morning. The mechanism for this relationship to the sleep–wake cycle is undetermined. The EEG shows bursts of polyspike

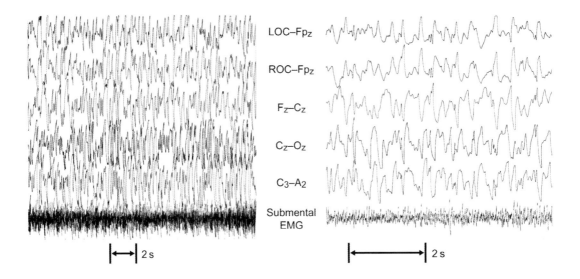

LOC–Fpz

ROC–Fpz

Fz–Cz

Cz–Oz

C3–A2

Submental EMG

2 s          2 s

**Figure 18.2**  Continuous spike and wave activity during non-rapid eye movement (NREM) sleep. This record shows generalized spike and wave activity during NREM sleep completely obliterating normal sleep rhythms. The fragment on the left is displayed at the conventional 30-s epoch per screen used in polysomnography, while the fragment on the right is displayed at a 10-s epoch per screen, thus showing better resolution of the wave-forms. See Figure 4.1 for explanations of the derivations displayed

and wave activity at a frequency of 3–5 Hz, somewhat faster than seen in typical childhood absence epilepsy. The seizures are usually well controlled with valproic acid therapy, but lifelong therapy is required.

*Epilepsy with generalized tonic–clonic seizures on awakening*

This familial syndrome is similar to juvenile myoclonic epilepsy but probably has a different genetic basis. Generalized tonic–clonic seizures occur on wakening from sleep at any time of the day.

*Epilepsy with continuous spike waves during slow-wave sleep*

This rare syndrome of uncertain cause commences in early childhood, most commonly at about the age of 4–5 years[14]. A number of seizure types can occur, including partial or generalized motor seizures during sleep and absence seizures during wakefulness. The essential feature is a diffuse 2–3-Hz spike and wave pattern occurring throughout NREM sleep and occupying at least 85% of slow-wave sleep (Figure 18.2). Generally no clinical disturbances of sleep occur. Regression of behavior, language and motor development accompanies the seizures. The epileptic component is self-limiting, with cessation of seizures and normalization of the EEG after some years. However, despite some improvement in neuropsychological function, more than half of patients remain with severe deficits.

## Effects of epilepsy on sleep

### Nocturnal generalized seizures

Generalized tonic–clonic seizures at night cause considerable disruption of sleep[15]. The seizures themselves cause shifts in sleep stage to either wake or light NREM sleep (stages 1 or 2). Compared with epileptic patients who have not experienced a seizure that night, total sleep time decreases, while wake time after sleep onset and the number of awakenings increase. These awakenings occur both linked to the seizure and independent of it. With primary generalized seizures, the awakenings occur predominantly after the seizure, whereas with secondary generalized seizures, the awakenings occur both before and afterwards. The most striking change in sleep architecture is an absolute and relative reduction in REM sleep in the order of 50%. Stage 2 NREM sleep, probably in compensation, is increased in duration. The reason why REM sleep is decreased following a seizure is unknown. It is possible that this is simply due to the presence of sleep disruption with frequent arousals, but other hypotheses include the possibility that seizures might affect the circadian pattern of sleep stage occurrence resulting in REM sleep delay, or that they may have a direct REM sleep-suppressant effect.

### Nocturnal partial seizures

The effects of partial seizures during sleep are similar to those of generalized seizures but less intense. REM sleep time decreases[6], especially after multiple seizures in a single night[15]. REM sleep latency is reported to increase. Sleep efficiency and percentage deep NREM sleep may decrease[6], but this has not been a consistent finding[15].

### Epilepsy without nocturnal seizures

Patients with generalized and temporal lobe epilepsies not experiencing seizures at the time show an increase in awakenings and wake time after sleep onset, compared with a non-epileptic control group. These effects are more marked in patients with temporal lobe compared with generalized epilepsy. The mechanism is uncertain, but such sleep fragmentation may increase the risk of further seizure activity.

### Interictal epileptic discharges

Focal IEDs in temporal lobe epilepsy are not associated with arousals[3]. However, bursts of generalized spike and wave activity during sleep unassociated with clinical ictal manifestations may cause arousals and could contribute to daytime sleepiness (Figure 18.3).

### Antiepileptic drugs

Antiepileptic drugs (Table 18.3) in general stabilize sleep rhythms[16–18]. Sleep latency decreases, awakenings become fewer and sleep efficiency improves. These changes may be due to better seizure control or alternatively the effect of the drugs themselves. An exception is phenytoin, which increases

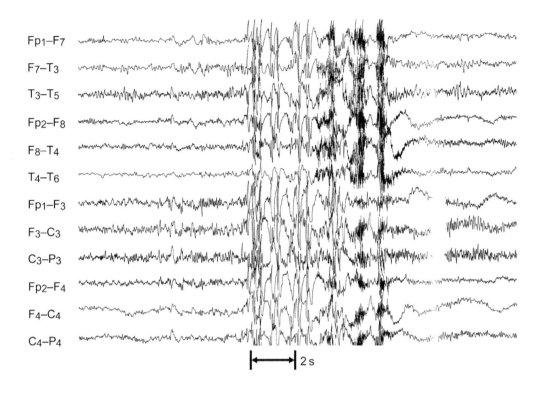

**Figure 18.3** Generalized spike and wave activity causing an arousal. This fragment shows a burst of generalized spike and wave activity arising out of non-rapid eye movement (NREM) sleep resulting in an arousal. See Figure 4.2 for location of the different electrodes

**Table 18.3** Anti-epileptic drugs and sleep

|  | Sleep latency | Wakenings | Sleep efficiency | Stage 2 NREM | Stages 3/4 NREM | REM sleep |
|---|---|---|---|---|---|---|
| Phenobarbital | ↓ | ↓ | ↑ | ↑ |  | ↓ |
| Phenytoin | ↓ | ↑ | ↓ | ↓ |  | ↓ |
| Carbamazepine |  |  | ↑ |  | ↑ | ↓ |
| Benzodiazepines | ↓ | ↓ |  | ↑ | ↓ | ↓ |
| Gabapentin |  | ↓ |  |  | ↑ | ↑ |
| Lamotrigine |  | ↓ |  | ↑ | ↓ | ↑ |

NREM, non-rapid eye movement; REM, rapid eye movement

awakenings and decreases sleep efficiency. The effects on sleep stages are less consistent and of uncertain clinical significance. Phenobarbital, carbamazepine and benzodiazepines decrease REM sleep, whereas REM sleep is enhanced by gabapentin and lamotrigine. Slow-wave sleep is increased by carbamazepine and gabapentin, but decreased by benzodiazepines and lamotrigine. Phenobarbital and benzodiazepines increase stage 2 NREM sleep, and in particular produce a higher frequency of sleep spindles. Valproic acid appears to have little effect on sleep patterns.

Many antiepileptic drugs (AEDs) can cause daytime sleepiness, especially phenobarbital, benzodiazepines and carbamazepine. Felbamate and lamotrigine can result in complaints of insomnia. Benzodiazepines and phenobarbital can aggravate obstructive sleep apnea syndrome, as can vagal nerve stimulation used to treat certain resistant seizure disorders[19].

## Daytime sleepiness and epilepsy

Epileptic patients frequently complain of sleepiness. In a study of 158 patients with seizure disorders, 28% had elevated scores on the Epworth sleepiness scale (ESS). When corrected for age and gender, this was significantly higher than in a control population with other types of neurological disease[20].

A number of factors may be responsible for daytime somnolence in epilepsy (Table 18.4). First, many AEDs are sedating, and this has usually been considered the most important factor. A study using the maintenance of wakefulness test showed that epileptic patients on AEDs were significantly sleepier than those who were untreated[21]. As

**Table 18.4** Factors responsible for sleepiness in epilepsy

| Antiepileptic drugs |
| --- |
| Nocturnal seizures |
| Primary sleep disorders (OSAs and RLS) |

OSAS, obstructive sleep apnea syndrome; RLS, restless legs syndrome

discussed above, epileptic seizures themselves can result in arousals and changes in sleep architecture. In a group of epileptic patients on stable medication, sleepiness measured by the ESS was greater in those with ongoing seizures compared with those who were seizure-free for at least a year[22]. Associated sleep disorders may also be important in the pathogenesis of sleepiness. Obstructive sleep apnea syndrome (OSAS) may be common in epileptic patients. In a study of 158 patients, sleepiness measured by the ESS correlated with symptoms of sleep-disordered breathing and restless legs syndrome, while AEDs, seizure frequency and the presence of nocturnal seizures did not significantly contribute[20].

These data underscore the importance of assessing for a primary sleep disorder before ascribing sleepiness in an epileptic patient to the effects of drugs or seizures. Additionally, OSAS may increase the frequency of seizures by fragmenting sleep, producing chronic sleep deprivation or inducing nocturnal hypoxemia. In some patients, the treatment of OSAS has appeared to reduce seizure frequency.

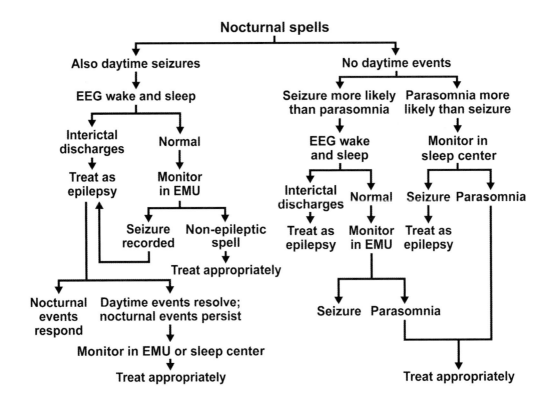

**Figure 18.4** Algorithm for the investigation of a patient with suspected nocturnal seizures. EEG, electroencephalogram; EMU, epilepsy monitoring unit

---

**Case 18.2**

A 52-year-old man presented with excessive daytime sleepiness present for about 10 years, but worsening in severity and interfering with his work as a bookkeeper. He had experienced complex partial seizures with secondary generalization since the age of 15 years. These had been reasonably well controlled for the preceding 10 years by 1200 mg carbamazepine daily with high therapeutic drug levels.

His last generalized seizure had occurred 5 years before presentation and partial seizures occurred about once every 9 months. His wife described snoring, especially when he slept on his back, and the patient was aware of occasional snort arousals. His wife had not observed apnea. His weight had increased by 15 lb over 10 years. Polysomnography revealed 42 obstructive apneas per hour with minimum desaturation of 79%. Nasal continuous positive airway pressure (CPAP) at

8 cmH$_2$O resulted in control of disordered breathing. After 1 month of CPAP use, the patient's sleepiness had resolved.

This case illustrates the importance of considering the presence of a sleep disorder in epileptic patients with sleepiness. For 10 years the patient's sleepiness had been ascribed to his use of carbamazepine, whereas it resolved entirely with treatment of OSAS.

### Sleep deprivation and epilepsy

Sleep deprivation can induce seizures, both in epileptic patients and occasionally in persons without a prior history of seizures. Thus, attention to sleep hygiene and achieving an adequate total sleep time is important in the behavioral management of epilepsy. In addition to seizures, interictal discharges may be precipitated by insufficient sleep. Sleep deprivation is widely used in EEG laboratories and epilepsy monitoring units as a method of inducing interictal discharges and seizures. The mechanism involved is uncertain, but most probably subsequent spikes and seizures occurring during sleep are due to increased amounts of rebound deep NREM sleep.

### Evaluation of the patient with suspected nocturnal seizures

Correct treatment depends on accurate distinction between nocturnal seizures and parasomnias (Figure 18.4). When seizures also occur during the day, the diagnosis is usually straightforward, especially if the interictal EEG is abnormal. However, difficulties may arise when the nocturnal spells appear to be different from the daytime seizures or when the events at night are

**Table 18.5** Headaches and sleep

| |
|---|
| Migraine |
|     arising from sleep |
|     relieved by sleep |
|     relation to sleepwalking |
| Cluster headache |
| Chronic paroxysmal hemicrania |
| Hypnic headache |
| Headache associated with sleep-disordered breathing |

unresponsive to seizure medication. When spells occur only at night and the clinician suspects that seizures are more likely than parasomnias, then a wake and sleep EEG, often preceded by sleep deprivation, may confirm the diagnosis. However, when this is normal, it is usually necessary to attempt a recording of the actual spell. Whether this should be done in a sleep laboratory or an epilepsy monitoring unit depends on the expertise and facilities available at each center. If parasomnias are more likely than seizures, the sleep laboratory may be the better site, but a full EEG montage with time-synchronized video monitoring will still be needed. In addition, the interpreter needs to be skilled in reading ictal EEG recordings. Collaboration between an epileptologist and a sleep specialist will result in the best outcome.

## SLEEP AND HEADACHES

Headaches represent another form of paroxysmal neurological disorder often closely associated with sleep (Table 18.5). Certain

377

types of headache arise only or predominantly from sleep, while others may be relieved by sleep. Sleep disorders, such as obstructive sleep apnea syndrome, may induce headaches, while headaches may result in sleep deprivation.

## Migraine

Migraine is a syndrome characterized by unilateral headaches, often pulsating, and associated with nausea and intolerance of light and sound. It may occur with or without sensory, predominantly visual, auras. Migraine headaches frequently arise from sleep, and appear most commonly to originate from REM sleep, both during the night[23] and during daytime naps[24]. In contrast, sleep is a well-recognized factor in terminating a migraine attack. In a prospective study of 310 patients, a higher percentage of patients obtained relief by sleeping than by quietly resting[23]. There is also a poorly understood relationship between arousal parasomnias and migraine, with sleepwalking occurring in 20–55% of migraineurs[25–27]. A history of sleepwalking and sleep terrors was more common in 100 patients with migraine than in control subjects[27].

## Cluster headaches

Cluster headaches are a predominantly male disease, characterized by excruciating bouts of unilateral face or head pain lasting 1–2 h and recurring between one and three times a day. Unilateral nasal blockage and conjunctival injection are common accompaniments. Episodic cluster headaches occur for weeks to months and then remit for a period of weeks to years, while chronic cluster headaches may occur for several years without remission. Attacks are especially common during the night, and have been related to REM sleep in the episodic[23,28] but not the chronic form[29]. In some patients, cluster headaches may be associated with REM-related obstructive apneas[30,31]. In studies of cluster-headache patients not selected for sleep symptoms, OSAS has been found in 31–60%[32]. Of 19 attacks recorded during polysomnography, eight (42%) were associated with oxyhemoglobin desaturation, five during REM and three during NREM sleep[31]. Improvement in cluster headaches has been reported with treatment of OSAS in a few patients[30,33]. Administration of oxygen is commonly used for the treatment of acute cluster headaches, also suggesting that hypoxemia may play a role in he pathogenesis for a subgroup of patients.

## Chronic paroxysmal hemicrania

This headache is common in middle-aged women, and may be a variant of cluster headaches. Attacks last a shorter period (10–20 min), and may recur more frequently over the course of a day. Unlike cluster headaches, they usually respond to indomethacin treatment. When the headaches occur at night, they appear to arise predominantly from REM sleep[34].

## Hypnic headache

Hypnic headache is a rare idiopathic condition, with episodes arising only from sleep and not having the clinical characteristics of other well-defined headache syndromes. The disorder affects middle-aged and older persons, with a mean age of onset of about 60 years[35]. Women are more affected than men, and about half of patients have other diurnal headache syndromes, especially migraine. Hypnic headaches wake the patient from sleep at a constant time, most commonly between 1 and 3 a.m. The headache is bilateral in two-thirds of patients, and has either a frontal or a diffuse localization. It is described as a dull pressure or, less commonly, as pulsating, sharp or stabbing. Nausea, photophobia and sonophobia are uncommon. The duration of the pain ranges from less than 30 min to more than 2 h. Nightly occurrence is common.

The timing of the headache as well as the occasional description of the pain commencing during a dream has led to the hypothesis that hypnic headaches may be a REM sleep-associated phenomenon. However, the only polysomnographic recording of a hypnic headache not associated with sleep-disordered breathing demonstrated an origin from stage 3 NREM sleep[36]. One patient with otherwise typical hypnic headaches was found on polysomnography to develop the headache during REM sleep-related obstructive apneas, and nasal CPAP relieved the headaches[37]. OSAS does not appear to underlie most hypnic headaches, and the underlying pathophysiology is not understood. Caffeine and indomethacin, either before sleep or after waking with the headache, have been reported as effective therapies[38]. Lithium may also be helpful, but side-effects often limit its use.

## Case 18.3

A 73-year-old man presented with a 4-year history of waking every night between 1:30 and 3:00 a.m. with a non-pulsating headache above the left eye lasting about an hour, and not associated with nausea or a visual disturbance. He believed that drinking a cup of tea relieved the pain. He did not report daytime headaches. He had a history of snoring and daytime sleepiness. A polysomnogram revealed OSAS, with 18 disordered breathing events per hour. He woke with a typical headache while in REM sleep, associated with oxyhemoglobin desaturation to 89%. He was treated with nasal CPAP which he used regularly, but the headaches continued. About 3 years after presentation they remitted spontaneously.

This case illustrates the complexity and uncertainties regarding hypnic headaches. Despite a headache being recorded during REM sleep at the time of sleep-disordered breathing, treatment with nasal CPAP did not help. Presumably the patient had a form of idiopathic hypnic headache which seemed to respond to self-medication with caffeine.

## Headache associated with sleep-disordered breathing

Early-morning headache is commonly accepted as a symptom of OSAS, but studies comparing the frequency of headache in OSAS with that in other sleep disorders have found similar frequencies[39,40]. However, headaches appear to be more common in patients with OSAS compared with groups without any sleep disorders[39,41]. Headaches are more frequent in snorers compared with non-snorers[42]. In a study of 19 patients with chronic headaches and a history of snoring, observed apneas or excessive daytime sleepiness[40], 17 were found to have OSAS. The headaches of 37% improved following nasal

CPAP therapy. Most responders had migraine or mixed headache.

These varying findings can best be reconciled by the results of a study of headaches in 80 consecutive OSAS patients compared with 22 controls with periodic limb movements of sleep causing a similar arousal frequency[33]. Headache frequency as a whole was not significantly different in the two groups, but 48% of patients in the OSAS group had headaches on awakening, compared with none in the control group. These headaches did not fulfil criteria for migraine or tension headaches. They were generally brief in duration, and located frontally, occipitally or globally. Severity of the awakening headache graded by a validated scale correlated with degree of oxyhemoglobin saturation but not with frequency of apneas and hypopneas alone. Nasal CPAP therapy resulted in a mean of 80% improvement in awakening headaches, but not in migraines or tension headaches. Thus OSAS should be considered in patients with awakening headaches, and appropriate tests performed. The most likely mechanism appears to be cerebral vasodilatation induced by either hypoxia or hypercapnia.

## REFERENCES

1. Malow BA, Selwa LM, Ross D, Aldrich MS. Lateralizing value of interictal spikes on overnight sleep-EEG studies in temporal lobe epilepsy. *Epilepsia* 1999;40:1587–92

2. Autret A, Laffont F, Roux S. Influence of waking and sleep stages on the inter-ictal paroxysmal activity in partial epilepsy with complex seizures. *Electroencephalogr Clin Neurophysiol* 1983;55:406–10

3. Malow BA, Lin X, Kushwaha R, Aldrich MS. Interictal spiking increases with sleep depth in temporal lobe epilepsy. *Epilepsia* 1998; 39:1309–16

4. Sammaritano M, Gigli GL, Gotman J. Interictal spiking during wakefulness and sleep and the localization of foci in temporal lobe epilepsy. *Neurology* 1991;41:290–1

5. Minecan D, Natarajan A, Marzec M, Malow B. Relationship of epileptic seizures to sleep stage and sleep depth. *Sleep* 2002;25:899–904

6. Bazil CW, Walczak TS. Effects of sleep and sleep stage on epileptic and nonepileptic seizures. *Epilepsia* 1997;38:56–62

7. Crespel A, Coubes P, Baldy-Moulinier M. Sleep influence on seizures and epilepsy effects on sleep in partial frontal and temporal lobe epilepsies. *Clin Neurophysiol* 2000;111:S54–9

8. Provini F, Plazzi G, Tinuper P, Vandi S, Lugaresi E, Montagna P. Nocturnal frontal lobe epilepsy. A clinical and polygraphic overview of 100 consecutive cases. *Brain* 1999;122:1017–31

9. Phillips HA, Scheffer IE, Berkovic SF, Hollway GE, Sutherland GR, Mulley JC. Localization of a gene for autosomal dominant nocturnal frontal lobe epilepsy to chromosome 20q13.2. *Nat Genet* 1995;10:117–18

10. Lugaresi E, Cirgnotta F, Montagna P. Nocturnal paroxysmal dystonia. *J Neurol Neurosurg Psychiatry* 1986;49:375–80

11. Meierkord H, Fish DR, Smith SJ, Scott CA, Shorvon SD, Marsden CD. Is nocturnal paroxysmal dystonia a form of frontal lobe epilepsy? *Mov Disord* 1992;7:38–42

12. Pedley TA, Guilleminault C. Episodic nocturnal wanderings responsive to anticonvulsant drug therapy. *Ann Neurol* 1977;2:30–5

13. Peled R, Lavie P. Paroxysmal awakenings from sleep associated with excessive day-

time somnolence: a form of nocturnal epilepsy. *Neurology* 1986;36:95–8

14. Tassinari CA, Meletti S, Rubboli G, Michelucci R. Electrical status epilepticus of sleep. In Dinner DS, Luders HO, eds. *Epilepsy and Sleep: Physiological and Clinical Relationships*. San Diego: Academic Press, 2001:156–73

15. Touchon J, Baldy-Moulinier M, Billiard M, Besset A, Cadilhac J. Sleep organization and epilepsy. In Degen R, Rodin EA, eds. *Epilepsy, Sleep and Sleep Deprivation*. Amsterdam: Elsevier, 1991:73–81

16. Declerck AC, Wauquier A. Influence of antiepileptic drugs on sleep patterns. In Degen R, Rodin EA, eds. *Epilepsy, Sleep and Sleep Deprivation*. Amsterdam: Elsevier, 1991:153–63

17. Placidi F, Scalise A, Marciani MG, Romigi A, Diomedi M, Gigli GL. Effect of antiepileptic drugs on sleep. *Clin Neurophysiol* 2000; 111:S115–19

18. Sammaritano M, Sherwin A. Effect of anticonvulsants on sleep. *Neurology* 2000; 54:S16–24

19. Malow BA, Edward SJ, Marzec M, Sagher O, Fromes G. Effects of vagus nerve stimulation on respiration during sleep: a pilot study. *Neurology* 2000;55:1450–4

20. Malow BA, Bowes RJ, Lin X. Predictors of sleepiness in epilepsy patients. *Sleep* 1997; 20:1105–10

21. Salinsky MC, Oken BS, Binder LM. Assessment of drowsiness in epilepsy patients receiving chronic antiepileptic drug therapy. *Epilepsia* 1996;31:181–7

22. Manni R, Tartara A. Evaluation of sleepiness in epilepsy. *Clin Neurophysiol* 2000; 111:S111–4

23. Dexter JD, Weitzman ED. The relationship of nocturnal headaches to sleep stage patterns. *Neurology* 1970;20:513–18

24. Dexter JD. The relationship between stage III + IV + REM sleep and arousals with migraine. *Headache* 1979;19:364–9

25. Barabas G, Ferrari M, Matthews WS. Childhood migraine and somnambulism. *Neurology* 1983;33:948–9

26. Preladier A, Guroud M, Dry J. Childhood migraine and somnambulism. *Headache* 1987;27:143–5

27. Dexter JD. The relationship between disorders of arousal from sleep and migraine [Abstract]. *Headache* 1986;26:322

28. Manzoni GC, Terzano MG, Moretti G, Cocchi M. Clinical observations on 76 cluster headache cases. *Eur Neurol* 1981; 20:88–94

29. Pfaffenrath V, Pollmann W, Ruther E, Lund R, Hajak G. Onset of nocturnal attacks of chronic cluster headache in relation to sleep stages. *Acta Neurol Scand* 1986;73:403–7

30. Buckle P, Kerr P, Kryger M. Nocturnal cluster headache associated with sleep apnea. A case report. *Sleep* 1993;16:487–9

31. Kudrow L, McGinty DJ, Phillips ER, Stevenson M. Sleep apnea in cluster headache. *Cephalalgia* 1984;4:33–8

32. Nobre ME, Filho PF, Dominici M. Cluster headache associated with sleep apnoea. *Cephalalgia* 2003;23:276–9

33. Loh NK, Dinner DS, Foldvary N, Skobieranda F, Yew WW. Do patients with obstructive sleep apnea wake up with headaches? *Arch Intern Med* 1999; 159:1765–8

34. Kayed K, Godtlibsen OB, Sjaastad O. Chronic paroxysmal hemicrania IV: 'REM sleep locked' nocturnal headache attacks. *Sleep* 1978;1:91–5

35. Dodick DW, Mosek AC, Campbell JK. The hypnic ('alarm clock') headache syndrome. *Cephalalgia* 1998;18:152–6

36. Arjona JAM, Jimenez-Jimenez FJ, Vela-Bueno A, Tallon-Barranco A. Hypnic headache associated with stage 3 slow wave sleep. *Headache* 2000;40:753–4

37. Dodick DW. Polysomnography in hypnic headache syndrome. *Headache* 2000;40:748–52

38. Dodick DW, Jones JM, Capobianco DJ. Hypnic headache: another indomethacin-responsive headache syndrome? *Headache* 2000;40:830–5

39. Aldrich MS, Chauncey JB. Are morning headaches part of obstructive sleep apnea syndrome? *Arch Intern Med* 1990;150:1265–7

40. Poceta JS, Dalessio DJ. Identification and treatment of sleep apnea in patients with chronic headache. *Headache* 1995;35:586–9

41. Ulfberg J, Carter N, Talback M, Edling C. Headache, snoring and sleep apnoea. *J Neurol* 1996;243:621–5

42. Jennum P, Hein HO, Suadicani P, Gyntelberg F. Headache and cognitive dysfunctions in snorers. A cross-sectional study of 3323 men aged 54 to 74 years: the Copenhagen Male Study. *Arch Neurol* 1994;51:937–42

# Index